AF449259

Anaesthetic and Extracorporeal Gas Transfer

KEITH L. DORRINGTON

Lincoln College, Oxford

CLARENDON PRESS · OXFORD
1989

Oxford University Press, Walton Street, Oxford OX2 6DP
Oxford New York Toronto
Delhi Bombay Calcutta Madras Karachi
Petaling Jaya Singapore Hong Kong Tokyo
Nairobi Dar es Salaam Cape Town
Melbourne Auckland
and associated companies in
Berlin Ibadan

Oxford is a trade mark of Oxford University Press

Published in the United States
by Oxford University Press, New York

British Library Cataloguing in Publication Data
Dorrington, Keith L.
Anaesthetic and extracorporeal gas transfer.
1. Medicine. Inhalation anaesthesia
I. Title
617.'962
ISBN 0–19–857632–3

Library of Congress Cataloging in Publication Data
Dorrington, Keith L.
Anaesthetic and extracorporeal gas transfer/Keith L. Dorrington.
p. cm. — (Oxford medical engineering series; 9)
Includes bibliographies.
1. Anesthesiology—Apparatus and instruments. 2. Artificial
respiration—Equipment and supplies. I. Series.
240 D716a]   RD78.8.D66   1989   617'.96—dc 19
ISBN 0–19–857632–3

Set by
Macmillan India Ltd, Bangalore 25
Printed and bound in
Great Britain by Biddles Ltd,
Guildford and King's Lynn

Preface

The aim of this book is to present a rigorous analysis of a wide range of gas transfer problems of common interest in anaesthesia and intensive care. The approach to the theoretical analyses which are undertaken is initially descriptive and historical, secondly frequently diagrammatic, and thirdly extensively mathematical. The level of mathematical complexity does not extend beyond the calculus of simple partial differential equations. Frequent use is made of experimental data for comparison with theory.

Clinicians will recognize and understand many of the solutions presented, especially in the first four chapters. The biomedical engineering student will find that little or no prior medical knowledge is expected. Fundamental physical principles have been revised, including the kinetic theory of gases, the first and second laws of thermodynamics, and the uniform laminar flow of a Newtonian liquid.

Many of the solutions are presented for the first time. The theoretical and experimental work of others is referred to within the text, and suggestions for further reading follow each chapter.

Some of the material presented here has been taught to third year Engineering undergraduates in Oxford and examined over the past three years in their Final Honour School. Problems are presented at the end of all but the first, introductory, chapter as exercises for the biomedical engineering student.

Lincoln College K. L. D.
April 1988

Acknowledgements

The preparation of this book has been made possible by the Rector and Fellows of Lincoln College through the provision of a Nuffield Medical Research Fellowship. I am indebted to Dr Michael E. Ward for first stimulating my interest in anaesthesia whilst I was still at medical school, and to Professor M. Keith Sykes and Dr John Edmonds-Seal for encouraging my entry into the specialty some years later. Dr Brian J. Bellhouse and Dr Jean-Patrice Gardaz introduced me to laboratory research in extracorporeal circulation. I am grateful to Dr John R. Lehane for being a stimulating co-author of two papers on medical breathing systems, the themes of which are presented in this book. Dr Peter J. D. Mayes has kindly given permission for me to publish his own numerical solutions to two problems in Chapter 6. Dr John Wells has made helpful suggestions, following a study of the contents. Mrs Daphne Robinson has typed much of the manuscript.

Permissions have been obtained from the following publishers for the use of diagrammatic material: Springer-Verlag GmbH and Co, Berlin, West Germany (Figures 1.2, 3.29, and 3.30); Professional and Scientific Publications Ltd, London, UK (figures 1.6, 2.10, 3.25, 3.26, and 3.28); Munksgaard Int. Pub., Copenhagen, Denmark (figure 2.14); Academic Press, London, UK (figures 2.29, 2.30, 2.31, and 3.12); British Medical Journal, London, UK (figure 2.36); Blackwell Scientific Publications Ltd, Oxford, UK (figure 3.10); Elsevier Science Publishing Co. Inc., New York, USA (figure 3.27); Williams and Wilkins Co., Baltimore, USA (figures 4.33 and 4.34); Canadian Anaesthetists' Society Journal, Toronto, Canada (figure 4.35); J. B. Lippincott Co., Philadelphia, USA (figure 5.2); Butterworth Scientific Ltd, Guildford, UK (figures 5.3, 5.4, and 5.5); and Macmillan Press Ltd., Basingstoke, UK (figures 5.14 and 5.17).

Finally, I thank my wife Marion for helping me to find time to write.

K.L.D.

Contents

1 Oxygen and carbon dioxide transport in the body

1.1 Introduction

The human body is an internal combustion engine. It tolerates innumerable solid and liquid fuels but its requirement for one gas is absolute: without oxygen we stall.

In certain respects this prime role for oxygen (O_2) is surprising. Early forms of life left the production line without a need for oxygen to sustain themselves. Examples of such *anaerobic* organisms alive today include yeasts and several disease-forming bacteria, for example that responsible for tetanus. Moreover, in high concentrations oxygen proves to be a poison even to us *aerobic* organisms, who cannot live without it; blindness in the newborn and lung damage at all ages are serious complications of exposure to excess.

The body's need for oxygen is not only absolute, it is also immediate. Because the body's useful reserve of oxygen, when breathing air, is only approximately six times its oxygen consumption per minute, survival after cessation of breathing is normally limited to a few minutes at most. It is no surprise then that we are equipped with a most elaborate control mechanism for the automatic maintenance of breathing as well as an aggressive conscious preoccupation with 'coming up for air' in situations in which our breathing is threatened.

In medical practice the patient's own preservation of breathing may be threatened by disease or interrupted by anaesthesia or surgery. In these situations, maintenance of respiration either via the patient's own lungs or via some totally artificial device becomes the first duty of the medical attendant. In the ABC of emergency first aid, A stands for airway and B stands for breathing (C stands for circulation), emphasizing the priority of restoring gas exchange before doing anything else to resuscitate the patient.

In virtually all anaesthetic procedures the patient's breathing is modified or maintained by the use of equipment relying for its safety on good engineering design and careful use. In the United States, 42 anaesthetics are commenced every minute, summing to 22 million annually. The corresponding annual sum for the United Kingdom is approximately 5 million. Of the American total, more than 2000 patients are known to die annually during anaesthesia as a result of equipment failure or human error.

The use of totally artificial lungs has led to a current worldwide sale of over 300 000 devices each year, mainly for use in the operating theatre during cardiac surgery when the patient's own lungs (and heart) temporarily cease to perform their usual functions, as the body's normal plumbing is purposefully deranged.

1.2   The respiratory quotient

We breathe in to supply ourselves with oxygen. We breathe out firstly because inspiration introduces some gases (notably nitrogen) which can dilute oxygen to dangerously low levels, and secondly to rid ourselves of one of the products of combustion, carbon dioxide (CO_2). We may also regard the other major product of combustion, water, as being exhausted almost entirely by the lungs and the upper airways, but in the reckoning of the body's total input/output water balance this relatively small amount of water is usually forgotten or hidden between the sums of larger volumes: drink, intravenous fluids, urine, and so on. Table 1.1 gives examples of two industrial and two physiological fuels with their associated products assuming total combustion with oxygen to CO_2 and water.

Palmitate is representative of a range of fatty acids which make up much of our diet; glucose is representative of the carbohydrate component of our food. It can be noted that the breakdown of both these fuels produces one molecule of water with every molecule of CO_2. The expiration of water vapour during breathing is approximately equal to this metabolic production of water unless the inspired air is itself highly saturated with water.

Table 1.1. *Combustion products of industrial and physiological fuels*

Fuel	Oxygen consumption	Combustion products	[1]CO_2/O_2
Methane[2]			
CH_4	$2O_2$	CO_2 and $2H_2O$	0.50
Heptane[3]			
C_7H_{16}	$11O_2$	$7CO_2$ and $8H_2O$	0.64
Palmitate[4]			
$C_{15}H_{31}COOH$	$23O_2$	$16CO_2$ and $16H_2O$	0.70
Glucose[5]			
$C_6H_{12}O_6$	$6O_2$	$6CO_2$ and $6H_2O$	1.00

[1] Molecular ratio of CO_2 production to O_2 consumption, known physiologically as the respiratory quotient, R.

[2] Forms approximately 95 per cent by volume of natural gas.

[3] A major component of petrol.

[4] A component of animal and vegetable fat; a representative of all fatty acids, which approximate to the formula $(CH_2)_n$.

[5] A dietary and therapeutic sugar; a representative of all carbohydrates, which approximate to the formula $(CH_2O)_n$.

The ratio of the number of molecules of CO_2 produced to the number of molecules of oxygen consumed during combustion is known in biological systems as the respiratory quotient and is denoted by R. Values of this ratio for the four fuels in Table 1.1 are given in the right hand column. The importance of R is that it defines for the natural lungs or any artificial lung the relative burden of exhausting CO_2 on the one hand and taking up oxygen on the other. Physiologists have tended to restrict the use of the term 'respiratory quotient' to refer only to the ratio of CO_2 production to oxygen consumption in the tissues. When referring to the ratio of CO_2 elimination and oxygen uptake by the lungs, the term 'respiratory exchange ratio' is preferred. Under steady state conditions these will, of course, usually be equal.

1.3　The Avogadro connection

In the stoichiometry* of metabolism we count molecules (Table 1.1); in the mechanics of breathing we are concerned with the convection and diffusion of volumes of gas. The quantitative relationship between molecular fractions and volume fractions of mixtures of gases and vapours is of such prime importance that we devote space to it at this early stage. For many readers this discussion will cover already familiar territory.

Not unlike some other expositors of outstanding discoveries, Amedeo Avogadro[†] died before his simple but brilliant conception became recognized. Born in Turin in 1776, he practiced as a lawyer for many years. From about 1800 he began to study physics and continued his career occupying chairs in physics off and on for most of his remaining life. In 1811 he published in French a paper which asserted that *equal volumes of all gases (under the same conditions of temperature and pressure) contain equal numbers of molecules*, a hypothesis which should have resolved the contemporary difficulties among chemists seeking to establish a consistent system of atomic weights. The fact that the hypothesis was ignored for 50 years has been attributed in part to Avogadro's clumsy nomenclature and in part to his lack of direct experimental evidence.

The argument used by Avogadro to justify his hypothesis was that it led to the simplest, and we presume therefore most rational, explanation for the formation of a range of gases from their more elemental constituents. Among his subjects were substances later to be of great interest to anaesthetists: ether, nitrous oxide, water vapour, ethyl chloride, CO_2 and alcohol. We shall examine some implications of the hypothesis for the molecular model of gases and consider to what extent we may expect it to be exact, and to what extent merely an approximation to the behaviour of real gases and vapours.

* from the Greek *stoikheion* element: 'measurement of the elements'.
[†] Lorenzo Romano Amedeo Carlo Avogadro di Quaregua e di Cerreto (1776–1856).

1.4   The squash court model of a gas

The Avogadro principle presupposes a gas to be particulate. We consider further the implications of assuming that the particles or molecules constituting a gas are in continuous motion and involved in collisions with the walls of their container and with each other. This so-called 'kinetic' theory of the gaseous phase of matter is at once extraordinarily simple yet powerfully predictive.

We regard (Fig. 1.1) the molecules of a gas to be like many highly elastic squash balls bouncing around off the floor, walls, and ceiling of a court. We consider their average velocity to be known, $\bar{c}$ m s^{-1} even though the range or distribution of velocities about this mean may be as yet obscure. Conceive

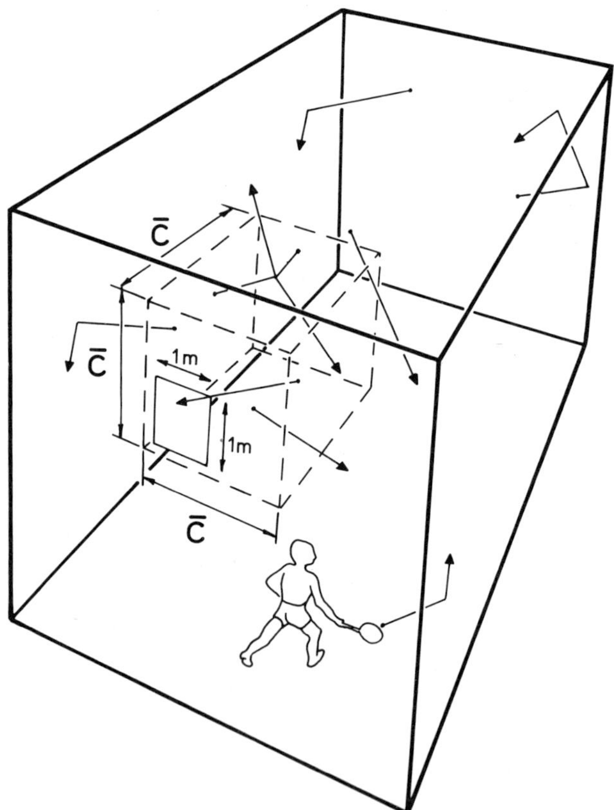

Fig. 1.1. Squash court model of a gas with a mean molecular velocity $\bar{c}$. The paths traversed in one second by nine molecules are represented; two molecules suffer a collision; four molecules are shown colliding with the walls of the court. An imaginary cubic cage of side $\bar{c}$ aids mathematical description (see text).

now an imaginary cubic cage (Fig. 1.1) within the court with dimensions $\bar{c} \times \bar{c} \times \bar{c}$ m, and consider the question: how many balls leave the cage in one second? We are not looking for an exact answer but one to an order of magnitude, that is, to within a factor of ten of the exact solution. You will note that in one second molecules travel, on average, a distance of $\bar{c}$ m. Since the cage has a side length of $\bar{c}$ and molecules rarely collide with each other, we must expect many, possibly most, of the molecules initially in the cage to cross its walls during the passage of one second. There will also be some molecules (Fig. 1.1) which will both enter the cage and leave it within the passage of a second. Considering all possibilities, we conclude that the number of molecules leaving the cage in one second is given to an order of magnitude by the number contained within the cage:

$$N \simeq n\bar{c}^3, \tag{1.1}$$

where n is the number of molecules per unit volume (m^3) and $\bar{c}^3$ is the volume of the cage.

It follows from eqn (1.1) that the number of molecules crossing from inside out across a single side of the cubic cage is $n\bar{c}^3/6$ and that, since each side of the cage has an area $\bar{c}^2$ m^2, the number crossing a single square metre on the side of the cage is given by

$$N \simeq \frac{n\bar{c}^3/6}{\bar{c}^2} = \frac{1}{6} n\bar{c}. \tag{1.2}$$

(A more rigorous analysis using calculus yields $n\bar{c}/4$.)

Consider now that one side of the imaginary cage lies adjacent to a wall of the court and the consequences of this on determining the pressure generated at the wall by the molecules which must now rebound into the cage rather than leave it. Molecules approaching the wall will do so with a velocity normal (at right angles) to the wall of the order of $\bar{c}$ and bounce away following collision with a similar, possibly the same, velocity. A molecule of mass m thus experiences a change of momentum of the order of $2m\bar{c}$. The pressure generated by approximately $n\bar{c}/6$ collisions per square metre per second (eqn (1.2)) each with an *impulse* of $2m\bar{c}$ is therefore

$$p \simeq \frac{n\bar{c}}{6} \times 2m\bar{c} = \frac{1}{3} nm\bar{c}^2. \tag{1.3}$$

A rigorous analysis which assumes perfectly elastic collisions at the wall yields an almost identical result with the mean of the squares of molecular velocities appearing in place of the square of the mean velocity:

$$p = \frac{1}{3} nm\overline{c^2}. \tag{1.4}$$

We have assumed in our model of a gas that molecules collide with each other much less frequently than they collide with the walls of their container. Consequently we do not expect their mean kinetic energy ($\overline{mc^2}/2$) to be a function of their density in the container ($\propto n$), but to be a function of temperature only. At constant temperature our model therefore predicts that p is proportional to n:

$$p \propto n \bigg|_{\text{temp. const.}} . \tag{1.5}$$

1.5   Boyle's law

Equation (1.5) is a statement of Boyle's law, an experimental finding that we owe to the English chemist Robert Boyle*. He found that at low densities all gases at the same temperature have a pressure which tends to be inversely related to volume (V):

$$\boxed{pV = \text{constant} \bigg|_{\text{temp. const.}}} . \tag{1.6}$$

The equivalence between eqns (1.5) and (1.6) is obvious when we note that the volume of a container of a fixed mass of gas must be inversely proportional to the number of molecules per unit volume:

$$V \propto 1/n. \tag{1.7}$$

Boyle's law, then, lends weight to the assumption in our model gas that the mean molecular kinetic energy ($\overline{mc^2}/2$) may be a function of nothing but temperature and is therefore a constant as long as the temperature remains unchanged:

$$\frac{1}{2}\overline{mc^2} = \text{constant} \bigg|_{\text{temp. const.}} . \tag{1.8}$$

If we now take eqn (1.4) in conjunction with Avogadro's law rather than Boyle's law, we discover an important corollary regarding the constant in eqn (1.8). For, if equal volumes of two different gases with molecular masses m_1 and m_2 do indeed contain equal numbers of molecules ($n_1 = n_2$) under the same conditions of temperature and pressure ($p_1 = p_2$), it follows from

* Robert Boyle, 1627–91, not to be confused with the later Henry Boyle of anaesthetic fame.

eqn (1.4) that

$$m_1 \overline{c_1^2} = m_2 \overline{c_2^2} \Big|_{\text{temp. const.}} , \qquad (1.9)$$

or

$$\frac{1}{2} m_1 \overline{c_1^2} = \frac{1}{2} m_2 \overline{c_2^2} \Big|_{\text{temp. const.}} . \qquad (1.10)$$

That is to say, the mean molecular kinetic energies of all gases at the same temperature are identical, and the constant in eqn (1.8) is the same for all gases.

It is a thorny question, about which thermodynamicists continue to debate, whether eqn (1.10) can be derived from the precepts of classical mechanics directly from the simple assumptions of our kinetic model. We shall not pursue the problem further here but rather draw one important conclusion of practical value for the solution of problems in respiration engineering. That is, because the Avogadro principle relates closely to Boyle's law (eqns (1.8) and (1.10)), to the extent that a gas deviates from Boyle's law we may expect it to deviate from Avogadro's law. In a mixture of gases, fractions by numbers of molecules will not always exactly equal fractions by volume.

1.6   Oxygen demand and CO_2 elimination: normal values

We have seen that Avogadro's law licences us to relate numbers of molecules directly to volumes of gas, if we maintain the same conditions of temperature and pressure. We have seen too that the relation is probably accurate to the same extent as Boyle's law is accurate for any particular gas and conditions of pressure and temperature. For oxygen and CO_2 at physiological conditions of pressure and temperature, Boyle's law holds to a fair degree of precision and for most calculations errors arising from assuming 'ideal' behaviour can be ignored.

In relation to Table 1.1, we noted that different fuels undergoing full combustion to CO_2 and water generate different molecular ratios, R, of CO_2 production to oxygen consumption. This respiratory quotient we can now see will equal the volume ratio of CO_2 production to oxygen consumption, so long as volume measurements are taken at the same pressure and temperature:

$$R = \frac{\text{Vol. of } CO_2 \text{ produced by combustion}}{\text{Vol. of oxygen consumed by combustion}} \Big|_{\substack{\text{same pressure} \\ \text{and temperature}}} . \qquad (1.11)$$

Thus whilst metabolizing fats (typified by palmitate for which $R = 0.7$) the molecular output of CO_2, and hence volume expired, is some 30 per cent less than the oxygen consumed. In these circumstances we breathe more in than we breathe out. Whilst consuming carbohydrate (typified by the sugar glucose for which $R = 1.0$), input and output volumes are equal. Under conditions of heavy exercise it is possible for R to rise well above unity to about 2, and in these circumstances of partial anaerobic respiration the expiration of CO_2 dominates breathing.

An unusual state of affairs can be established in which the respiratory quotient 'seen' by the body's own lungs can be reduced to zero ($R = 0$) by arranging for an extracorporeal lung to remove from the blood the whole of the body's metabolic production of CO_2, whilst performing little or no oxygen transfer via the device. In this situation the patient is, in effect, breathing in oxygen via their own lungs whilst having to breathe out nothing. The lungs can indeed be motionless, or *apnoeic*, whilst the uptake of oxygen occurs by *steady convection* from the nose or mouth down into the lungs. The method can be shown to function only in the steady state when the patient breathes a very high concentration of oxygen. This technique of extra-corporeal CO_2 removal ($ECCO_2R$) with apnoeic oxygenation (AO) which reduces R to zero for the patient's own lungs is currently under appraisal as a treatment for some forms of respiratory failure.

At rest, the normal adult consumes approximately 250 ml (STPD*) of oxygen every minute. In these circumstances, and with a normal mixed diet, the respiratory quotient takes values close to 0.8 and consequently the volume of CO_2 expired from the lungs is approximately $0.8 \times 250 = 200$ ml (STPD) per minute.

Oxygen consumption (and CO_2 elimination) is one of several physiological variables which varies approximately with the surface area of living or-ganisms, and is consequently roughly related to the two-thirds power of the organism's volume (assuming similarities of shape) and mass (assuming similarities of mean density). Thus an infant of mass 7 kg when compared with an adult of 70 kg has a relative mass of 0.1 but an oxygen requirement, not one tenth of the adult's $250\,\mathrm{ml\,min^{-1}}$, but nearer $0.1^{2/3} \times 250 = 54\,\mathrm{ml\,min^{-1}}$. This is more than double what might be expected ($25\,\mathrm{ml\,min^{-1}}$) if the oxygen consumption were assumed to be proportional to mass alone, and becomes a very important consideration when working with human infants and even smaller animals.

1.7   Airway architecture and the composition of alveolar gas

The importance of the respiratory exchange ratio is not limited to the information it gives about the relative flows of gas to and from the lungs.

* Standard Temperature and Pressure, Dry: 0 °C (273.15 K) and 1 atmosphere ($= 1.013$ bar $= 101.3$ kPa $= 760$ mm Hg). Because gas volumes are strong functions of temperature, pressure, and degree of saturation with water vapour, a reference is mandatory. This is one of several used in medical and engineering literature. STP is often written as a shorthand for STPD.

Because blood equilibrates with the gas in the terminal *alveoli* of the airways, R plays a role in dictating the relative concentrations in the blood of oxygen and CO_2.

The natural airways commence at the nostrils or *nares* (when nose breathing) and the lips (when mouth breathing). The alternative nasal and oral airways act to humidify inspired gas and together with the *pharynx*, where they converge, contain the airways' initial defences against infection and contamination. The pharynx communicates with the *larynx* in which the vocal cords guard over entry to the *trachea*. From the trachea the airways divide to form some 23 generations (Fig. 1.2), terminating in approximately 8 million ($\simeq 2^{23}$) *alveolar sacs*. The initial 16 generations (comprising *bronchi, bronchioles,* and *terminal bronchioles*) represent an *anatomical dead space* in which no gas exchange occurs directly between the airways and blood; the final 7 generations (comprising *respiratory bronchioles, alveolar ducts,* and *alveolar sacs*) carry, as they spread out, ever increasing numbers of alveoli in which gas exchange occurs with capillary blood. In the adult there are some 300 million alveoli each with a diameter of approximately 0.3 mm, providing a total gas exchange area of 50–100 m^2: the area is widely remembered in the medical profession as being 'about the area of a tennis court'!*

Alveolar gas is in close proximity to blood in the lung capillaries as depicted in Fig. 1.3. It is separated from blood by a composite membrane some 0.5 μm thick, across which there is a rapid diffusion of oxygen into the blood and CO_2 into the alveolar gas. At the level of the alveoli there is little tidal movement of gas with inspiration and expiration; the larger proximal airways are predominantly *convecting* paths, but the smaller distal airways are predominantly *diffusing* paths for gas transport. The composition of alveolar gas is both fairly constant from breath to breath and in close equilibrium with blood leaving the lung capillaries (end capillary blood) due to its proximity to this blood across an alveolar membrane with a low resistance to diffusion of both oxygen and CO_2.

In Fig. 1.4 we illustrate the derivation of the *alveolar gas equation* which relates the concentrations of oxygen and CO_2 in alveolar gas and, by extension, in blood itself. In this derivation (and throughout this text) we make use of the concept of *partial pressure* of a gas mixed in amongst others: it is that pressure which would be exerted by that gas alone, in its same container, were the molecules of all the other gases present to be selectively removed. Attributed to Dalton† is a *law of partial pressures* which states that the total pressure of a mixture of gases equals the sum of the partial pressures of its constituent gases; this is readily seen to accord with the kinetic theory of

---

* The area of a tennis court is in fact 260.75 m^2.
† John Dalton 1766–1844.

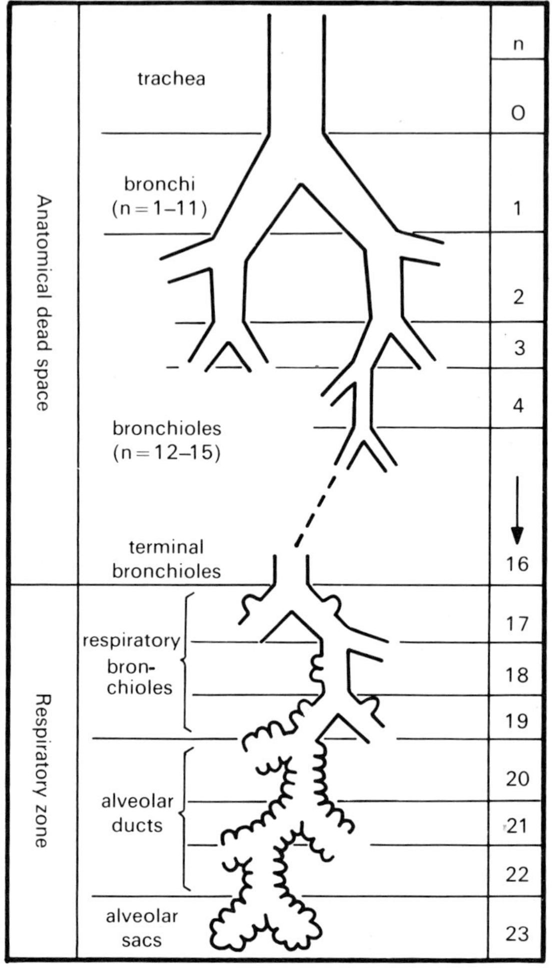

Fig. 1.2. The divisions of the airways according to Weibel (1963. *Morphometry of the human lung,* Chapter X. Springer-Verlag, Berlin.)

gases (eqn (1.4)) in which each molecule of a gas makes its isolated contribution to the pressure of the whole, unaffected by its neighbours.

Consequent upon Boyle's law (eqn (1.6)), we can further see that the partial pressure of a gas in a mixture is proportional to its fraction by volume in the mixture when each volume fraction is measured at the same total pressure of the mixture. In Fig. 1.4 we depict volume fractions of a bolus of inspired gas making its way on inspiration towards an alveolus (a), and the volume fractions of a bolus of expired gas leaving the alveolus on expiration (b).

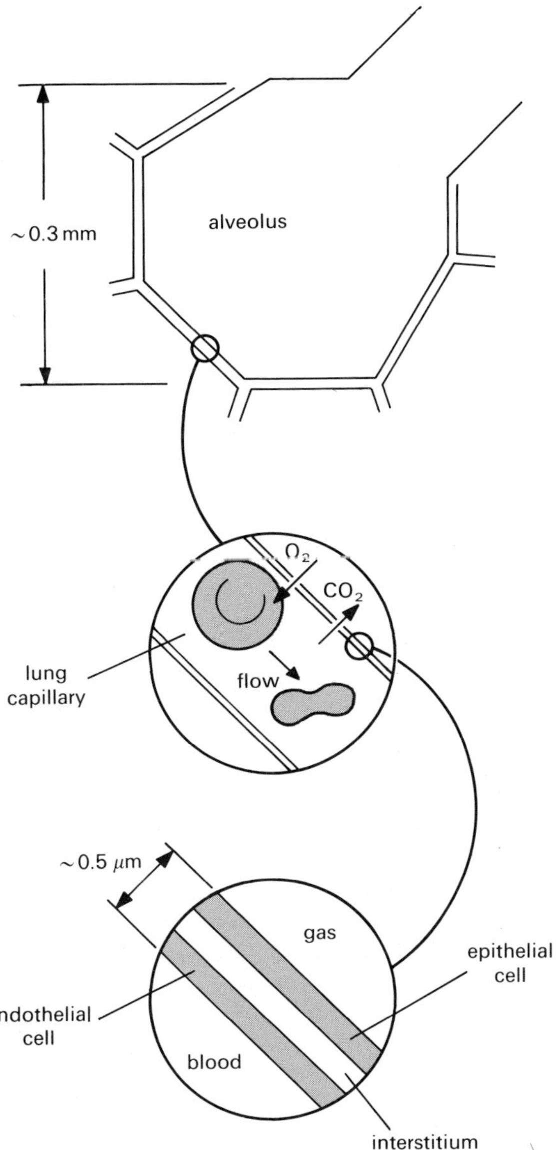

Fig. 1.3. Illustration of the proximity of alveolar gas to blood flowing in lung capillaries. As blood passes the alveolus, oxygen is received from alveolar gas and CO$_2$ given up by the blood. Oxygen and CO$_2$ diffuse across a composite membrane some 0.5 μm thick, lined on both the gas side and blood side with living cells. The diameter of the lung capillaries is of the order of the diameter of red cells.

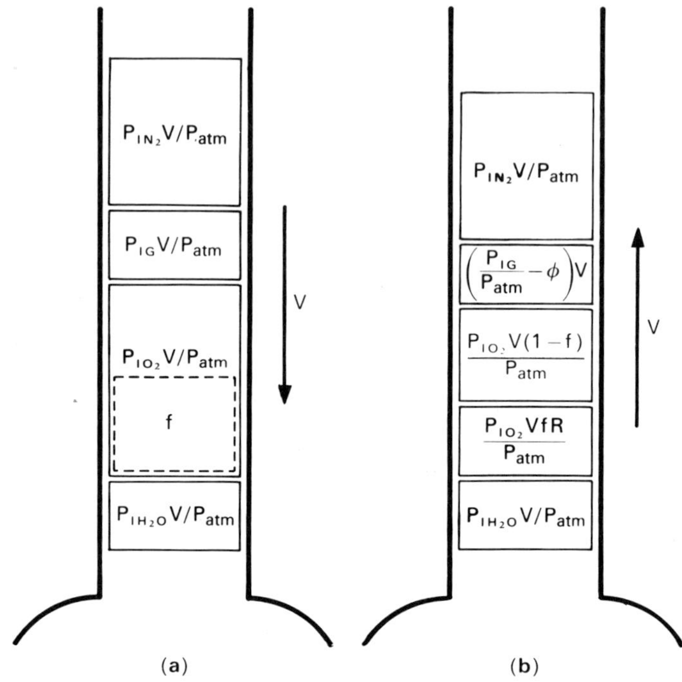

Fig. 1.4. The derivation of the alveolar gas equation. On inspiration (a) a bolus of volume V moves towards an alveolus and is composed of nitrogen N_2, an anaesthetic gas G, oxygen O_2, and water vapour H_2O. The cycle of breathing is completed during expiration (b) by the passage of a bolus of gas of volume V' away from the alveolus (see text).

The inspired bolus has volume V and is at atmospheric pressure P_{atm}. (Inspiratory and expiratory excursions cause alveolar pressure to differ only minimally from ambient pressure.) The bolus we take to be composed of nitrogen, oxygen, water vapour*, and an unspecified third gas G (which may usefully stand for an anaesthetic vapour). We represent the inspired partial pressures of these gases respectively by P_{IN_2}, P_{IO_2}, P_{IH_2O}, and P_{IG}, recognizing from Dalton's law that

$$P_{IN_2} + P_{IO_2} + P_{IH_2O} + P_{IG} = P_{atm}. \tag{1.12}$$

The volumes of nitrogen, oxygen, water vapour and G entering the alveolus are consequently $P_{IN_2}V/P_{atm}$, $P_{IO_2}V/P_{atm}$, $P_{IH_2O}V/P_{atm}$, and $P_{IG}V/P_{atm}$ (Fig. 1.4a).

---

* Probably virtually fully saturated, having passed the wet mucous lining of the upper airways.

The expired bolus has a volume V' and is a sample of alveolar gas (Fig. 1.4b). In leaving the alveolus it returns the alveolus to exactly the same state in which it found itself before the bolus V entered (Fig. 1.4a). We calculate the volume V' by accounting for the changes which occur during the course of the one cycle of inspiration and expiration. We assume that a fraction f of the oxygen in the inspired bolus exchanges with blood yielding a volume of CO_2 equal to $R f P_{IO_2} V / P_{atm}$; that a fraction ϕ of the total bolus V is an absorbed volume (ϕV) of the unspecified gas G; and that no nitrogen is either taken up by or removed from the blood. The expired bolus volume V' is therefore related to the inspired bolus volume V by

$$V' = V[(1-f)P_{IO_2}/P_{atm} + R f P_{IO_2}/P_{atm} + P_{IN_2}/P_{atm}$$
$$+ P_{IH_2O}/P_{atm} + P_{IG}/P_{atm} - \phi].* \tag{1.13}$$

Combining eqns (1.12) and (1.13) we find

$$V' = V[1 - f(1-R)P_{IO_2}/P_{atm} - \phi], \tag{1.14}$$

and defining P_{IO_2}/P_{atm} as the *inspired oxygen fraction*, F_{IO_2}, we have

$$V' = V[1 - f(1-R)F_{IO_2} - \phi]. \tag{1.15}$$

The composition of the gas in the expired bolus V' is the same as that of alveolar gas since the bolus is a sample of alveolar gas. We use a subscript A to denote alveolar partial pressures and are now in a position to express alveolar volume fractions of oxygen and CO_2 from Fig. 1.4(b) and eqn (1.15):

$$\frac{P_{AO_2}}{P_{atm}} = \frac{(1-f)P_{IO_2}V/P_{atm}}{V[1-f(1-R)F_{IO_2}-\phi]} = \frac{(1-f)F_{IO_2}}{[1-f(1-R)F_{IO_2}-\phi]}, \tag{1.16}$$

and

$$\frac{P_{ACO_2}}{P_{atm}} = \frac{R f P_{IO_2}V/P_{atm}}{V[1-f(1-R)F_{IO_2}-\phi]} = \frac{R f F_{IO_2}}{[1-f(1-R)F_{IO_2}-\phi]}, \tag{1.17}$$

Solving now for the unknown fraction f of inspired oxygen which participates in exchange with the blood, we divide eqn (1.16) by eqn (1.17):

$$\frac{P_{AO_2}}{P_{ACO_2}} = \frac{(1-f)}{R f}, \tag{1.18}$$

from which

$$f = \frac{(P_{ACO_2}/R)}{P_{AO_2} + (P_{ACO_2}/R)}. \tag{1.19}$$

* Inspired and expired volumes of water vapour have here been assumed to be equal. If both inspired volume V and expired volume V' are saturated with water vapour at the same temperature, and $V' \neq V$, this assumption is invalid. Deviations from this assumption for this and other reasons can be taken into account in terms of the variable ϕ.

By substitution of eqn (1.19) in eqn (1.16) or (1.17) we obtain finally

$$P_{AO_2} = \frac{P_{IO_2}}{(1-\phi)} - \frac{P_{ACO_2}}{R}\left(1 - F_{IO_2}\frac{(1-R)}{(1-\phi)}\right) \qquad (1.20)$$

Equation (1.20) is one form of the alveolar gas equation. In the steady state, breathing air (F_{IO_2} approximately equal to 0.2), the equation reduces to

$$P_{AO_2} = P_{IO_2} - \frac{P_{ACO_2}}{R}[1 - 0.2(1-R)], \qquad (1.21)$$

and taking as a representative value $R = 0.8$:

$$P_{AO_2} = P_{IO_2} - 1.20 P_{ACO_2}. \qquad (1.22)$$

For many purposes it is accurate enough to adopt the approximation

$$P_{AO_2} \simeq P_{IO_2} - P_{ACO_2}. \qquad (1.23)$$

In the steady state, with a subject breathing ever greater concentrations of oxygen ($F_{IO_2} \to 1$), eqn (1.23) tends towards an exact form of eqn (1.20) since $[1 - F_{IO_2}(1-R)]/R \to 1$ as $F_{IO_2} \to 1$.

The alveolar gas equation predicts a precise relationship between the partial pressures of oxygen and CO_2 in the alveoli as a function of the respiratory quotient, the inspired oxygen fraction, and the fractional uptake by the lung ϕ of any gas other than oxygen which may be exchanged across the alveolar–blood interface. Some caution must be exercised in the interpretation of this equation for several reasons, one of which is that it takes no account of variations with time in the composition of alveolar gas. We expect gas exchange to and from the alveoli to be contributed to both by tidal movements of convection (with inspiration and expiration) and by the process of diffusion within the airways. In setting up the model of Fig. 1.4 we have assumed nothing about the mechanism whereby gas enters and leaves the alveolus, but only that the expired gas is a sample of alveolar gas.

It is clearly possible to envisage a situation in which the composition of alveolar gas varies markedly throughout the inspiratory cycle. If gas flow into and out of the alveolus was entirely tidal and the alveolus volume after inspiration equalled the volume V of the inspired bolus, then for a brief moment immediately following inspiration the alveolar gas would have a composition identical to that of inspired gas ($P_{ACO_2} = 0$, $P_{AO_2} = P_{IO_2}$). The alveolar gas composition would change with time between inspiration and expiration, only attaining that predicted by eqn (1.20) immediately before expiration.

In normal breathing, the composition of alveolar gas varies little with time, and with the oscillatory pattern of breathing in and out, because the volume of each breath in (called the *tidal* volume) is substantially smaller than the volume of gas in the alveoli. The normal tidal volume for quiet breathing in an adult is about 500 ml. The volume of the anatomical dead space (Fig. 1.2) is approximately 150 ml and so only $500 - 150 = 350$ ml of fresh gas in each breath reaches the respiratory zone. This zone (virtually the whole volume of which is alveolar) has a volume during quiet breathing of around 3000 ml*. Consequently the useful part of the tidal volume is normally not much more than 10 per cent of the total alveolar volume and changes in the composition of alveolar gas with time are correspondingly small. When these small changes are taken into consideration, we must regard eqn (1.20) as strictly valid for alveolar gas only during expiration.

1.8   Alveolar oxygen and CO_2 partial pressures: normal values

Under normal circumstances the body's respiratory control mechanisms are dominated by a drive to maintain the partial pressure of CO_2 in arterial blood (P_{aCO_2}[†]) close to 5.3 kPa. When we speak of a partial pressure of a gas (in this case CO_2) in a liquid (in this case blood) we are referring to that partial pressure of the gas in the gas phase with which the liquid would be in equilibrium at a gas–liquid interface. This partial pressure of a gas in a liquid is thus only indirectly a measure of the concentration of the gas molecules in the liquid, a relationship which will be clarified later in relation to oxygen and CO_2 in the blood.

Now, *arterial* blood is that blood leaving the left side of the heart immediately following its departure from the lungs and it is therefore usually nearly equilibrated with alveolar gas. In the normal state, the arterial and the alveolar partial pressures of CO_2 (and oxygen) are nearly equal and we have

$$P_{ACO_2} \simeq P_{aCO_2} \simeq 5.3\,\text{kPa}. \tag{1.24}$$

Under these conditions, and when breathing air which is either saturated with water vapour or becomes saturated in its passage through the upper airways ($P_{IH_2O} \doteq 6.3\,\text{kPa}$ at body temperature, $37\,^{\circ}\text{C}$), eqn (1.22) predicts[‡]

$$P_{AO_2} = P_{IO_2} - 1.20 \times 5.3$$

$$= 0.21(100 - 6.3) - 6.4$$

$$= 19.7 - 6.4$$

$$= 13.3\,\text{kPa}. \tag{1.25}$$

---

* The full excursion of total lung volume in the adult from the deepest expiration to deepest inspiration is approximately from 1500 to 6000 ml.

[†] small subscript a denotes 'arterial'.

[‡] taking the volume fraction of dry air to be 0.21, and atmospheric pressure to be 100 kPa.

The normal range for measured P_{aO_2} in young adults is variably given as 12.0–14.7 kPa, suggesting that the alveolar partial pressure predicted by eqn (1.22) does indeed give a good estimate of a normal arterial partial pressure for oxygen.

In Fig. 1.5 the alveolar gas eqn (1.20) is plotted for three values of F_{IO_2} and three values of R (ϕ is zero), with P_{ACO_2} as ordinate and P_{AO_2} as the abscissa. We see that at each value of F_{IO_2} different respiratory quotients are represented by a family of straight lines fanning out from a point which gives the composition of the inspired gas ($P_{AO_2} = F_{IO_2}P_{atm}$; $P_{ACO_2} = 0$). The normal alveolar gas composition whilst breathing air ($F_{IO_2} = 0.2$) is depicted.

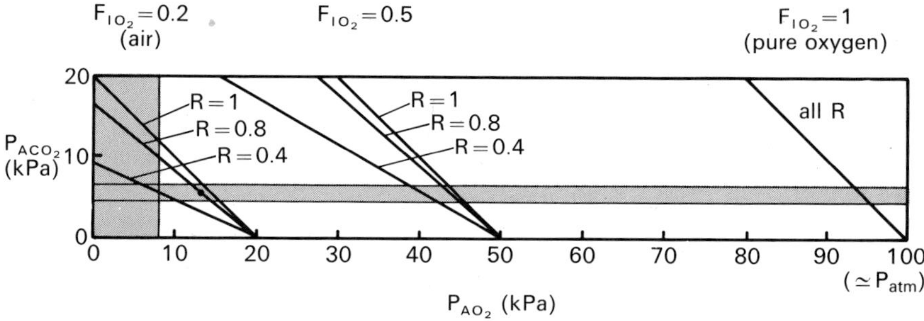

Fig. 1.5. A plot of the alveolar gas equation (eqn 1.20) for three values of inspired oxygen fraction F_{IO_2} and three values of respiratory quotient R. The horizontal shaded region represents the normal limits within which the body maintains the arterial CO_2 partial pressure ($P_{aCO_2} \simeq P_{ACO_2}$). The vertical shaded area represents the region in which the body responds particularly actively to a low arterial oxygen partial pressure ($P_{aO_2} \simeq P_{AO_2}$) to avoid hypoxia. The normal values of alveolar partial pressure breathing air at sea level are located by a dot on the line $R = 0.8$ for $F_{IO_2} = 0.2$ (see text).

The horizontal shaded area in Fig. 1.5 locates the narrow range ($\simeq 4.5$–6.5 kPa) within which the body's respiratory control mechanism attempts to maintain the arterial partial pressure of CO_2 ($P_{aCO_2} \simeq P_{ACO_2}$) by varying the *ventilation* (depth and rate of breathing). The manner in which changes in ventilation give rise to changes in P_{AO_2} will be examined in section 1.10. Under normal circumstances the P_{aCO_2} has a much more profound influence on this control mechanism than P_{aO_2}. However, if the P_{aO_2} (usually $\simeq P_{AO_2}$) falls below about 8 kPa, the mechanism begins to respond more actively to the P_{aO_2} than P_{aCO_2}. With impending *hypoxia** the threat to life from lack of oxygen overrides the risks of *hypo* or *hypercapnia*[†]. We can see from Fig. 1.5 that air breathing is a relatively precarious state in the sense that

---

* low oxygen concentration in the blood. The term is sometimes used more specifically to denote low availability of oxygen in the cells of living tissues.
[†] low and high CO_2 concentrations respectively in the blood.

it doesn't take an enormous rise in P_{ACO_2} to shift the operating condition into the risk zone $P_{AO_2} < 8\,kPa$.

As one ascends to altitude the origin of the fan of curves for air breathing shifts horizontally to the left taking with it the normal operating point which meets the region $P_{AO_2} \leq 8\,kPa$ when the inspired oxygen tension (P_{IO_2}) reaches approximately 15 kPa. This corresponds with the barometric P_{O_2} at an altitude of approximately 3000 m. Above this altitude it becomes necessary to hyperventilate in order to reduce P_{ACO_2} (sliding down the appropriate alveolar gas line in Fig. 1.5) to maintain a tolerable P_{AO_2}, until the body is able to make longer term adjustments to altitude.

1.9   Experimental validation of the alveolar gas equation

As mentioned earlier, an unusual state of affairs can be established in which the pulmonary respiratory quotient can be varied in the range $R = 0$ to $R \simeq 1$ by arranging for an extracorporeal lung to remove from the blood varying amounts of the body's metabolic production of CO_2. According to eqn (1.20) (setting $\phi = 0$ here), if R is varied using this technique constant values of P_{AO_2} and P_{ACO_2} (and hence constant values of P_{aO_2} and P_{aCO_2} to which they are closely related) can only be maintained if F_{IO_2} is suitably adjusted. Recalling that $P_{IO_2} = F_{IO_2} \times P_{atm}$, and rearranging eqn (1.20) we obtain

$$F_{IO_2} = \frac{P_{ACO_2} + RP_{AO_2}}{(1-R)P_{ACO_2} + RP_{atm}}. \tag{1.26}$$

In experiments performed in lambs using extracorporeal CO_2 removal, Gattinoni et al. (Gattinoni, L. *et al.* (1978) *British Journal of Anaesthesia* **50**, 753–7) have measured the steady F_{IO_2} required to maintain a P_{aO_2} of 10.43 kPa and a P_{aCO_2} of 4.66 kPa. Their results are compared in Fig. 1.6 with eqn (1.26) and excellent agreement is achieved by setting $P_{AO_2} = 14.91$ and $P_{ACO_2} = P_{aCO_2}$. The alveolar–arterial oxygen pressure difference ($P_{AO_2} - P_{aO_2}$) predicted by this correlation was similar to control values. The data provide strong support for the validity of eqn (1.20).

1.10   Ventilation and the body's control of blood gas concentrations

The study of the body's control of breathing has fascinated physiologists for many years and continues to be loaded with mystery. We are still largely ignorant of how breathing is profoundly modified to supply the demands of vigorous exercise, for example, which in fit adults may increase the requirement for oxygen to up to 15 times normal ($\simeq 4\,l\,min^{-1}$) and the production of CO_2 to some 30 times ($\simeq 8\,l\,min^{-1}$).

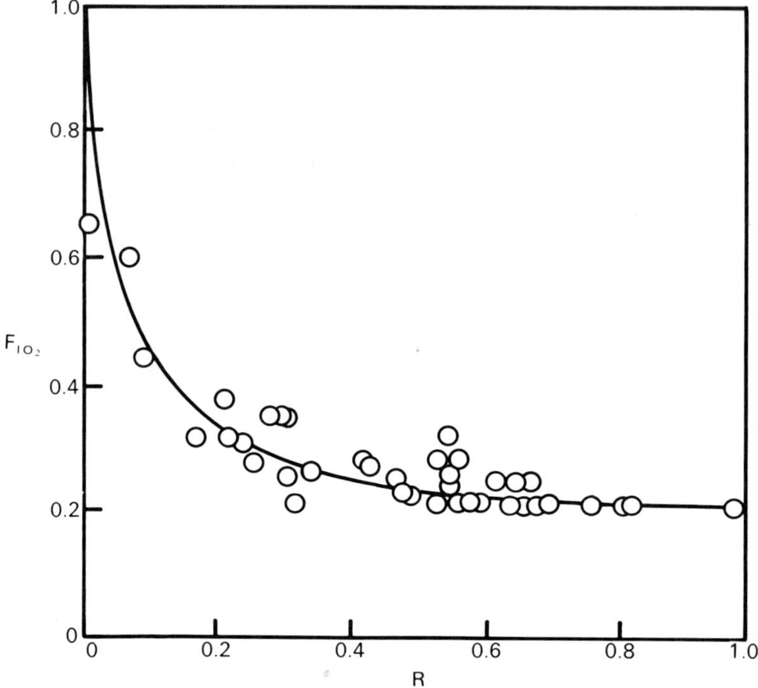

Fig. 1.6. Measurements in lambs, during extracorporeal CO_2 removal, of the inspired dry oxygen fraction F_{IO_2} required to maintain steady blood gases (P_{aO_2} = 10.43 kPa; P_{aCO_2} = 4.66 kPa) for different values of pulmonary respiratory quotient R. These are compared with the relationship between F_{IO_2} and R predicted by the alveolar gas equation (eqn 1.26) obtaining minimum sum of squares with P_{AO_2} = 14.91 kPa and P_{aCO_2} = 4.66 kPa. F_{IO_2} is stated as a fraction of dry inspired gas. (Redrawn from *British Journal of Anaesthesia*, with permission.)

From an engineering point of view, we shall regard the body's respiratory control system (Fig. 1.7) as sensing two main variables (P_{aCO_2} and P_{aO_2}) in order to control only one (ventilation). On the arterial side of the circulation there are sensors (known as chemoreceptors) in the brain and in the neck and chest, which respond to changes in the partial pressures of CO_2 and oxygen in the arterial blood. The *central* chemoreceptors, those in the brain, respond primarily to changes in arterial CO_2 partial pressure, P_{aCO_2}, and they do so indirectly by sensing changes in the hydrogen ion concentration ($[H^+]$), itself related to P_{aCO_2}. The *peripheral* chemoreceptors, those in the neck and chest, act differently. They respond mainly to changes in arterial oxygen partial pressure, P_{aO_2}, but also to some extent to P_{aCO_2}. In fact about 30 per cent of the ventilatory response to change in P_{aCO_2} normally comes from the peripheral receptors and the remaining 70 per cent from the central

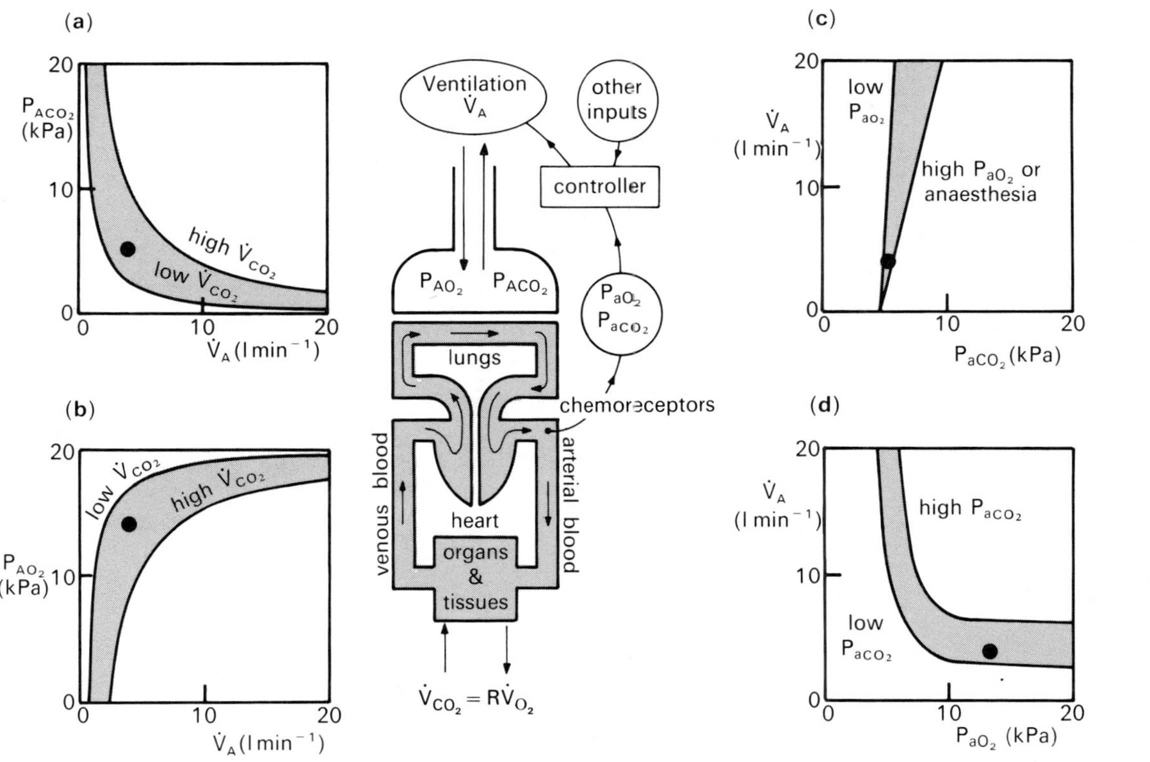

Fig. 1.7. The body's respiratory control system. Chemoreceptors on the arterial side of the circulation detect changes in arterial oxygen and CO_2 partial pressures (P_{aO_2}, P_{aCO_2}) which are used as feedback signals to control a single variable, ventilation. The system response ($P_{ACO_2} \simeq P_{aCO_2}$, $P_{AO_2} \simeq P_{aO_2}$) to changes in alveolar ventilation $\dot{V}_A$ is plotted in (a) and (b) (eqns 1.32 and 1.34) for high and low values of metabolic generation of CO_2 ($\dot{V}_{CO_2} = 400$ and 100 ml min⁻¹). The controller response is variable from person to person but represented typically in (c) and (d). It will be noted that there is a steep ventilatory response to changes in P_{aCO_2} but little response to changes in P_{aO_2} unless $P_{aO_2} < 8$ kPa. The solid point on all graphs locates normal conditions in the adult at rest.

receptors.* Information from these sensors and other sources is processed by a central respiratory controller in the brain. We shall outline the algorithm of this processor for controlling ventilation, but first consider how it is that changes in ventilation can serve to change P_{aCO_2} and P_{aO_2}.

Ventilation is the product of the tidal volume (volume of one breath in) V_T and the respiratory rate r (number of breaths per minute):

$$\dot{V} = V_T r. \tag{1.27}$$

It is the total volume of gas inspired over unit time and consequently is sometimes referred to as the *minute volume*. Of the total tidal volume, a sizeable fraction enters the anatomical dead space V_D ($\simeq 150$ ml of the upper airways) and is subsequently expired devoid of CO_2. Only the remainder reaches the alveoli. The *alveolar ventilation*, the effective ventilation for the exhausting of CO_2, is thus given by

$$\dot{V}_A = (V_T - V_D)r. \tag{1.28}$$

For a normal adult V_T and r at rest are about 500 ml and 12 min^{-1} respectively. The alveolar ventilation in these circumstances becomes

$$\dot{V}_A = (500 - 150) \times 12$$

$$= 4200 \text{ ml min}^{-1}$$

$$\simeq 4 \text{ l min}^{-1}. \tag{1.29}$$

It is the expiration of alveolar gas which transports CO_2 out of the body and since the fraction by volume of CO_2 in alveolar gas is P_{ACO_2}/P_{atm}, the body's rate of production of CO_2, $\dot{V}_{CO_2}$, must be given by

$$\dot{V}_{CO_2} = \left(\frac{P_{ACO_2}}{P_{atm}}\right)\dot{V}_A, \tag{1.30}$$

or substituting from eqs (1.27) and (1.28),

$$\dot{V}_{CO_2} = \left(\frac{P_{ACO_2}}{P_{atm}}\right)\left(1 - \frac{V_D}{V_T}\right)\dot{V}. \tag{1.31}$$

The relationship between P_{ACO_2} and $\dot{V}_A$ (eqn (1.30)) is a simple inverse relationship appearing as a rectangular hyperbola on a plot of P_{ACO_2} against $\dot{V}_A$ (Fig. 1.7(a)):

$$\boxed{P_{ACO_2} = \frac{(P_{atm}\dot{V}_{CO_2})}{\dot{V}_A}}. \tag{1.32}$$

For the normal adult at rest $\dot{V}_{CO_2} \simeq 0.2 \text{ l min}^{-1}$, and with $P_{atm} = 100 \text{ kPa}$ eqn

---

* These percentages depend upon the speed with which changes in P_{aCO_2} occur. Peripheral receptors can respond to more sudden changes than can central receptors.

(1.32) becomes

$$P_{ACO_2} = 20/\dot{V}_A \; kPa \tag{1.33}$$

where $\dot{V}_A$ is in units of $l\,min^{-1}$. For $\dot{V}_A = 4\,l\,min^{-1}$ this yields the expected normal value $P_{ACO_2} = 5\;kPa$.

In Fig. 1.7(a) we plot this normal operating point and also the $P_{ACO_2} - \dot{V}_A$ relationship for a high value of $\dot{V}_{CO_2}$ ($\simeq 0.4\,l\,min^{-1}$) and a low value of $\dot{V}_{CO_2}$ at rest ($\simeq 0.1\,l\,min^{-1}$). The high value might be observed, for example, during exercise; the low value could be seen during deep anaesthesia. The relationship between total ventilation $\dot{V}$ and P_{ACO_2} is complicated by the need to account for the dead space (eqn (1.31)). It is not a simple inverse relationship because the ratio of dead space to tidal volume V_D/V_T will itself vary with $\dot{V}$. For this reason we have chosen to plot only $\dot{V}_A$ in Fig. 1.7.

The alveolar oxygen partial pressure P_{AO_2} is dictated from the P_{ACO_2} by the alveolar gas equation (eqn (1.20)). Assuming a respiratory quotient of 0.8 the alveolar gas equation becomes

$$P_{AO_2} = P_{IO_2} - 1.2\,P_{ACO_2}, \tag{1.22}$$

and for air breathing (assuming a high degree of saturation with water vapour) $P_{IO_2} \simeq 20\;kPa$. In Fig. 1.7(b) we plot the result of combining eqns (1.22) and (1.32) to yield the P_{AO_2} as a function of $\dot{V}_A$:

$$P_{AO_2} = 20 - 1.2\frac{(P_{atm}\,\dot{V}_{CO_2})}{\dot{V}_A}\;kPa. \tag{1.34}$$

For the normal values $P_{atm} = 100\;kPa$, $\dot{V}_{CO_2} = 0.2\,l\,min^{-1}$, $\dot{V}_A = 4\,l\,min^{-1}$ eqn (1.34) gives

$$P_{AO_2} = 20 - 1.2\frac{(100 \times 0.2)}{4}$$

$$= 14\;kPa, \tag{1.35}$$

as expected. This normal operating point is plotted in Fig. 1.7(b) as well as the $P_{AO_2} - \dot{V}_A$ relationship for both the high and low values of $\dot{V}_{CO_2}$ represented in Fig. 1.7(a).

Figures 1.7(a) and (b) summarize then the response of the lungs to changes in alveolar ventilation. In the healthy subject the arterial partial pressures of oxygen and CO_2 are nearly equal to the alveolar partial pressures because good equilibration occurs as blood passes through lung capillaries, separated from alveolar gas by only a thin membrane which is permeable to the gases (Fig. 1.3). Figures 1.7(a) and (b) are therefore in effect plots of P_{aCO_2} and P_{aO_2} against $\dot{V}_A$ and represent the system response to changes in the input variable, ventilation. We now examine the algorithm of the controller of breathing to see how it responds to feedback signals of P_{aO_2} and P_{aCO_2} (from the chemo-receptors) to induce changes in ventilation.

In relation to Fig. 1.5 we noted that the controller attempts to maintain the P_{aCO_2} within a very narrow range, but that it is only influenced to any great degree by the P_{aO_2} if its value falls below about 8 kPa. The mechanism behind this response is depicted in Figs. 1.7(c) and (d). These figures show the results of experiments in which subjects have breathed different concentrations of oxygen and CO_2 in such a manner that only one of the two variables P_{aCO_2} and P_{aO_2} is altered at any one time. The ventilation generated by the subjects is then plotted as a function of these arterial partial pressures.

The very marked response of the controller to changes in P_{aCO_2} is apparent from the extremely steep and highly linear response lines of Fig. 1.7(c). The CO_2 response and oxygen response are interrelated in such a manner that hypoxia (low P_{aO_2}) generates an even steeper CO_2 response line than for normal or high P_{aO_2}. Many drugs and anaesthetic agents depress the ventilatory response in such a way that their effect is represented by a decrease in gradient of the CO_2 response line (Fig. 1.7(c)). The fan of CO_2 response lines for different P_{aO_2} has been found to display the interesting property of having a single origin on the horizontal axis. The reason for this is not clear.

The ventilatory response of the controller to P_{aO_2} is shown in Fig. 1.7(d). There is little response for values of P_{aO_2} in the normal range but a marked increase in ventilation is generated as the P_{aO_2} falls below about 8 kPa. The steep rise in the response curves at low P_{aO_2} is thought to be asymptotic to a vertical line at about $P_{aO_2} = 4$ kPa. A family of oxygen response curves can be plotted for different values of P_{aCO_2} in accord with Fig. 1.7(c). Those for high P_{aCO_2} lie above those for low P_{aCO_2}. It has also been discovered that quite independently of changes in P_{aCO_2}, exercise itself can raise or lower the oxygen response curve. The mechanism for this response of the controller is unknown.

In summary, the body's respiratory control system depends upon detection of P_{aCO_2} and P_{aO_2} for control of ventilation. The system response to changes in ventilation is predictable from eqn (1.32) and the alveolar gas equation. This response generates Fig. 1.7(a) and (b). The controller algorithm can be measured by experiment and its response to the arterial CO_2 and oxygen partial pressures is depicted in Figs. 1.7(c) and (d). Many other factors influence the pattern of breathing. Effects of anaesthesia and exercise have been noted. Speech, laughter, sneezing, hiccuping, sighing and eating all involve involuntary changes in breathing. In addition, we are all familiar with its voluntary control: 'take deep breaths in and out Mr Jones'.

1.11   Oxygen and CO_2 carriage in the blood

The blood forms the main motorway system round the body for the transport of fuels, building materials, waste products, weapons and messages. It is a liquid, yet 40 per cent of the volume of blood is occupied by living cells, each being a vehicle with its own specific cargo. By far the largest fleet of these vehicles are the red cells (erythrocytes) which number around 5×10^{12} per litre of blood and are responsible for its characteristic red colour. The main role of the red cell is to assist in the transport of oxygen and CO_2 around the body: oxygen as a fuel from the lungs to the organs and tissues, CO_2 as a waste product from the organs and tissues to the lungs (Fig. 1.7).

The other major groups of cells in the blood are white cells and platelets. White cells variably number around 5×10^9 per litre and participate in the body's defences. These cells are of considerable importance to the designer of artificial blood handling devices such as extracorporeal lungs because they may be stimulated to action as blood comes into contact with engineering materials which are foreign to the body. Once activated in this way the white cells become capable of damaging the body's own organs and tissues through a misguided response to the quite unphysiological stimulus. The design engineer must attempt to minimize these effects by choosing appropriate materials, usually polymers, for the construction of artificial lungs.

Platelets number approximately 2×10^{11} per litre and participate in the coagulation of blood, a protective mechanism for preventing leakage from blood vessels. These cells too are of importance in the context of extra-corporeal devices for two main reasons. Firstly, all known engineering materials encourage the process of coagulation, which is undesirable and may be disastrous in extracorporeal lungs. Without the use of anticoagulant drugs extracorporeal bypass would rarely be feasible at present. Secondly, at least some platelets are consumed or damaged by foreign surfaces and this may lead to such a deficiency of platelets in the patient that uncontrollable bleeding occurs. This may be either during the bypass procedure itself or afterwards, in the period before the body's own manufacture of platelets has caught up with the loss. Whenever a patient's blood is made to flow through an extracorporeal circuit the aim must be to control the coagulation mechanism, to prevent at one extreme clotting up of the circuit and at the other extreme spontaneous bleeding inside the patient.

If blood were simply water we should easily be able to calculate the concentration C of a gas transported in the blood from a knowledge of the partial pressure P of the gas with which the blood has been equilibrated:

$$C = \alpha P, \tag{1.36}$$

where α is known as the solubility coefficient and remains a constant over wide ranges of concentration. Equation (1.36) expresses Henry's law*. It assumes constant temperature, and is widely applicable to gases dissolved in liquids, though each gas–liquid pair has a specific value for α.

We choose to express gas concentrations in liquid in ml (STP) per 100 ml, that is in ml of gas per 100 ml of liquid where the gas volume is referred to

---

* William Henry 1774–1836, an English chemist.

Standard Temperature (0 °C) and Pressure (1 atm = 101.3 kPa). These units may be written in the shorthand form ml(STP)%. Since we express partial pressure P in kPa, the units of the solubility coefficient α (eqn (1.36)) will be ml(STP)% kPa^{-1}.

For oxygen in water at 37 °C, α is equal to 0.023 ml(STP)% kPa^{-1}. If blood were simply water the concentration of oxygen in arterial blood with $P_{aO_2} = 13$ kPa (a normal value for air breathing) would be $0.023 \times 13 = 0.3$ ml(STP)%. We earlier gave a normal oxygen consumption for an adult of 250 ml(STP)min^{-1}, and bearing in mind that the blood flow through the heart and lungs (the *cardiac output*) is normally around 5 l min^{-1} we can calculate that 5 litres of water would be grossly inadequate to carry 250 ml(STP) of oxygen every minute. The maximum oxygen carriage would in fact be

$$\frac{0.3 \text{ ml(STP)\%}}{100} \times 5000 \text{ ml min}^{-1} = 15 \text{ ml(STP)min}^{-1}, \qquad (1.37)$$

which is only 6 per cent of the required 250 ml(STP) min^{-1}. It is for this reason that we have evolved a far more effective means of transporting oxygen than would be provided by water alone.

CO_2 is more soluble in water than oxygen but can still not be dissolved in sufficient quantities to obviate the need for a special transport system of its own. For CO_2 in water at 37 °C, α is equal to 0.52 ml(STP)% kPa^{-1}. The normal partial pressure of CO_2 in venous blood (arriving at the lungs ready to offload CO_2) is $P_{vCO_2} = 6$ kPa. Again, assuming blood to be water, it would carry to the lungs

$$\frac{0.52 \times 6}{100} \times 5000 \simeq 150 \text{ ml(STP) min}^{-1} \qquad (1.38)$$

of CO_2. Since the normal metabolic production of CO_2 by the body is around 200 ml(STP) min^{-1} this too falls short of meeting the body's requirements.

In Figs. 1.8(a) and (b) the dissolved oxygen and CO_2 in blood is plotted according to Henry's law (eqn (1.36)) for comparison with the total concentration of the two gases carried by blood. Concentration C is plotted as a function of partial pressure P for the ranges of P of practical interest in respiration engineering. Exposure to high concentrations of oxygen commonly occurs in medical practice, if only for short periods of time, and so P_{O_2} values in blood are frequently experienced in virtually the whole range, 0–100 kPa; physiological CO_2 partial pressures rarely extend beyond the range 0–20 kPa. The dissolved concentrations of the two gases in blood are equal to their dissolved concentrations in water to the accuracy with which we have given α above.

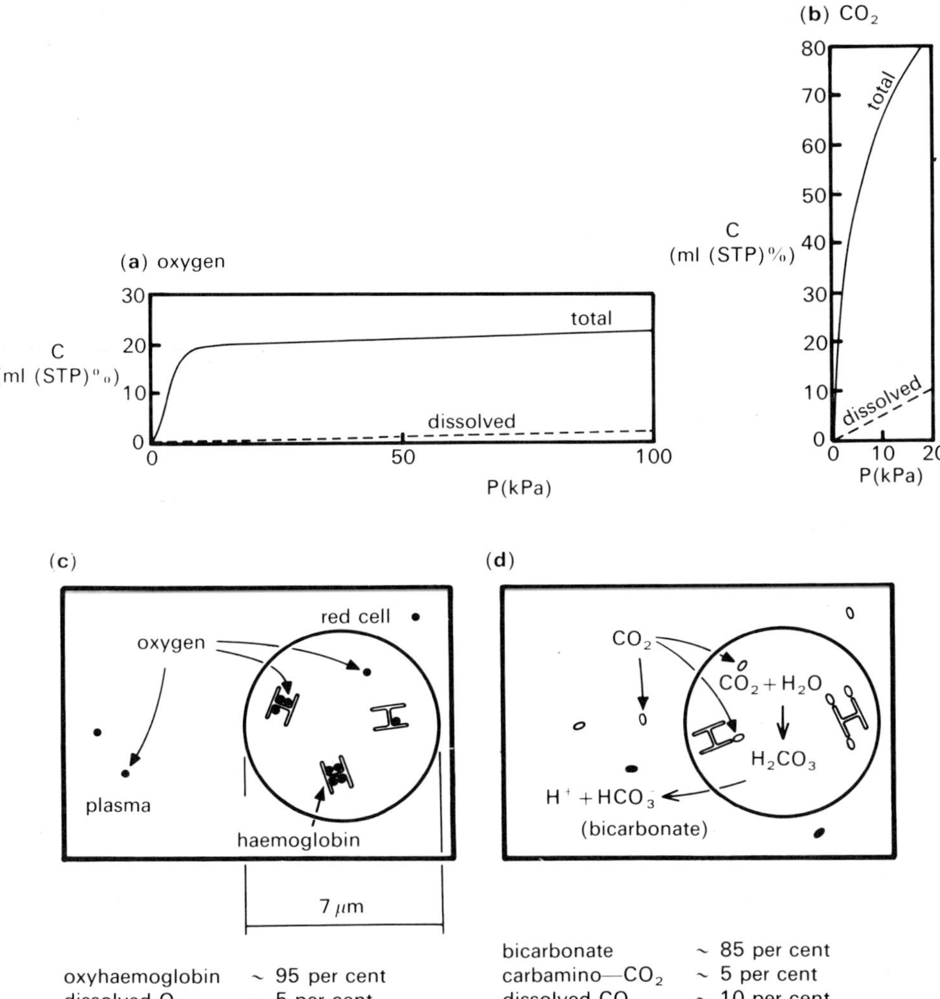

oxyhaemoglobin   ~ 95 per cent
dissolved O$_2$ ~ 5 per cent

bicarbonate   ~ 85 per cent
carbamino—CO$_2$ ~ 5 per cent
dissolved CO$_2$ ~ 10 per cent

Fig. 1.8. Oxygen and CO$_2$ carriage in the blood. The oxygen (a) and CO$_2$ (b) dissociation curves give the concentration C of the respective gases in blood as a function of partial pressure P. A small proportion of C is contributed by dissolved gas (dashed lines) plotted according to Henry's law (eqn 1.36). Oxygen is carried in two forms (c) whereas CO$_2$ is carried in three forms (d).

Most oxygen carried in the blood is bound to haemoglobin, forming oxyhaemoglobin, a molecule of molecular weight 67 000 amu* which occupies the red cells (Fig. 1.8(c)). Each molecule of haemoglobin binds up to four molecules of oxygen, the mean number depending upon the P_{O_2} in the blood.

* atomic mass unit: based on the standard of assigning a molecular weight of 12 amu to the isotope ^{12}carbon.

Full *saturation* of haemoglobin is said to occur when the full quota of four molecules of oxygen are bound or *associated* with each haemoglobin molecule in a sample of blood. A plot of the percentage saturation of haemoglobin against P_{O_2} is termed the *oxyhaemoglobin dissociation curve* and would be obtained from Fig. 1.8(a) from the difference between the C–P curve for the total oxygen carriage and the dissolved oxygen. Association between oxygen and haemoglobin is almost complete at a P_{O_2} of about 15 kPa and above this value the oxyhaemoglobin dissociation curve has a flat plateau. The continuing gentle upward slope of the C–P curve for the total oxygen carriage (Fig. 1.8(a)) derives from the increasing contribution to the total of the dissolved oxygen within the water of both blood cells and the 60 per cent of the volume of blood outside its cells known as *plasma*.

The fraction of oxygen carried in the dissolved form clearly varies markedly with P_{O_2} but is always small. At $P_{O_2} = 15$ kPa it forms approximately 1 per cent of the total, whereas at $P_{O_2} = 100$ kPa its contribution is nearer 10 per cent. The distinction between dissolved and associated oxygen is of considerable importance in respiration engineering when we attempt to model the oxygen transfer of artificial lungs (chapter 5). Only the dissolved oxygen has a mobility within cells and plasma sufficient to allow us to regard it as a diffusible species. Oxygen associated with haemoglobin is by contrast imprisoned within the red cells and must be regarded as a convected species largely unable to move by diffusion.

CO_2 is carried in the blood in three forms: dissolved, as bicarbonate, and as carbamino—CO_2 (Fig. 1.8(d)). The dissolved CO_2 in cells and plasma can be seen from Fig. 1.8(b) to contribute around 10 per cent. The greater bulk of the CO_2 is carried as bicarbonate which is formed by a reaction of CO_2 with water, first to produce carbonic acid (H_2CO_3) and then bicarbonate (HCO_3^-):*

$$CO_2 + H_2O \rightleftharpoons H_2CO_3 \rightleftharpoons H^+ + HCO_3^-. \tag{1.39}$$

The first reaction is normally both slow (half-time of the order of 1 min) and at equilibrium produces only about one molecule of H_2CO_3 for every 1000 molecules of CO_2 present in solution. Both reactions occur in water, but would make only a small contribution to helping to transport CO_2.

In blood the reaction forming H_2CO_3 from CO_2 is greatly speeded up by the presence inside red cells of an enzyme called carbonic anhydrase. The presence of this mechanism, together with the presence in both cells and plasma of molecules which will bind hydrogen ions, H^+, (see right-hand side of reaction (1.39)) causes the sequence of reactions forming bicarbonate from

---

* This is more correctly represented as

$$CO_2 + 2H_2O \rightleftharpoons H_2O + H_2CO_3 \rightleftharpoons H_3O^+ + HCO_3^-,$$

where H_3O^+ is the hydronium ion.

CO_2 to be both speeded up and predisposed towards the right, allowing large amounts of bicarbonate to form rapidly from dissolved CO_2 as CO_2 enters the blood from the organs and tissues. The reverse sequence of events occurs in the lungs where CO_2 is offloaded and the concentration of bicarbonate rapidly decreases.

Carbamino—CO_2 is formed when CO_2 becomes bound to the terminal amine group ($—NH_2$) of protein molecules in both cells and plasma:

$$\text{Protein}—NH_2 + CO_2 \rightleftharpoons \text{Protein}—NH—COOH. \qquad (1.40)$$

Approximately 5 per cent of the CO_2 carried by blood is in the form of carbamino—CO_2. Most of it is in fact bound to haemoglobin in the red cells and haemoglobin has evolved a remarkable facility whereby reaction (1.40) is strongly encouraged to move to the right as haemoglobin dissociates from oxygen. In other words the haemoglobin molecule can bind more CO_2 if it binds less oxygen. Accordingly, as blood passes through the organs and tissues it gives up oxygen for combustion and in so doing enables itself to carry away more CO_2 than would otherwise be possible. This is known as the Haldane* effect and explains why, even though carbamino—CO_2 may form only 5 per cent of the CO_2 carried in blood, it may account for around 30 per cent of the arterio–venous difference in CO_2 carriage as blood passes through the organs and tissues. Though it is a small fraction of the total CO_2 carried in blood, carbamino—CO_2 is nevertheless a major contributor to its transport around the body[†]. This Haldane effect would appear graphically in Fig. 1.8(b) as a slight displacement of the $C–P$ curve for CO_2 for different values of P_{O_2}, with the curve shifted to the right for high P_{O_2} and to the left for low P_{O_2}.

There is a similar displacement of the oxygen dissociation curve (Fig. 1.8(a)) as the P_{CO_2} changes, termed the Bohr[‡] effect. This phenomenon is also an artful feature of the haemoglobin molecule, whereby it adjusts its affinity for oxygen molecules according to how much CO_2 is bound to it in such a way that picking up CO_2 encourages it to offload oxygen. The Bohr effect appears as a shift to the right of the $C–P$ curve for oxygen (Fig. 1.8(a)) for high values of P_{CO_2} and a shift to the left for low values of P_{CO_2}.

The Bohr effect and the Haldane effect act synergistically to enhance the performance of the blood's transport system for oxygen and CO_2. In Fig. 1.9, the approximate normal arterial and venous partial pressures for oxygen and CO_2 are plotted on the respective dissociation curves with the Bohr and Haldane effects shown as shifts in these curves. It will be noted that the depicted arteriovenous differences in CO_2 and oxygen concentrations are 4

---

* John Scott Haldane (1860–1936), Oxford physiologist.
† The contributions of differences between arterial and venous blood of CO_2 concentration are normally approximately as follows: dissolved CO_2 = 10 per cent, bicarbonate = 60 per cent, carbamino—CO_2 = 30 per cent.
‡ Christian Bohr (1855–1911), Scandinavian physiologist.

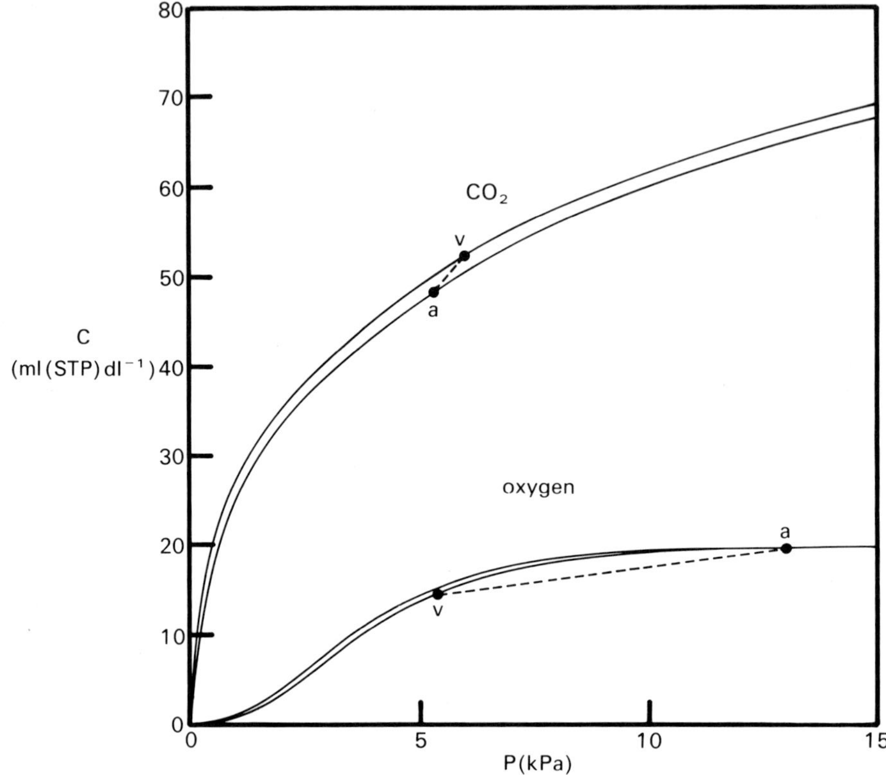

Fig. 1.9. Approximate content–partial pressure relationships for oxygen and CO_2 in blood with arterial and venous conditions labelled. The shift of the oxygen curve due to changes in pH and P_{CO_2} is known as the Bohr effect. The shift of the CO_2 curve due to changes in P_{O_2} is known as the Haldane effect.

and 5 ml(STP)% respectively, consistent with a respiratory quotient of

$$R = 4/5 = 0.8. \tag{1.41}$$

The arteriovenous oxygen difference is also consistent with an oxygen consumption by the body of $250\ \text{ml(STP)}\,\text{min}^{-1}$ being delivered by a cardiac output of $5\,\text{l}\,\text{min}^{-1}$:

$$250\ \text{ml(STP)}\,\text{min}^{-1} = 5\ \text{ml(STP)}\% \times 5\,\text{l}\,\text{min}^{-1} \times 10. \tag{1.42}$$

It is of practical interest that although a much greater extraction of CO_2 from venous blood than normal (4 ml(STP)%) can be accomplished artificially by moving further towards the origin down the CO_2 dissociation curve, it is impossible (except under hyperbaric conditions) to deliver significantly more oxygen to venous blood than is delivered physiologically (5 ml(STP)%). This arises because the oxygen dissociation curve reaches an almost flat plateau (Fig. 1.8(a)) at high values of partial pressure. A consequence of this observation is that the whole of a patient's metabolic production of CO_2 ($\simeq 200$ ml(STP)min^{-1}) can be removed using an extracorporeal lung with a relatively small blood flow* ($\simeq 1$–2 l min^{-1}). If we wish to deliver via an extracorporeal lung a patient's whole oxygen requirement ($\simeq 250$ ml(STP)min^{-1}), the blood flow in the bypass circuit needs to be approximately equal to the normal cardiac output ($\simeq 5$ l min^{-1}). These differences between removal from blood of CO_2 and delivery to blood of oxygen have important implications for the way extracorporeal lungs may be used in intensive care, where one of their future roles may be for CO_2 removal alone.

An elementary understanding of the way oxygen and CO_2 are transported in the body forms an important foundation for the medical engineer working on respiratory problems.

Further reading

Avogadro, A. (1811). D'une manière de déterminer les masses relatives des molécules élémentaires des corps, et les proportions selon lesquelles elles entrent dans ces combinaisons. *Journal de Physique et de Chimie* **73**, 58–76.

Christiansen, J., Douglas, C. G., and Haldane, J. S. (1914). The adsorption and dissociation of carbon dioxide by human blood. *Journal of Physiology* **48**, 244–71. (Description of the physiological significance of the Haldane effect.)

Dorrington, K. L. (1988). Extracorporeal gas exchange in acute respiratory failure. *British Medical Journal* **296**, 151–2.

Henry, W. (1803). Experiments on the quantity of gases absorbed by water, at different temperatures, and under different pressures. *Philosophical Transactions of the Royal Society* **93**, 29–42.

Meyer, K. H. and Gottlieb-Billroth, H. (1921). Theorie der Narkose durch Inhalationsanästhetika. *Zeitschrift für physiologische Chemie* **112**, 55–79. (Confirmation of the theory of H. H. Meyer (1899) and Overton (1901) regarding the lipid solubility characteristics of anaesthetics.)

Nunn, J. F. (1987). *Applied Respiratory Physiology* (3rd edn). Butterworths, London.

Riley, R. L., Lilienthal, J. L., Proemmel, D. D., and Franke, R. E. (1946). On the determination of the physiologically effective pressures of oxygen and carbon dioxide in alveolar air. *American Journal of Physiology* **147**, 191–8.

Sears, F. W. (1969). *Thermodynamics*, Chapters 11–14. Addison-Wesley, Reading, Massachusetts.

---

* The limit on just how great an arteriovenous difference in CO_2 concentration (and hence how small a blood flow) can be tolerated is probably defined by red cell damage induced by changes in hydrogen ion concentration as CO_2 is extracted from blood, not by arrival at the origin of the CO_2 dissociation curve.

Webster, N. R. and Nunn, J. F. (1988). Molecular structure of free radicals and their importance in biological reactions. *British Journal of Anaesthesia* **60**, 98–108. (Toxicity of high concentrations of oxygen.)

West, J. B. (1985). *Respiratory Physiology: the Essentials* (3rd edn). Williams and Wilkins, Baltimore, Maryland.

Whipp, B. J. (ed.) (1987). *The Control of Breathing in Man*. Manchester University Press, Manchester.

2 Medical breathing systems

2.1 Introduction

A *breathing system* is an arrangement of ducting which directs respiratory gases from their supply to a subject in such a manner as to permit *control* over the composition of the inspired gas. Non-medical breathing systems are important in extremes of environment to divers, mountaineers, pilots and astronauts, and arguably the simplest breathing system is one familiar to most who visit the seaside as children: the snorkel. Some form of medical breathing system is probably experienced by a majority of patients admitted to hospital, predominantly those undergoing surgery.

Breathing systems invariably represent the link between a continuous supply of fresh gases and the intermittent inspiratory demand of the subject, who usually spends more time breathing out than breathing in. The performance of all the breathing systems we shall examine in the following sections depends on this oscillatory pattern of demand.

Apart from preventing the user from inhaling neat water, the control offered by a snorkel over the composition of inspired gas is somewhat limited; simply stated, the longer the snorkel the more CO_2 is rebreathed with each breath and the more difficult it is to breathe through it. Consider a diver (Fig. 2.1) who expires breaths each with a *tidal volume*, V_T. His expired breath when out of water normally has a CO_2 volume fraction, F_{ECO_2}, around 0.05. Whilst breathing through a snorkel with volume V_D he suffers the disadvantage of having a rebreathe (at the beginning of each inspiration) the gas expired into the snorkel with the preceding breath*. The volume of gas leaving the diver which now escapes to the atmosphere is reduced to $V_T - V_D$. Now if the diver were to continue taking the same sized breath and expire the same volume of CO_2 per breath whilst snorkel diving, the expired CO_2 fraction F'_{ECO_2} under these conditions would need to be

$$F'_{ECO_2} = \frac{V_T}{(V_T - V_D)} \times F_{ECO_2}. \tag{2.1}$$

In practice the respiratory control system is so intolerant of sudden hypercapnia (the alveolar and arterial P_{CO_2} would rise with F'_{ECO_2}) that the diver would increase depth (V_T) and rate (r) of breathing (i.e., *ventilation*, $\dot{V} = V_T r$) to compensate for the added *dead space* of the snorkel and thereby keep $F'_{ECO_2} \simeq F_{ECO_2}$.

---

* We assume here that the swimmer follows the common practice of breathing both in and out through the snorkel. Nasal expiration via a face mask is clearly possible, but leads to condensation on the mask.

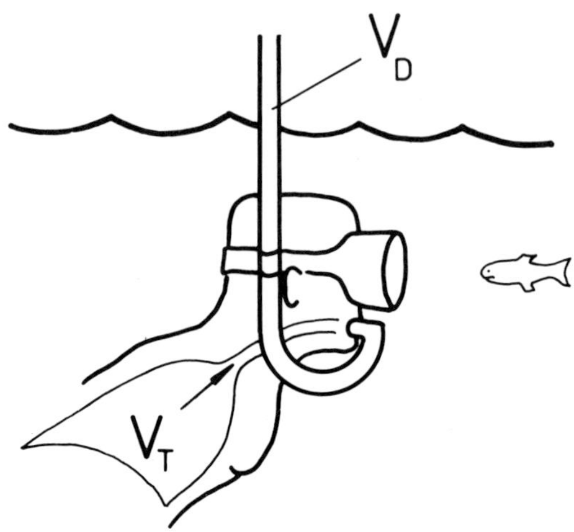

Fig. 2.1. The snorkel is probably the simplest breathing system. It illustrates the problem of rebreathing CO_2 from a dead space volume V_D. V_T is the tidal volume.

A useful way of defining the tendency of a system to produce *rebreathing* is indeed to calculate the ratio of the ventilation required whilst breathing through the system ($\dot{V}$) to that in the absence of the system ($\dot{V}_0$) for identical values of F_{ECO_2} in both cases. This ratio ($\dot{V}/\dot{V}_0$) we call the *rebreathing index*. It can be examined usefully as a function of the design variables of the system.

For the case of the snorkel we have the simple relationship

$$(V_T - V_D)r = V_{T0}\,r_0, \tag{2.2}$$

where V_{T0} and r_0 are the tidal volume and respiratory rate in the absence of a snorkel. Since $\dot{V} = V_T r$ and $\dot{V}_0 = V_{T0}\,r_0$ we write

$$\dot{V} - V_D r = \dot{V}_0$$

or

$$\frac{\dot{V}}{\dot{V}_0} = 1 + \left(\frac{V_D r}{\dot{V}_0}\right). \tag{2.3}$$

This simple relationship is plotted in Fig. 2.2. One conclusion of interest from this analysis is that for given values of V_D and $\dot{V}_0$ the rebreathing index of the snorkel is smaller as r is reduced. This is entirely to be expected since for a given ventilation, $V_T r$, fewer larger breaths involve fewer excursions of the dead space volume than many smaller breaths.

Unlike the snorkel, some breathing systems have the characteristic that however much the user increases his ventilation $\dot{V}$ he may be unable to achieve the same F_{ECO_2} with the system as he had breathing with his normal

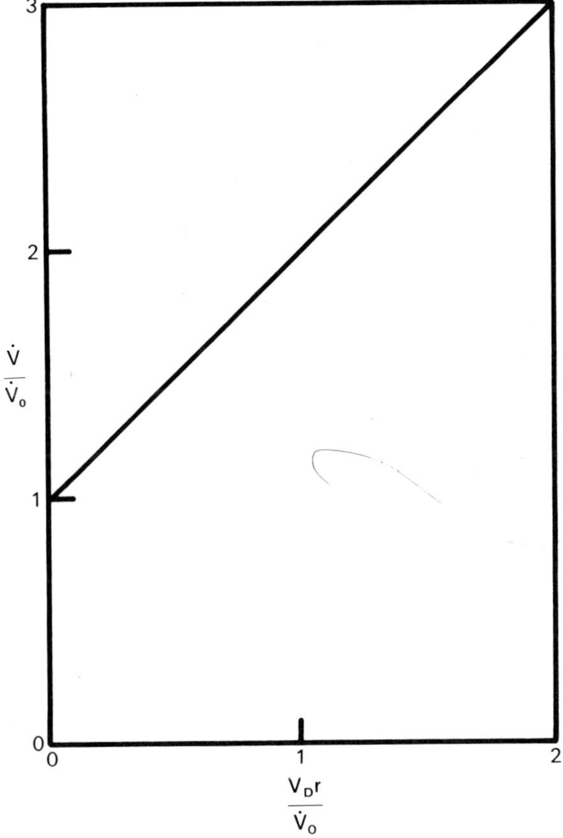

Fig. 2.2. The rebreathing index ($\dot{V}/\dot{V}_0$) for the snorkel of volume V_{D}. r is the respiratory rate during snorkel breathing and $\dot{V}_0$ is the normal ventilation in the absence of the snorkel ($V_{\mathrm{D}} = 0$).

ventilation $\dot{V}_0$ without it. In these cases the rebreathing index becomes indeterminate, and an alternative useful indicator of the tendency of CO_2 to accumulate is the ratio $F'_{\mathrm{ECO_2}}/F_{\mathrm{ECO_2}}$ of the expired CO_2 fractions with and without the breathing system for identical values of ventilation $\dot{V}_0$ in both cases. This ratio we call the *CO_2 retention index.*

For the case of the snorkel, assuming constant CO_2 elimination with and without the system, we have

$$F'_{\mathrm{ECO_2}}(V_{\mathrm{T}} - V_{\mathrm{D}})r = F_{\mathrm{ECO_2}} V_{\mathrm{T0}} r_0, \tag{2.4}$$

and for identical values of ventilation in the two cases

$$V_{\mathrm{T}}r = V_{\mathrm{T0}}r_0 = \dot{V}_0. \tag{2.5}$$

The CO_2 retention index for the snorkel is thus

$$\frac{F'_{ECO_2}}{F_{ECO_2}} = \frac{1}{1-(V_D/V_T)}.$$

(2.6)

This relationship is plotted in Fig. 2.3. We shall see later that, whereas the rebreathing index is most valuable in expressing the performance of a system used during spontaneous ventilation, the CO_2 retention index becomes a more useful measure of the performance of a breathing system used during mechanical ventilation where the patient's ventilation is controlled not by the patient but by a machine.

The simple example of snorkel breathing illustrates the importance of dead space in a breathing system. If there is no axial mixing along a duct between

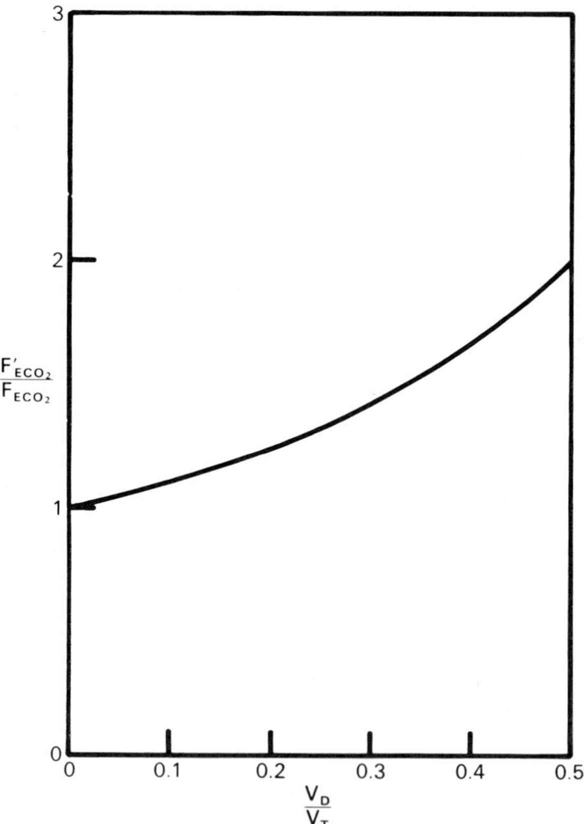

Fig. 2.3. The CO_2 retention index (F'_{ECO_2}/F_{ECO_2}) for snorkel of volume V_D. V_T is the tidal volume.

dead space gas and fresh gas, maintenance of life becomes impossible when the dead space volume exceeds the tidal volume. We shall see in chapter 4 that, where axial mixing (often termed axial dispersion) occurs in a breathing system, adequate expiration of CO_2 may be maintained even when the tidal volume is smaller than the dead space. This state of affairs can only be achieved at high frequencies of ventilation and it is axiomatic to the analyses of breathing systems in this chapter that axial mixing may be regarded as absent.

With anaesthetic breathing systems not only do we wish to avoid the patient rebreathing a large proportion of CO_2, we also aim to keep only the patient anaesthetized, not his attendants. Systems may therefore need to be free of leaks. In addition, even in non-anaesthetic concentrations anaesthetic agents may have a somewhat objectionable pungent odour (for example, ether) or adverse sequelae with chronic exposure (for example, bone marrow depression with nitrous oxide), and medical attendants now need to be protected from excessive exposure to exhaust gases. This clearly has a bearing on the design of medical breathing systems.

2.2 The variable-concentration oxygen mask

The frequent need to increase the inspired oxygen fraction (F_{IO_2}) of a spontaneously breathing patient can be met using a simple form of mask to which oxygen is delivered and through which, simply via some holes, the patient may also entrain air and expire (Fig. 2.4(a)). The masks are termed *variable-concentration* masks because the inspired oxygen concentration depends upon the fresh gas flow to the mask. We model such a breathing system by assuming a volumetric oxygen fresh gas flow $\dot{V}_{FG}$ into a mask which has a reservoir volume V_m. The patient's breathing is modelled simply by assuming that both inspiration and expiration occur at constant flows $\dot{V}_I$ and $\dot{V}_E$, with their duration having a ratio t_I/t_E which is variable (Fig. 2.4(b)). Since the respiratory quotient is usually close to one, the error in assuming that the inspired and expired volumes are identical is small and we neglect it here (for $R = 0.8$, oxygen consumption $= 250\ \mathrm{ml\ min}^{-1}$, $\dot{V} = 6000\ \mathrm{ml\ min}^{-1}$, the error will be $\simeq 1$ per cent). For equal inspired and expired volumes we have

$$\dot{V}_I t_I = \dot{V}_E t_E \qquad (2.7)$$

and the areas under the inspiratory and expiratory regions of the breathing curve (Fig. 2.4(b)) are identical.

We consider the composition of inspired gas. During inspiration the oxygen line supplies to the mask a volume $\dot{V}_{FG} t_I$. If $\dot{V}_I > \dot{V}_{FG}$ we may presume that all of this oxygen is inspired. The composition of the remaining inspired gas will depend on a number of factors including the mask's reservoir volume V_m and the proximity to the nose and/or the mouth of the air holes in the

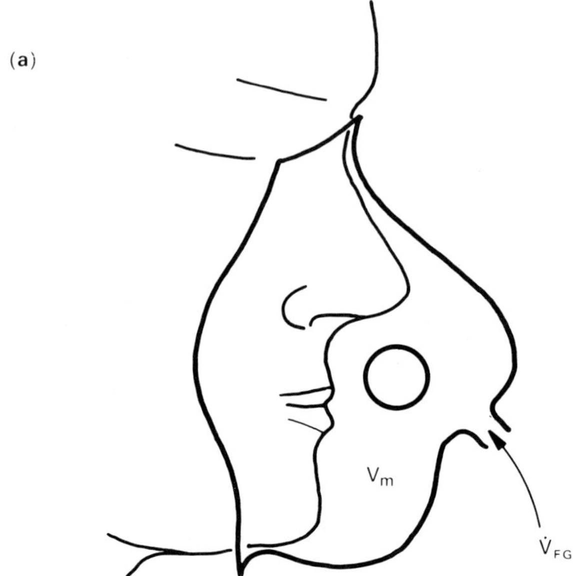

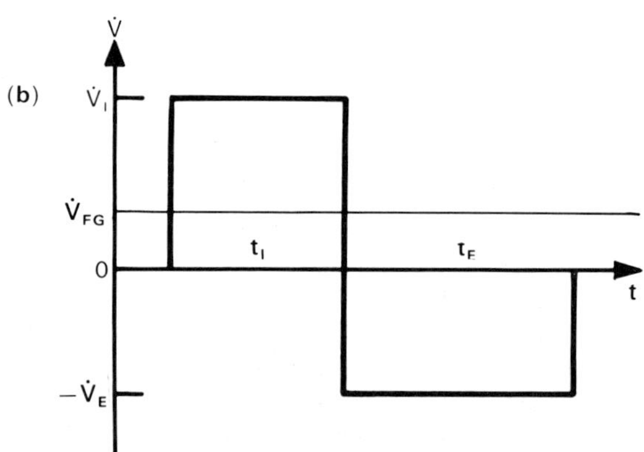

Fig. 2.4. The variable-concentration oxygen mask (a) produces an inspired oxygen fraction which varies with the fresh gas flow of oxygen $\dot{V}_{FG}$ to the mask and with the mask volume V_m. The patient's breathing is modelled here (b) by assuming constant inspiratory and expiratory flows, respectively, of duration t_I and t_E.

mask. We shall examine two extreme cases to delineate the full range of behaviour that may be expected from this kind of mask (Fig. 2.5).

Firstly, assume that the mask volume is small, the air holes lie close to the nose, and consequently the remaining inspired gas is entirely entrained air

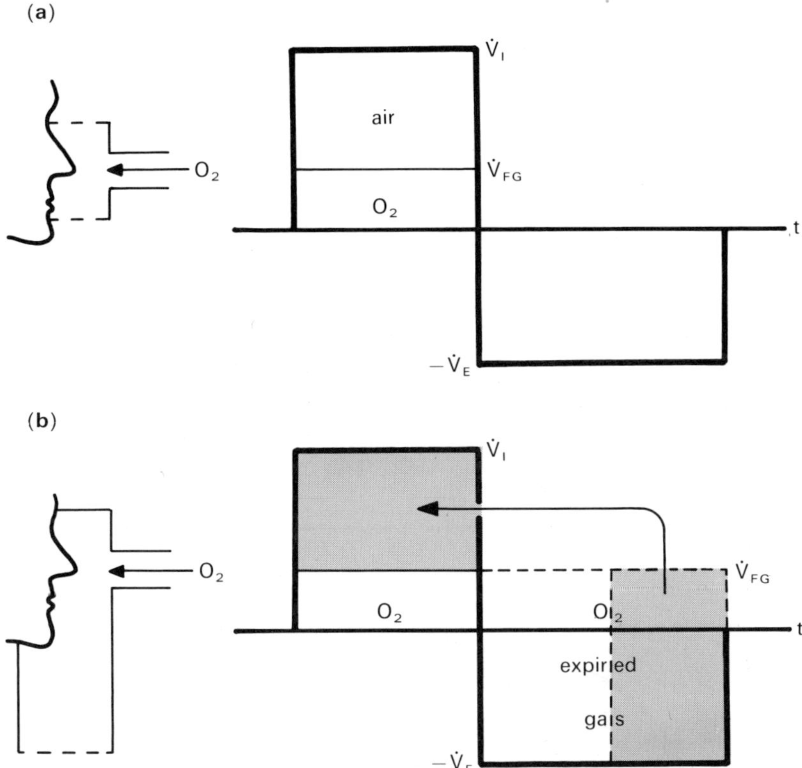

Fig. 2.5. The variable-concentration oxygen mask has a rebreathing index which depends upon the mask volume V_m. The two extreme cases are (a) $V_m \to 0$ and (b) $V_m \to \infty$. In (a), the patient inspires a mixture of all the oxygen delivered to the mask during inspiration ($\dot{V}_{FG}t_I$) plus entrained fresh air (($\dot{V}_I - \dot{V}_{FG})t_I$); there is no rebreathing. In (b) the inspired breath is composed of all the oxygen delivered to the mask during inspiration ($\dot{V}_{FG}t_I$) plus gas (shaded) from the reservoir of the mask. This gas is in turn a sample of a mixture of a volume $V_E t_E$ of expired gas plus the oxygen delivered to the mask during expiration ($\dot{V}_{FG}t_E$).

(Fig. 2.5(a)). The inspired oxygen fraction is then given by

$$F_{IO_2} = \frac{\dot{V}_{FG} + 0.2(\dot{V}_I - \dot{V}_{FG})}{\dot{V}_I}$$

$$= 0.2 + 0.8(\dot{V}_{FG}/\dot{V}_I). \tag{2.8}$$

The ventilation $\dot{V}$ is related to the inspiratory flow $\dot{V}_I$ by

$$\dot{V} = \dot{V}_I \frac{t_I}{(t_I + t_E)}$$

$$= \dot{V}_I/(1 + t_E/t_I). \tag{2.9}$$

Since there is no rebreathing with this system, the rebreathing index is given by

$$\dot{V}/\dot{V}_0 = 1. \tag{2.10}$$

Using eqns (2.9) and (2.10) we may therefore express F_{IO_2} (eqn 2.8) in terms of the clinically useful ratio $\dot{V}_{FG}/\dot{V}_0$:

$$F_{IO_2} = 0.2 + \frac{0.8(\dot{V}_{FG}/\dot{V}_0)}{(1 + t_E/t_I)}. \tag{2.11}$$

Equation (2.11) is plotted in Fig. 2.6 (line a) with t_E/t_I set equal to 1. The equation is valid and the plot is linear up to $\dot{V}_{FG}/\dot{V}_0 = 2$ beyond which F_{IO_2} remains equal to 1, which it clearly cannot exceed. The constant rebreathing index for this small volume mask (eqn (2.10)) is plotted in Fig. 2.7 (line a) for comparison with the case of the large volume mask discussed below.

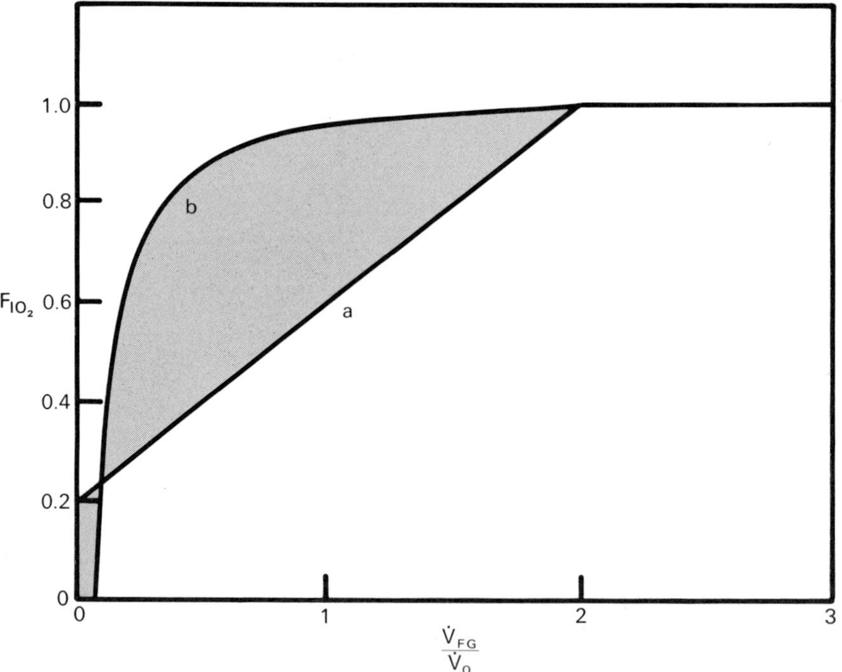

Fig. 2.6. Variable-concentration oxygen masks: the inspired oxygen fraction as a function of $\dot{V}_{FG}/\dot{V}_0$. $\dot{V}_{FG}$ is the fresh gas (oxygen) flow and $\dot{V}_0$ is the ventilation in the absence of rebreathing ($F_{IO_2} = 1$) for the same expired CO_2 fraction F_{ECO_2} (see text). (a) Small mask $V_m \to 0$ (eqn (2.11)), (b) large mask $V_m \to \infty$ (eqn (2.20)). Both cases have been plotted for $t_E/t_I = 1$. Curve b has been plotted also assuming $\dot{V}_{O_2} = 250$ ml min^{-1}, $\dot{V}_0 = 6000$ ml min^{-1}. Curves for masks of intermediate volume will lie in the shaded region between the two extremes.

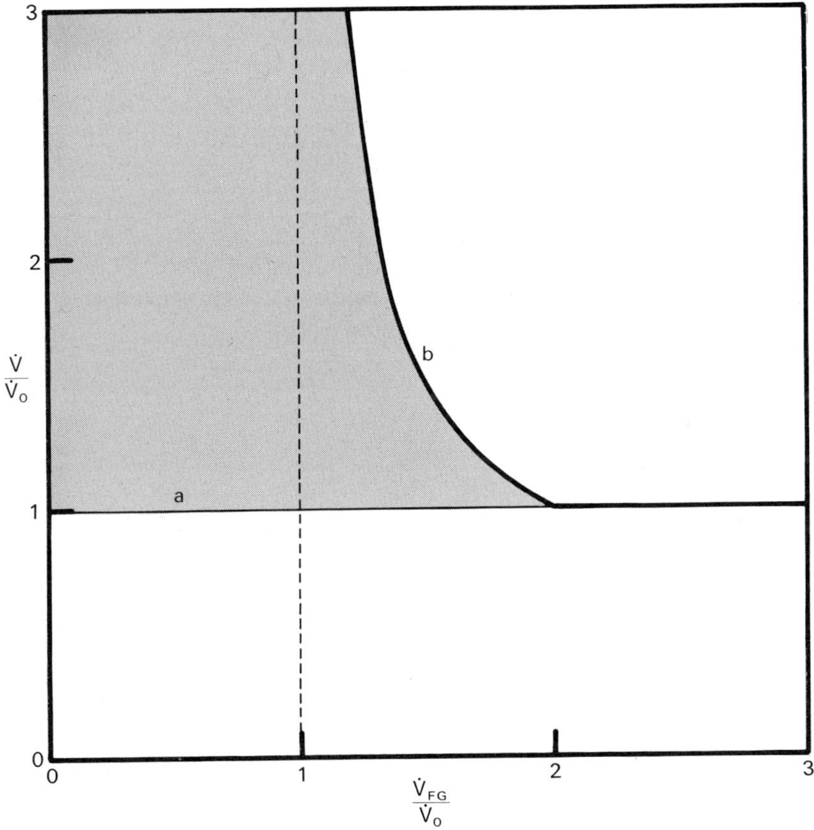

Fig. 2.7. Variable-concentration oxygen masks: the rebreathing index as a function of $\dot{V}_{FG}/\dot{V}_0$. $\dot{V}_{FG}$ is the fresh gas (oxygen) flow and $\dot{V}_0$ is the ventilation in the absence of rebreathing ($F_{IO_2} = 1$) for the same expired CO_2 fraction F_{ECO_2} (see text). (a) small mask $V_m \rightarrow 0$ (eqn (2.10)), (b) large mask $V_m \rightarrow \infty$ (eqn (2.21)) assuming $t_I/t_E = 1$. Curves for masks of intermediate volume will lie in the shaded region between the two extremes.

For our second extreme case we assume that the mask volume is large but fresh gas is still delivered close to the nose. The air holes lie distant from the nose and consequently no entrained air is inspired (Fig. 2.5(b)). Again the patient breathes a volume $\dot{V}_{FG} t_I$ of pure oxygen from the supply line. The remaining gas breathed is from the reservoir of the mask, and in the absence of detailed information regarding streaming of flow through the mask we assume this gas to be a perfect mixture of the expired gas (volume $\dot{V}_E t_E$) and the pure oxygen delivered to the mask during the previous expiration (volume $\dot{V}_{FG} t_E$). Denoting the oxygen fraction of expired gas as F_{EO_2} we deduce the inspired oxygen fraction for this case to be

$$F_{IO_2} \equiv \frac{\dot{V}_{FG} + (\dot{V}_I - \dot{V}_{FG})(\dot{V}_{FG} + F_{EO_2}\dot{V}_E)/(\dot{V}_{FG} + \dot{V}_E)}{\dot{V}_I}. \tag{2.12}$$

The inspired and expired oxygen fractions are related (to the extent that eqn(2.7) is valid) by the equation

$$(F_{IO_2} - F_{EO_2})\,\dot{V} = \dot{V}_{O_2}, \tag{2.13}$$

where $\dot{V}_{O_2}$ is the oxygen consumption per minute of the patient. A typical value for an adult male is 250 ml min^{-1} (chapter 1). We make use of eqns (2.7) and (2.13) to eliminate $\dot{V}_E$ and F_{EO_2} from eqn (2.12):

$$F_{IO_2} = 1 - \left(\frac{\dot{V}}{\dot{V}_{FG}} - \frac{1}{(1 + t_E/t_I)}\right)\frac{\dot{V}_{O_2}}{\dot{V}}. \tag{2.14}$$

The rebreathing index for the large volume mask can be calculated by recalling that the inspired gas (Fig. 2.5(b)) comprises a volume of pure oxygen $\dot{V}_{FG}\,t_I$ direct from the fresh gas supply, together with a volume $(\dot{V}_I - \dot{V}_{FG})\,t_I$ taken from an assumed perfect mixture of expired gas $(\dot{V}_E\,t_E)$ and the pure oxygen delivered to the mask during the previous expiration $(\dot{V}_{FG}\,t_E)$. If F_{ECO_2} is the fraction of CO_2 in expired gas, then the inspired CO_2 fraction will be given by

$$F_{ICO_2} = \frac{(\dot{V}_I - \dot{V}_{FG})\,F_{ECO_2}\,\dot{V}_E/(\dot{V}_E + \dot{V}_{FG})}{\dot{V}_I}. \tag{2.15}$$

If the production per minute of CO_2 is $\dot{V}_{CO_2}$ then the mean inspired and expired CO_2 fractions are given (to the extent that eqn (2.7) is valid) by

$$(F_{ECO_2} - F_{ICO_2})\,\dot{V} = \dot{V}_{CO_2}. \tag{2.16}$$

We eliminate F_{ICO_2} from the left-hand side of eqn (2.15) by substitution from eqns (2.7) and (2.9) to leave us an expression for F_{ECO_2}:

$$F_{ECO_2} = \frac{[1 + (1 + t_I/t_E)(\dot{V}/\dot{V}_{FG})]}{(1 + t_I/t_E)} \times \frac{\dot{V}_{CO_2}}{\dot{V}}. \tag{2.17}$$

Now in the absence of rebreathing, with a ventilation $\dot{V}_0$, the expired CO_2 fraction (eqn (2.16) with $F_{ICO_2} = 0$) would be

$$F_{ECO_2} = \frac{\dot{V}_{CO_2}}{\dot{V}_0}, \tag{2.18}$$

and for F_{ECO_2} to be identical both with (eqn (2.17)) and without (eqn (2.18)) rebreathing, the ventilations $\dot{V}$ and $\dot{V}_0$ for the two respective cases will be related by

$$\frac{\dot{V}}{\dot{V}_0} = \frac{[1 + (1 + t_I/t_E)(\dot{V}/\dot{V}_{FG})]}{(1 + t_I/t_E)}. \tag{2.19}$$

Equation (2.19) may now be incorporated into eqn (2.14) to express F_{IO_2} as a function of $\dot{V}_{FG}/\dot{V}_0$:

$$F_{IO_2} = 1 - \left[\frac{\dot{V}_0}{\dot{V}_{FG}}(1 + t_I/t_E) - \frac{t_I}{t_E} \right] \frac{\dot{V}_{O_2}}{\dot{V}_0}. \tag{2.20}$$

This result is plotted in Fig. 2.6 (line b) for the case $t_I/t_E = 1$, $\dot{V}_{O_2} = 250\ \mathrm{ml\ min}^{-1}$, $\dot{V}_0 = 6000\ \mathrm{ml\ min}^{-1}$. We note that through most of the plot F_{IO_2} for the large volume mask is higher than that for the small volume mask at an equivalent fresh gas flow.

The rebreathing index can similarly be expressed as a function of $\dot{V}_{FG}/\dot{V}_0$ by rearrangement of eqn (2.19)

$$\frac{\dot{V}}{\dot{V}_0} = \frac{1}{(1 + t_I/t_E)} \frac{(\dot{V}_{FG}/\dot{V}_0)}{[(\dot{V}_{FG}/\dot{V}_0) - 1]}. \tag{2.21}$$

Equation (2.21) is plotted in Fig. 2.7 (line b) for the case $t_I/t_E = 1$. We note that $\dot{V}_{FG}/\dot{V}_0 = 1$ is an asymptote, reminding us that however much rebreathing is attempted a patient will be quite unable to maintain normocapnia (normal F_{ECO_2}) if a large mask is supplied only with the normal volume flow they require in the absence of a mask ($\dot{V}_0$).

When $t_I/t_E = 1$ and $\dot{V}_{FG}/\dot{V}_0$ takes values greater than 2, eqn (2.20) predicts a value of F_{IO_2} greater than 1 and eqn (2.21) yields $\dot{V}/\dot{V}_0 < 1$. The solution then corresponds with a negative F_{ICO_2} which is clearly impossible. The upper limit for $\dot{V}_{FG}/\dot{V}_0$ for which these solutions are valid is therefore (setting $F_{IO_2} = 1$ in eqn (2.20))

$$\frac{\dot{V}_{FG}}{\dot{V}_0} = \frac{(1 + t_I/t_E)}{t_I/t_E}. \tag{2.22}$$

When $\dot{V}_{FG}/\dot{V}_0$ exceeds this value, both F_{IO_2} and $\dot{V}/\dot{V}_0$ are equal to 1. The reader may find it informative to compare Fig. 2.7 with the rebreathing index obtained for an oxygen tent (in effect another 'large volume oxygen mask') in answer to problem 1 at the end of the chapter.

We have seen that the rebreathing index cannot be defined for the large volume mask for $\dot{V}_{FG}/\dot{V}_0 < 1$. We conclude its analysis by deriving the CO_2 retention index which can be defined for all fresh gas flows. For identical values of ventilation with and without the mask, eqns (2.17) and (2.18) predict the ratio of F_{ECO_2} values to be

$$\frac{F'_{ECO_2}}{F_{ECO_2}} = \frac{1}{(1 + t_I/t_E)} + \frac{\dot{V}_0}{\dot{V}_{FG}}. \tag{2.23}$$

The solution is plotted in Fig. 2.8 for the case $t_I/t_E = 1$.

What are the practical implications of our analysis of variable-concentration oxygen masks? At first sight (Fig. 2.6), the large-reservoir mask would seem to offer a high efficiency of oxygen delivery, producing high F_{IO_2} at

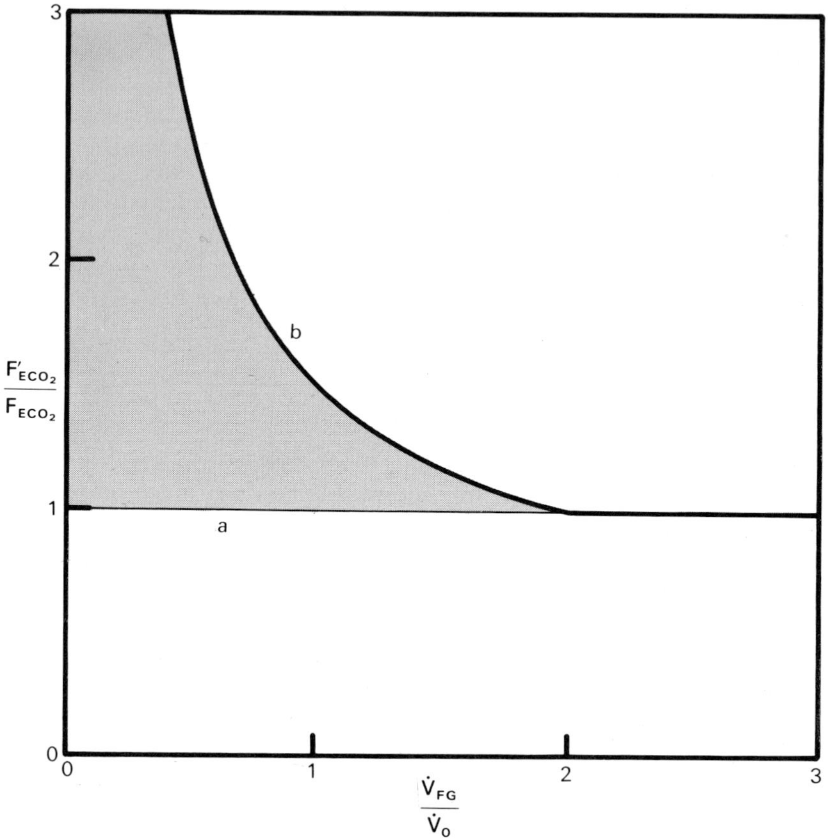

Fig. 2.8. Variable-concentration masks: the CO_2 retention index as a function of $\dot{V}_{FG}/\dot{V}_0$. F'_{ECO_2} and F_{ECO_2} are the expired CO_2 fractions, respectively, with and without the mask, measured for the same ventilation V_0. (a) Small mask (b) large mask (eqn (2.23)) assuming $t_I/t_E = 1$.

relatively low fresh gas flows. Such a system might be attractive to a mountaineer for whom carriage of oxygen involves transport of heavy cylinders. But the price to be paid for this relative efficiency is the effort and distress of increased ventilation (Fig. 2.7).

What degree of increase in ventilation are we capable of? During extreme exertion an athlete may attain a ventilation approximately 15 times his ventilation at rest, but with rebreathing at rest even relatively small increases in ventilation may be quite distressing. Furthermore, the resistance to flow generated by breathing systems limits hyperventilation quite stringently.

Assuming that a 50 per cent increase of ventilation is tolerable ($\dot{V}/\dot{V}_0 = 1.5$) Fig. 2.7 predicts $\dot{V}_{FG}/\dot{V}_0 = 1.5$ and Fig. 2.6 gives $F_{IO_2} = 0.98$. For the same F_{IO_2} the small volume mask would require a flow (Fig. 2.6) of $\dot{V}_{FG}/\dot{V}_0 = 1.97$.

However, such high values of F_{IO_2} are rarely needed. At the top of Everest (8848 m) the normal atmospheric pressure is approximately 33 kPa and the inspired P_{O_2} of moist air is about 5.7 kPa ($=0.21 \times (33 - 6)$*). Though Everest has been climbed without oxygen most climbers are unable to function under these conditions. However, only a moderate increase in F_{IO_2} is required to give an acceptable P_{IO_2}: for example, at $F_{IO_2} = 0.6$ the P_{IO_2} becomes $0.6 \, (33 - 6) = 16.2$ kPa, which would prove quite adequate. The small volume mask can deliver an F_{IO_2} of 0.6 at $\dot{V}_{FG}/\dot{V}_0 = 1$. It would be necessary to be at even higher altitudes than that of Everest to benefit from efficiency of gas-handling by using the large volume mask.

In clinical practice, where variable-concentration masks are used, they tend to be small volume masks ($\simeq 100$ ml) and are conventionally run with $\dot{V}_{FG} = 4 \, \mathrm{l\,min}^{-1}$ unless otherwise directed. Assuming again a value for $\dot{V}_0$ of $6 \, \mathrm{l\,min}^{-1}$ Fig. 2.6 predicts an F_{IO_2} of around 0.5.

Our analysis of the large volume mask appears to have demonstrated no advantages in its use in terms of efficiency yet in the next section we shall see that this device is in fact virtually identical to one of the most widely used anaesthetic breathing systems. It has merits which may outweigh what is actually its notable inefficiency in gas-handling.

2.3   Ayre's T-piece and the Bain system

In 1937 Ayre described an anaesthetic breathing system in which fresh gas was delivered at a T-shaped junction to a reservoir tube issuing from a face mask (Fig. 2.9(a)). The novel advantage of this arrangement was that, unlike several devices in use at the time, rebreathing could be largely eliminated simply by providing a high yet realistic fresh gas flow at the T-piece. The system used its gas supply to purge itself. Moreover, it achieved this without incorporating any one-way valves, which introduce resistance to flow and which are prone to mechanical failure.

This breathing system and some very similar members of the same family are now widely used in hospital practice to deliver anaesthetic gas to patients undergoing surgery. The anaesthetic mixture of gases can be delivered at the inlet to the T-piece (arrowed) close to a mask over the patient's face (or a tube directly entering the trachea). Both the expired gas and excess anaesthetic gas are free to leave the system by convection down the long reservoir tube. If it is desired to keep the system totally sealed, then an extension to this tube (a 'scavenging' tube) may be attached to carry the gases out of the operating theatre to the open air or some form of absorption device.

The Ayre T-piece system may be modified in a simple manner (Fig. 2.9(b)) to allow it to be used for assisting the patient's own respiratory efforts. The

* the partial pressure of water vapour at 37 °C is 6.3 ($\simeq 6$) kPa.

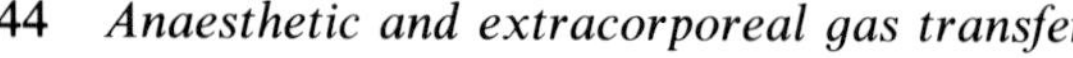

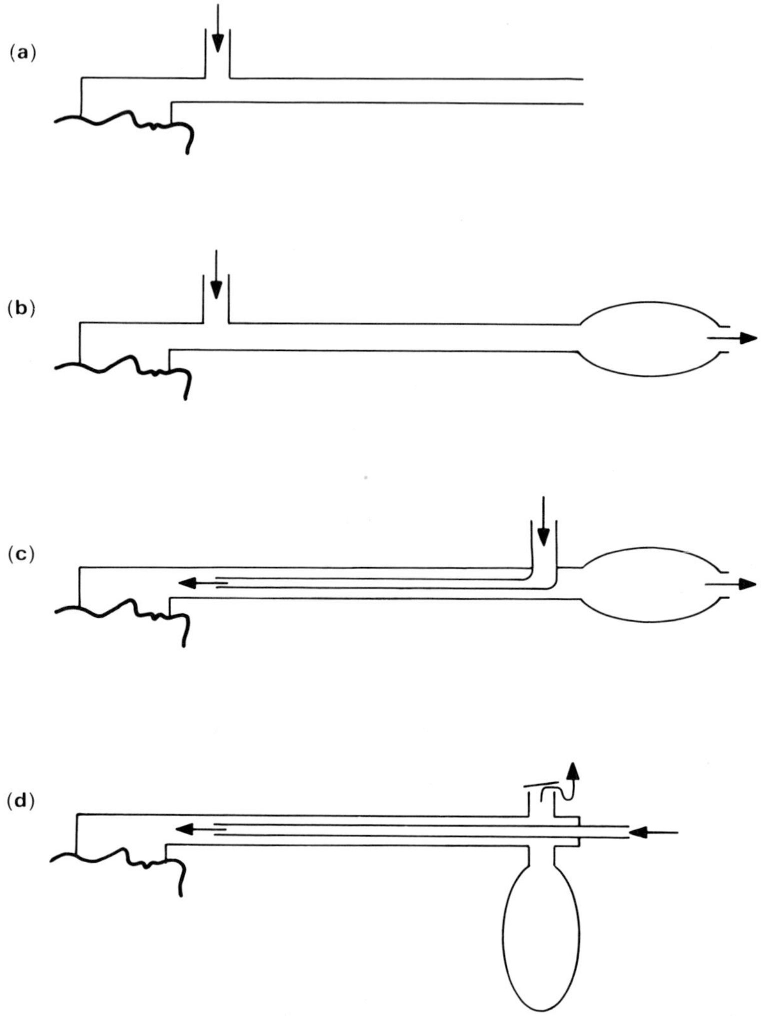

Fig. 2.9. T-piece breathing systems, now widely used in anaesthetic practice. These are, in effect, masks (Fig. 2.5(b)) with long extensions acting as a reservoir of gas. (a) As originally described by Ayre in 1937; (b) with the addition of a collapsible bag on the expiratory limb (Jackson Rees modification, 1950); (c) and (d) as modified to a coaxial form by Bain and Spoerel in 1972, and usually incorporating an expiratory valve above a hanging bag.

addition of a collapsible rubber bag to the reservoir tube is known as the Jackson Rees modification of Ayre's T-piece and makes it possible for the anaesthetist to ventilate the patient artificially by hand. This is achieved by partially or intermittently occluding the outlet hole of the bag whilst squeezing the bag with each breath to raise the pressure within the system and drive gas into the patient. Indeed many mechanical ventilators are in effect robots which perform these two functions automatically: occluding the outlet to a T-piece system during the inspiratory phase of a breathing cycle and at the same time squeezing a bag or bellows to inflate the patient via the reservoir tube (Fig. 4.16(b) and (c)).

A further modification has led to a third member of this family of T-piece breathing systems (Fig. 2.9(c) and (d)). Because fresh gas can be supplied under pressure to such a system, it can be delivered via a relatively narrow high-resistance tube running down the centre of the reservoir tube. This coaxial arrangement, known as the Bain system, was first described in 1972, and has the advantage of requiring only one tube to be connected to the patient for both the delivery and removal of anaesthetic gases. The system is usually arranged with a hanging bag and an expiratory valve (Fig. 2.9(d)).

The behaviour of T-piece systems becomes easy to understand when we compare Fig. 2.9(a) with Fig. 2.5(b) and note that what we have earlier termed a 'large-reservoir' face mask is similar to the T-piece system. Recall that although we considered the mask of Fig. 2.5(b) to be one with a large (reservoir) volume, we assumed throughout our analysis of its behaviour that fresh gas was delivered close to the nose so that all fresh gas arriving in the mask during inspiration was immediately available to be inspired by the patient.

T-piece systems all aim to achieve this goal (Fig. 2.9) of making fresh gas available for immediate inspiration whilst also providing a reservoir from which further gas can be recruited if the patient's inspiratory flow exceeds the flow of fresh gas into the T.

There is one major difference between the practical use of T-piece systems and the use we initially envisaged for the large reservoir oxygen mask of Fig. 2.5(b). We assumed the oxygen mask to be supplied only with pure oxygen and assessed its ability to provide a variable inspired oxygen fraction in relation to its rebreathing characteristics. Since no entrained air was permitted to reach the patient, the inspired gas was always a mixture of just oxygen and CO_2 (Figs. 2.5 and 2.6), making it virtually useless as a mask for any value of F_{IO_2} less than about 0.98. In contrast to this T-piece systems are always supplied with anaesthetic gases already mixed to the desired proportions before their arrival at the T. No attempt is usually made to use the breathing system itself as a means of adjusting the proportions of constituent gases in the anaesthetic mixture arriving at the patient.

Figure 2.10 is a plot of the rebreathing index of a T-piece system measured during experiments with awake volunteers by Willis, Pender and Mapleson (Willis, B. A., Pender, J. W. and Mapleson, W. W. (1975). *British Journal of Anaesthesia* **47**, 1239–45. Fig. 6). The data are means from measurements on six subjects. Note that the rebreathing index $\dot{V}/\dot{V}_0$ is plotted as a function of the ratio $\dot{V}_{FG}/\dot{V}_0$ of the fresh gas flow delivered at the T to the ventilation in

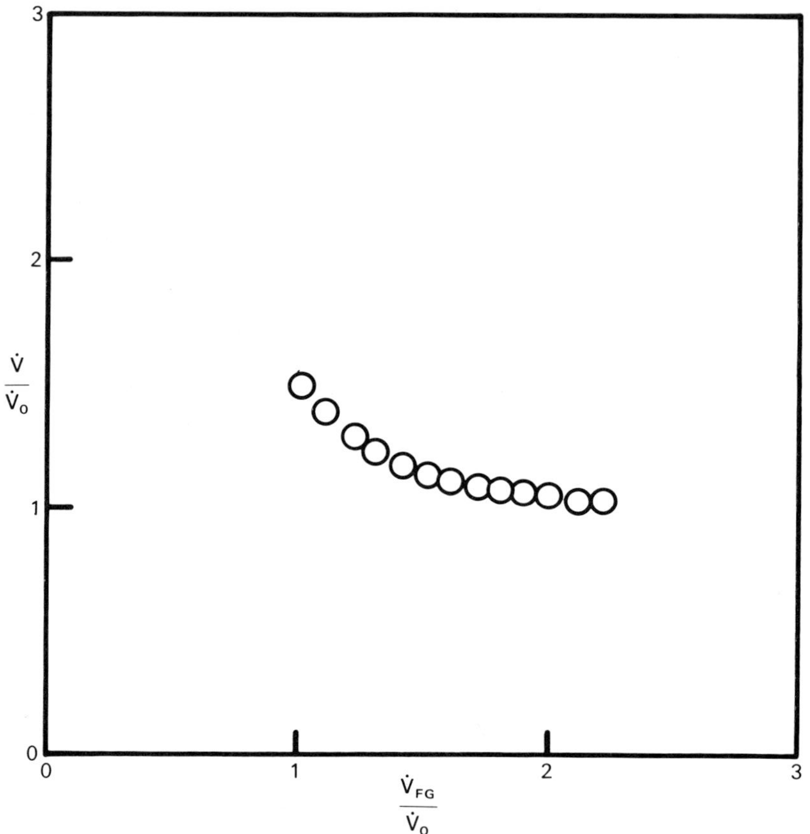

Fig. 2.10. The rebreathing index of a T-piece system as measured in six awake volunteers (see text). (Redrawn from the *British Journal of Anaesthesia* with permission.)

the absence of rebreathing ($\dot{V}_{FG} \rightarrow \infty$). Direct comparison is therefore appropriate with Fig. 2.7, where the rebreathing index for the functionally identical oxygen mask was plotted assuming that the patient's expired (and hence alveolar) CO_2 fraction (F_{ECO_2}) remains constant for all degrees of rebreathing.

We can see that agreement between theory (Fig. 2.7) and experiment (Fig. 2.10) is poor. The theory does seem to predict the observed elimination of rebreathing ($\dot{V}/\dot{V}_0 \rightarrow 1$) at $\dot{V}_{FG}/\dot{V}_0 \simeq 2$, but the predicted massive rise in the rebreathing index at $\dot{V}_{FG}/\dot{V}_0 = 1$ is not followed. In fact the measured rebreathing index for this fresh gas flow is approximately 1.5. What is the explanation for the lack of agreement?

One reason for the measured rebreathing index being less than that predicted is that our theory assumed a constant F_{ECO_2} which is never exactly realized in practice. We assumed that as $\dot{V}_{FG}$ is reduced, so $\dot{V}$ would rise to allow the patient's P_{ACO_2} and hence F_{ECO_2} to remain constant. Were this actually true the patient would be displaying a vertical ventilatory response line on a plot of ventilation against P_{aCO_2} (Fig. 1.7(c)). What actually happens as $\dot{V}$ rises is that the body's respiratory control mechanisms permit a rise in P_{aCO_2} (and hence P_{ACO_2} and F_{ECO_2}) according to the gradient of the response line. This gradient is therefore of importance in interpreting experimental data of the kind we are discussing, and since it is a function of P_{aO_2} (Fig. 1.7(c)) it is unfortunate that no information is given regarding the composition of the fresh gas used to generate the data of Fig. 2.10. However, even with quite a marked rise in P_{aCO_2} (say 30 per cent) we would not expect a resulting error of more than about 30 per cent in the rebreathing index. Some other factor must account for the major lack of agreement between theory and experiment.

We earlier illustrated the concept of respiratory dead space by considering breathing through a snorkel, but have subsequently assumed that dead space is absent from the breathing systems we have examined. We have assumed in effect that the fresh gas delivered to the system arrives in the immediate proximity of the site where oxygen and CO_2 are exchanged with the patient, that is, the alveoli. Figure 2.11(a) illustrates the error incurred in making this assumption. The fresh gas delivered to a breathing system (in this case a T-piece) is never immediately available for gas exchange in the lungs because it is always separated from the alveoli of the patient's lungs by a region of dead space, V_D. This dead space has two components: the equipment dead space V_{DE} and the anatomical dead space V_{DA}

$$V_D = V_{DE} + V_{DA}. \tag{2.24}$$

This total dead space volume may be a large proportion of each tidal volume. In the normal adult the anatomical dead space alone (Fig. 1.2) is approximately 150 ml, which itself forms 30 per cent of a normal resting tidal volume of 500 ml. The addition of equipment dead space (Fig. 2.11(a)) even for a closely fitting face mask may easily bring V_D up to 50 per cent of V_T during breathing at rest.

We now take into account the influence of a sizeable dead space in deriving the theoretical rebreathing index of the T-piece system. As previously, we model the pattern of breathing using constant inspiratory and expiratory flows $\dot{V}_I$ and $\dot{V}_E$ with durations t_I and t_E respectively. We again assume equal inspiratory and expiratory volumes (eqn (2.7)).

Figure 2.11(b) depicts the respiratory waveform for a subject who breathes through a T-piece for which the total dead space is V_D, with a fresh gas flow exceeding the inspiratory flow. In this situation rebreathing is minimized: the dead space gas is necessarily rebreathed along with its content of CO_2 but the remaining inspired gas is pure fresh gas. For a CO_2 elimination from the

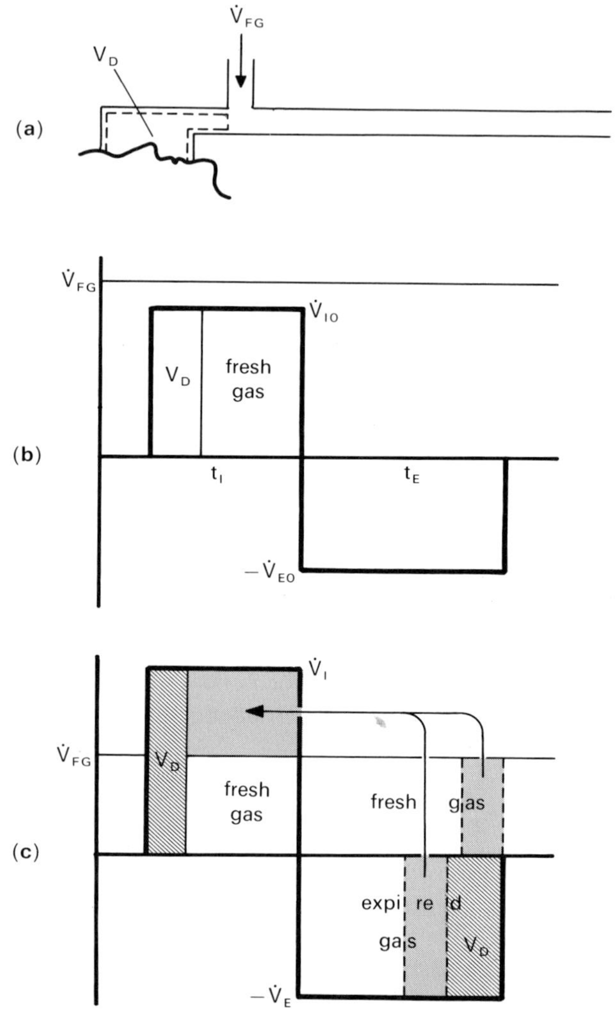

Fig. 2.11. Derivation of the rebreathing index (eqn. (2.30)) for a T-piece system (a) in which the dead space V_D is a sizeable fraction of the tidal volume; (b) the respiratory waveform when there is minimum rebreathing ($\dot{V}_{FG} > \dot{V}_{IO}$); (c) the respiratory waveform in the presence of rebreathing from the expiratory limb of the system ($\dot{V}_{FG} < \dot{V}_{IO}$). The respiratory rate is assumed to be the same in (b) and (c).

patient of $\dot{V}_{CO_2}$ we thus obtain

$$F_{ECO_2}(\dot{V}_0 - V_D r) = \dot{V}_{CO_2}, \tag{2.25}$$

where $\dot{V}_0$ is the ventilation at this minimum rebreathing ($= \dot{V}_{IO} t_I r$) and r is the respiratory rate. To find the rebreathing index for this system we wish to calculate at low fresh gas flows ($\dot{V}_{FG} < \dot{V}_{IO}$) the ventilation $\dot{V}$ necessary to keep F_{ECO_2} constant. We assume that r remains constant and that ventilation ($V_T r$) increases by changing V_T alone.

As $\dot{V}_{FG}$ falls below V_{IO} the inspired breath becomes a mixture of three components (Fig. 2.11(c)). First to be inspired is the dead space gas of volume V_D at a flow $\dot{V}_I$ and thus over a time $V_D/\dot{V}_I$. This dead space gas was expired by the patient during the previous cycle of breathing. Then a mixture is inspired of fresh gas (volume $\dot{V}_{FG}(t_I - V_D/\dot{V}_I)$) and reservoir gas (volume $\dot{V}_I - \dot{V}_{FG})(t_I - V_D/\dot{V}_I))$. This reservoir gas is itself a sample (Fig. 2.11(c)) from a mixture (assumed perfect*) of the expired gas (volume $\dot{V}_E t_E$) and the pure fresh gas delivered to the mask during the previous expiration (volume $\dot{V}_{FG} t_E$). Hence, the inspired CO_2 fraction will be given by

$$F_{ICO_2} \dot{V}_I t_I = V_D F_{ECO_2} + (\dot{V}_I - \dot{V}_{FG})(t_I - V_D/\dot{V}_I)\frac{F_{ECO_2} \dot{V}_E}{(\dot{V}_E + \dot{V}_{FG})}. \qquad (2.26)$$

For $V_D = 0$ this reduces to eqn (2.15) as expected.

The mean inspired and expired CO_2 fractions will be related (to the extent that eqn (2.7) is valid) by

$$(F_{ECO_2} - F_{ICO_2})\dot{V} = \dot{V}_{CO_2}. \qquad (2.16)$$

We eliminate F_{ICO_2} from the left-hand side of eqn (2.16) by substitution from eqns (2.26), (2.7) and (2.9):

$$F_{ECO_2} = \frac{[1 + (1 + t_I/t_E)(\dot{V}/\dot{V}_{FG})]}{[1 + t_I/t_E - V_D/(\dot{V}t_E)]} \times \frac{\dot{V}_{CO_2}}{\dot{V}}. \qquad (2.27)$$

For $V_D = 0$ this reduces to eqn (2.17) as expected. Equation (2.25) gives us an expression for F_{ECO_2} under conditions of minimum rebreathing (Fig. 2.11(b)). In fact eqn (2.27) reduces to eqn (2.25) when we set $\dot{V}_{FG} = \dot{V}_I$. For F_{ECO_2} to be identical both with (eqn (2.27)) and without (eqn (2.25)) rebreathing in excess of the dead space, the ventilations $\dot{V}$ and $\dot{V}_0$ for two respective cases will be related by

$$\frac{\dot{V}}{\dot{V}_0} = \frac{1}{(1 + t_I/t_E)} \times \frac{(\dot{V}_{FG}/\dot{V}_0)[1 + (V_D/\dot{V}_0)(t_I/t_E)/(t_I + t_E)]}{[(\dot{V}_{FG}/\dot{V}_0) - 1 + (V_D/\dot{V}_0)/(t_I + t_E)]}. \qquad (2.28)$$

For $V_D = 0$ this reduces to eqn (2.21) as expected.

During minimum rebreathing (Fig. 2.11(b)) the ventilation $\dot{V}_0$ is related to the tidal volume V_{TO} by

$$V_{TO} = \dot{V}_0(t_I + t_E). \qquad (2.29)$$

---

* The stratification of gas along a long thin reservoir tube will in general not lead to perfect mixing. In the particular case considered here, however, the presence of constant flows filling the reservoir during expiration, $\dot{V}_E$ and $\dot{V}_{FG}$, produces a uniform mixture within the tube even if axial mixing does not occur. The more general case is analysed in Chapter 4 for both mechanical and spontaneous ventilation.

Substituting from eqn (2.29) into eqn (2.28) we get

$$\frac{\dot{V}}{\dot{V}_0} = \frac{1}{(1+t_{\mathrm{I}}/t_{\mathrm{E}})} \times \frac{(\dot{V}_{\mathrm{FG}}/\dot{V}_0)[1+(V_{\mathrm{D}}/V_{\mathrm{T0}})(t_{\mathrm{I}}/t_{\mathrm{E}})]}{[(\dot{V}_{\mathrm{FG}}/\dot{V}_0)-1+(V_{\mathrm{D}}/V_{\mathrm{T0}})]}. \tag{2.30}$$

We now have an expression for the rebreathing index as a function of three ratios. In addition to the ratios $\dot{V}_{\mathrm{FG}}/\dot{V}_0$ and $t_{\mathrm{I}}/t_{\mathrm{E}}$ appearing in eqn (2.21) we have a measure of the dead space volume V_{D} expressed as a ratio of V_{D} to the tidal volume during minimum rebreathing V_{T0}. We commented earlier that V_{D} may easily equal 50 per cent of the normal resting tidal volume of 500 ml. This means that $V_{\mathrm{D}}/V_{\mathrm{T0}}$ may make an appreciable change to the rebreathing index for any given value of $\dot{V}_{\mathrm{FG}}/\dot{V}_0$.

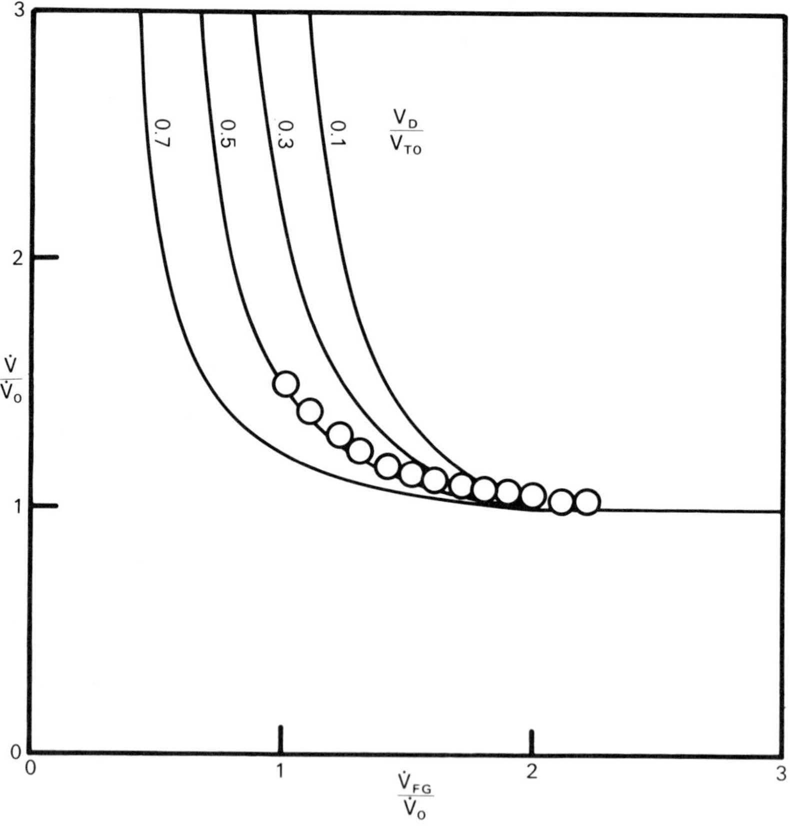

Fig. 2.12. The measured rebreathing index of a T-piece system (as in Fig. (2.10)) compared with theoretical prediction (eqn (2.30)) for four different values of ratio of the dead space volume V_{D} to the tidal volume when there is minimum rebreathing V_{T0}. $t_{\mathrm{I}}/t_{\mathrm{E}} = 1$ throughout.

Figure (2.12) compares the experimental data of Willis, Pender and Mapleson (Fig. 2.10) with plots of eqn (2.30) for four different values of $V_\mathrm{D}/V_\mathrm{T0}$. Inspiratory and expiratory times are equal ($t_1/t_\mathrm{E} = 1$). Agreement is fair for $V_\mathrm{D}/V_\mathrm{T0} = 0.5$.

The effect on the rebreathing index of varying the ratio of inspiratory time to expiratory time (t_1/t_E) is much less pronounced than the effect of varying $V_\mathrm{D}/V_\mathrm{T0}$. Figure 2.13 repeats the data of Figs. (2.10) and (2.12), this time compared with eqn (2.30) for four different values of t_1/t_E over the range of physiological interest. ($V_\mathrm{D}/V_\mathrm{T0}$ has been held constant at 0.5.) There is a suggestion from this plot that the experimental data can best be modelled for an I:E ratio somewhat less than 1.

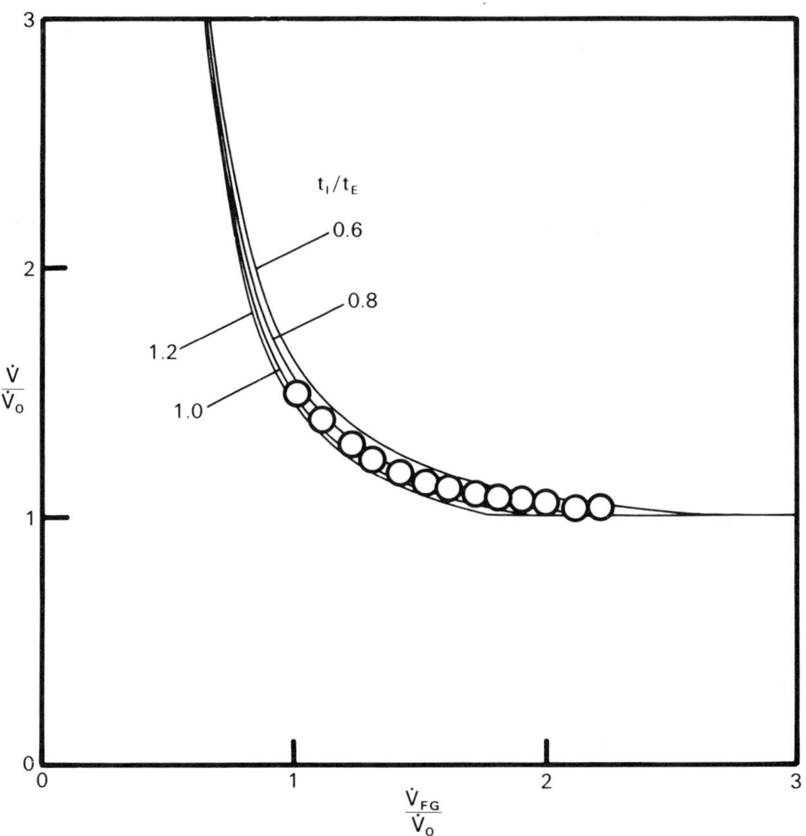

Fig. 2.13. The measured rebreathing index of a T-piece system (as in Fig. (2.10)) compared with the theoretical prediction (eqn. 2.30)) for four different values of the ratio of inspiratory time to expiratory time (t_1/t_E). $V_\mathrm{D}/V_\mathrm{T0} = 0.5$ throughout.

Our analysis so far of medical breathing systems has assumed a square-wave respiratory waveform which we can only expect to be an approximation to the physiological pattern of breathing (Figs. 2.4, 2.5 and 2.11). Further refinement of our theoretical analysis would require us to model normal breathing more closely, but the rewards of introducing further complexity may be limited. Figure 2.14 is a plot of the respiratory waveform measured in anaesthetized adults by Jonsson and Zetterström (Jonsson, L. O. and Zetterström, H. (1985). *Acta Anaesthesiologica Scandinavica* **29**, 309–14). Data from twelve individuals has been normalized by expressing inspiratory and expiratory flows as percentages of the maximum inspiratory flow for each patient; similarly the time scale is normalized to represent percentages of complete cycles. The I : E ratio is 0.85. The shape of the inspiratory part of the cycle is very similar to the shape of the expiratory part of the cycle and this tends to be a feature of the breathing of anaesthetized subjects which contrasts with the breathing of people who are awake. In awake subjects, there is a tendency for a pause in breathing to occur towards the end of expiration, delaying the next inspiration. This 'end-expiratory pause' may have quite a large influence on the measurement of the rebreathing index of a

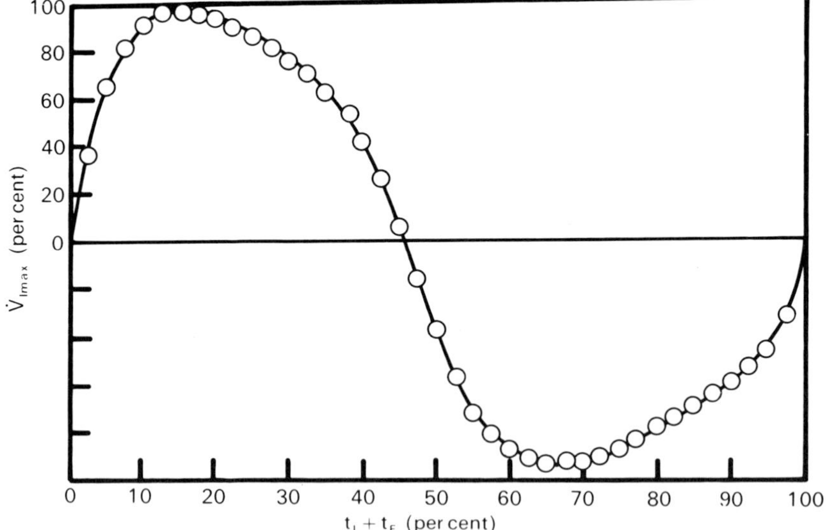

Fig. 2.14. The respiratory flow–time waveform of adult patients, anaesthetized with halothane in a nitrous oxide–oxygen mixture, breathing spontaneously through an endotracheal tube. Data are means of measurements on 12 patients. The data have been normalized by plotting flows as a percentage of each patient's maximum inspiratory flow and by plotting times as a percentage of the duration of each patient's breathing cycle. (Redrawn from *Acta Anaesthesiologica Scandinavica*, with permission.)

system and we shall examine some aspects of this towards the end of this chapter. Figure 2.14 does suggest, however, that the use of a square waveform in modelling breathing may be a satisfactory approximation in many applications.

2.4 The fixed-concentration (HAFOE) oxygen mask

It is sometimes desirable in clinical practice to be able to administer to a patient via a mask a known constant concentration of oxygen accurate to within a few per cent. The need arises for two reasons. Firstly, there are patients for whom an inspired oxygen fraction F_{IO_2} above some maximum value may prove harmful. Secondly, there are patients for whom an accurately determined F_{IO_2} permits the most beneficial interpretation of blood tests which measure the arterial oxygen partial pressure, P_{aO_2}. Some patients will fall into both categories.

We showed in the previous section that it is impossible to design a simple reservoir mask which can provide an F_{IO_2} which does not vary with both the oxygen flow ($\dot{V}_{FG}$) and the pattern of breathing ($\dot{V}_I$ and t_I/t_E), except for the trivial case $F_{IO_2} = 1$. Yet it remains desirable to make use of some kind of simple face mask which is supplied only with oxygen and which has a performance not varying with $\dot{V}_{FG}$, $\dot{V}_I$ and t_I/t_E.

The current solution to this problem was introduced into clinical practice in 1960 by Campbell, following the suggestion made to him by Nunn that the 'Venturi' principle might be used to mix oxygen with air. The concept is illustrated in Fig. 2.15. A high velocity jet of pure oxygen is delivered in the centre of a duct into which air can be entrained by the friction between the oxygen and the air with which it comes into contact. Turbulence within the duct mixes the oxygen with the air and the mixture is delivered to the mask. We shall show that the composition of the mixture may be expected to be independent of the flow of fresh gas (oxygen) $\dot{V}_{FG}$ delivered to the jet.

The total flow of the mixture is chosen to exceed the maximum inspiratory flow ($\dot{V}_I$) of any patient expected to use the mask so that in no circumstances will further dilution occur by entrainment of more air into the mask via the holes near the patient's nose and mouth. Campbell named the principle of this design of mask one of High Air Flow with Oxygen Enrichment (HAFOE), a name which emphasizes the two components of the principle; that oxygen is used to enrich air to achieve the desired F_{IO_2}, and that a high flow delivered at the patient's face prevents further dilution of the mixture when the patient takes a deep breath in.

The masks are, however, more popularly known as Venturi masks, taking the name of a nineteenth century Italian physicist*. Yet the use of this name is

---

* GB Venturi (1746–1822).

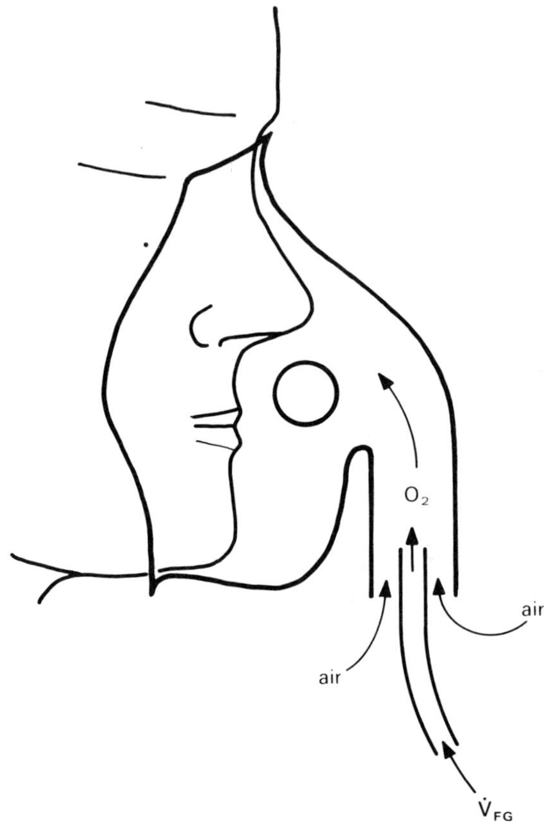

Fig. 2.15. The fixed-concentration oxygen mask produces an inspired oxygen fraction which is largely independent of the fresh gas flow of oxygen $\dot{V}_{FG}$ to the mask. Entrained air is enriched by a central jet of oxygen and the mixed gas enters the face-piece of the mask at high flow.

in one sense inappropriate. The Venturi principle is usually taken to refer to the observation that the pressure in a fluid stream is lower in a narrow section of pipe than in a broader section, and in fact venturi is now taken to refer to a constriction in a pipe introduced for the purpose of measuring the pressure or exerting suction via a hole in the narrow part of the pipe. However, entrainment of air does not require a constriction of any sort in the ducting of a HAFOE mask. But as we shall show in the next section, the introduction of a true venturi into the design can make the mask more resistant to stalling due to back pressure from the face-piece.

We examine the performance of the entrainment duct with the aid of Fig. 2.16. Our aim is to predict the composition of the mixed gas leaving the duct and entering the mask. Oxygen is delivered to the duct at a steady

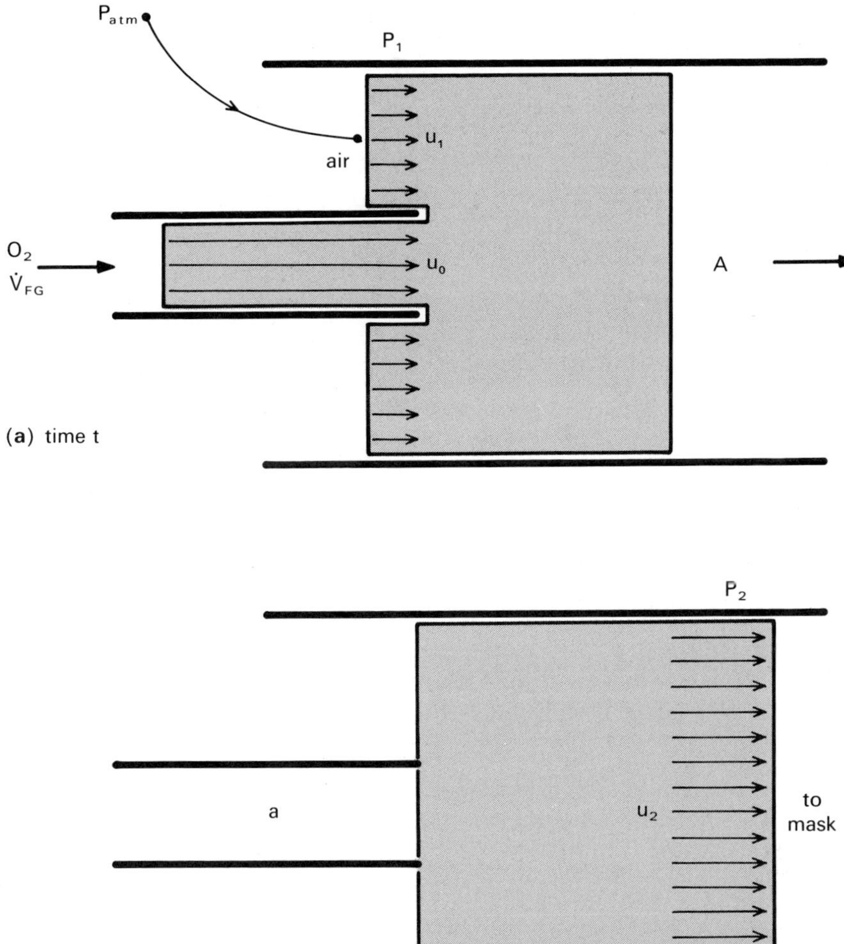

Fig. 2.16. The entrainment duct of the HAFOE mask. A fixed mass of gas is shaded and depicted at times t (a) and $t + 1$ s (b). Application of Newton's second law (in the form of the momentum equation) to this fixed mass allows us to predict the composition of the downstream mixture of air and oxygen, and hence F_{IO_2} for the mask.

volume flow $\dot{V}_{FG}$ in a jet with high velocity u_0 and cross-sectional area a ($\dot{V}_{FG} = u_0 a$). We ignore for the purposes of this analysis any variation of velocity across the individual flow sections. Also at the entry section to the duct there is flowing parallel to the oxygen jet, with a steady velocity u_1, the atmospheric air which is entrained into the duct at a volume flow $u_1(A - a)$ where A is the cross-sectional area of the outer ducting. This air is entrained from the surrounding atmosphere because of frictional or viscous shear between the high velocity jet of oxygen and the slower air which borders on the jet. We avoid examining the mechanism of this shear in detail by considering the flow of mixed oxygen and air only where it has attained a uniform velocity u_2 across the downstream section of area A.

The outline of a fixed mass (and hence volume; see below) of gas is depicted by the shaded box in Figs. 2.16(a) and (b), before and after the passage of one second respectively. We apply Newton's second law of motion to this mass of gas. We denote the pressures across the inlet and outlet sections of the duct p_1 and p_2 respectively, and we ignore boundary shear forces on our volume element. The difference between forces in the direction of flow on either side of the volume element must equal the rate of change of momentum of the mass of gas:

$$(p_1 - p_2)A = \rho_2 u_2^2 A - \rho_0 u_0^2 a - \rho_1 u_1^2 (A - a), \qquad (2.31)$$

where ρ_0 is the oxygen density, ρ_1 the density of air, and ρ_2 the density of the mixture leaving the duct. Continuity in inlet and outlet mass flows requires

$$\rho_0 u_0 a + \rho_1 u_1 (A - a) = \rho_2 u_2 A. \qquad (2.32)$$

What is the relationship between ρ_2 and the inlet densities ρ_0 and ρ_1? Assuming constant pressure and temperature during the mixing of the oxygen and air, it follows from Dalton's law of partial pressures* that the volume of the mixture will equal the sum of the volumes of component oxygen and air:

$$u_0 a + u_1 (A - a) = u_2 A. \qquad (2.33)$$

We may make use of eqn (2.33) despite the assumption in its derivation that pressure remains constant during the passage of gas through the duct, because the pressure changes occurring in a system of the kind we are considering are small relative to those required to produce sizeable changes in the density of individual gases. It can be shown that this claim is equivalent to the assumption that all flow velocities remain an order of magnitude smaller than the velocity of sound. Some readers will recognize this to be equivalent to the condition $M \ll 1$, where M is the Mach number.

The aim of our theoretical examination is to relate the flows of oxygen and air in order to calculate the composition of mixed gas entering the mask. Within three eqns (2.31–2.33) we have five unknowns: u_1, u_2, p_1, p_2 and ρ_2. The number of unknown parameters reduces to four when we note that the duct exit discharges to the mask at atmospheric pressure $p_2 = P_{atm}$. The complete solution to the problem then requires a fourth equation relating the inlet pressure p_1 to atmospheric pressure. Assuming incompressible steady

---

* and in turn from Avogadro's law. See chapter 1.

flow without friction for the entrained air, we may write Bernoulli's equation[†] along the streamline depicted in Fig. 2.16(a) relating the pressure of stationary atmospheric air to the pressure p_1 at the entry section:

$$\frac{P_{\text{atm}}}{\rho_1} = \frac{p_1}{\rho_1} + \frac{u_1^2}{2}. \tag{2.34}$$

Substitute for ρ_2, u_2 and p_1 respectively from eqns (2.32), (2.33) and (2.34) into eqn (2.31):

$$\left(P_{\text{atm}} - \frac{\rho_1 u_1^2}{2} - P_{\text{atm}} \right) A =$$

$$[\rho_0 u_0 a + \rho_1 u_1 (A - a)] \frac{[u_0 a + u_1 (A - a)]}{A} - \rho_0 u_0^2 a - \rho_1 u_1^2 (A - a)$$

or

$$-\frac{\rho_1 u_1^2}{2} \times A^2 = \rho_0 u_0^2 a^2 + \rho_1 u_1 u_0 a (A - a) +$$

$$\rho_0 u_0 u_1 a (A - a) + \rho_1 u_1^2 (A - a)^2 - \rho_0 u_0^2 a A - \rho_1 u_1^2 (A - a) A.$$

Collection of terms leads to the result

$$\rho_1 u_1^2 \left[\frac{A^2}{2a(A - a)} \right] = (\rho_1 u_1 - \rho_0 u_0)(u_1 - u_0). \tag{2.35}$$

If we initially regard ρ_0 and ρ_1 as equal, eqn (2.35) is easily solved by taking square roots on each side of the equation:

$$u_1 \frac{A}{\sqrt{2a(A - a)}} = \pm (u_1 - u_0) \tag{2.36}$$

A credible solution requires $u_0 > u_1$ and corresponds with the negative sign on the right-hand side of eqn (2.36), which yields the solution

$$\frac{u_1}{u_0} = \frac{\sqrt{2a(A - a)/A^2}}{1 + \sqrt{2a(A - a)/A^2}} \tag{2.37}$$

In terms of the flows of oxygen ($\dot{V}_{\text{FG}} = u_0 a$) and entrained air $\dot{V}_{\text{AIR}} = u_1 (A - a)$ eqn (2.37) can be written

$$\frac{\dot{V}_{\text{AIR}}}{\dot{V}_{\text{FG}}} = \frac{(A - a)}{a} \left(\frac{\sqrt{2a(A - a)/A^2}}{1 + \sqrt{2a(A - a)/A^2}} \right). \tag{2.38}$$

[†] In the form used here ignoring gravitational terms, Bernoulli's equation is the simplest integrated form of Newton's second law of motion applied to a mass element of inviscid incompressible fluid moving in steady flow, with velocity u at a distance s along its path through the surrounding fluid, with only pressure and acceleration terms: $-\mathrm{d}p/\mathrm{d}s = \rho u \, \mathrm{d}u/\mathrm{d}s$. Readers unfamiliar with Bernoulli's equation will find further explanation in any basic fluid mechanics text.

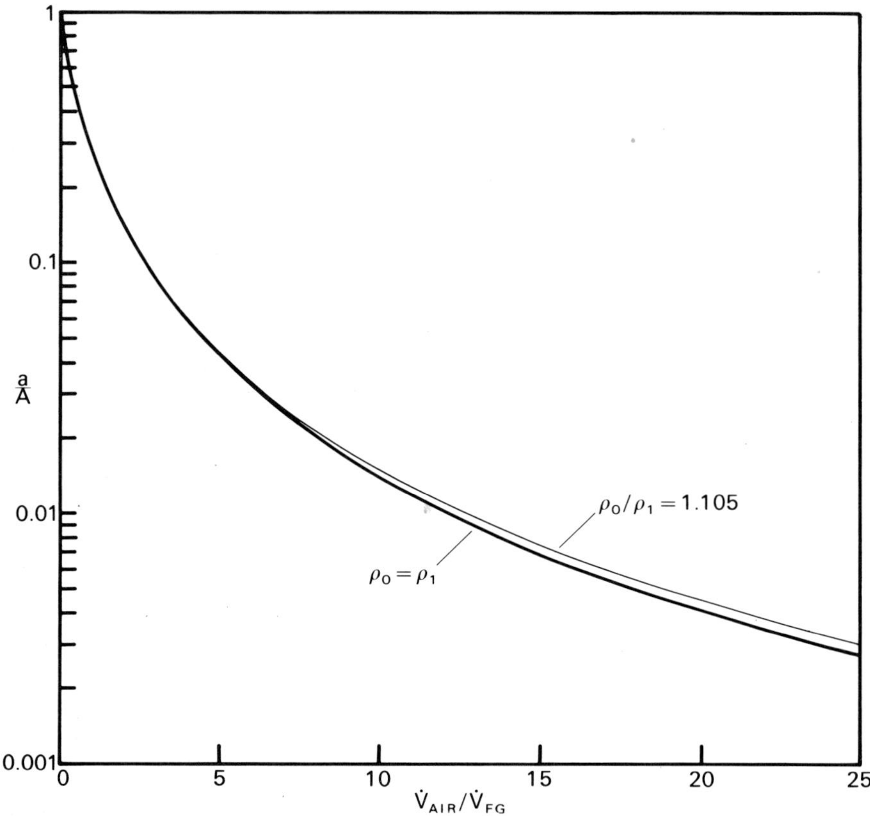

Fig. 2.17. The relative area of a/A of the oxygen jet in the entrainment duct of the HAFQE mask plotted as a function of the ratio of air flow to oxygen flow entering the duct. a/A is plotted on a logarithmic scale to encompass the wide range of relative areas in the clinically useful range. The curve for a precise oxygen to air density ratio ($\rho_0/\rho_1 = 1.105$) is virtually indistinguishable from that assuming equal densities ($\rho_0 = \rho_1$, eqn (2.38)).

Equation (2.38) is plotted in Fig. 2.17. The relative area of the oxygen jet a/A is plotted as a function of the relative entrainment of air $\dot{V}_{AIR}/\dot{V}_{FG}$. A log–linear format is used to demonstrate the large range required in the relative area to obtain an air entrainment in the clinically useful range. This range may be defined with the aid of Fig. 2.18, which relates the relative jet area to the oxygen fraction of the oxygen–air mixture leaving the entrainment duct. This figure is constructed using the relationship

$$F_{IO_2} = \frac{1 + 0.2(\dot{V}_{AIR}/\dot{V}_{FG})}{1 + (\dot{V}_{AIR}/\dot{V}_{FG})}, \tag{2.39}$$

which takes 0.2 as the oxygen volume fraction of air. Clinical indications for

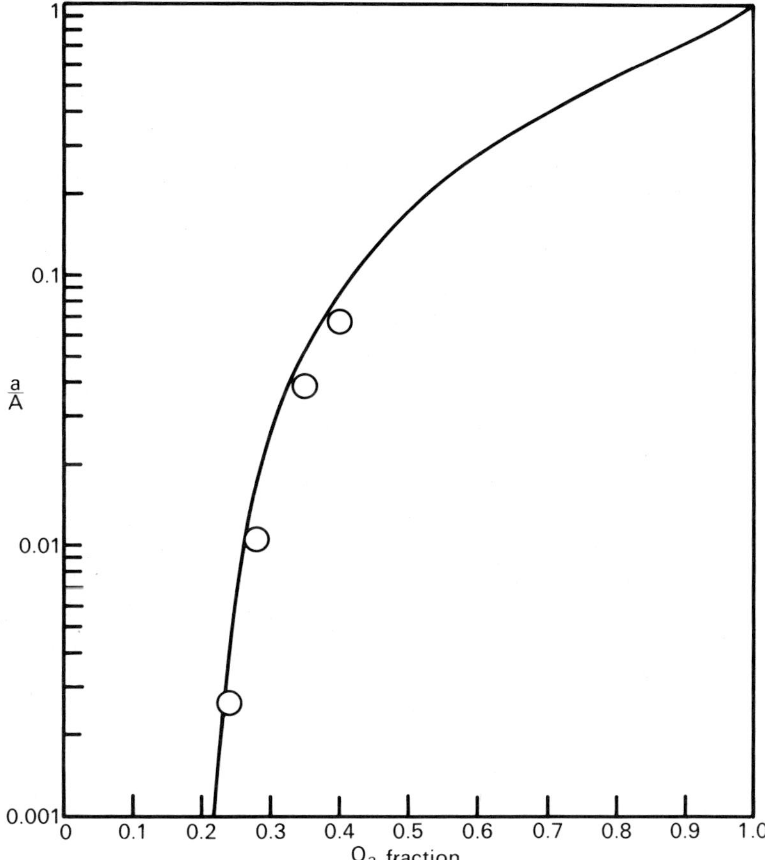

Fig. 2.18. The relative area a/A of the oxygen jet in the entrainment duct of the HAFOE mask plotted as a function of F_{IO_2} according to eqns (2.38) and (2.39). Data points represent measured areas from commercially available masks (Ventimask Mks 2 and 3) rated by the manufacturer (Vickers Medical) at F_{IO_2} values 0.24, 0.28, 0.35 and 0.40.

constant concentration oxygen masks tend to be in the range of F_{IO_2} 0.24–0.60. Figure 2.18 shows that to achieve this a range of relative jet areas is needed from 0.005–0.3.

You may ask: what error has been entailed in Figs. (2.17) and (2.18) by the assumption that the densities of oxygen and air have been assumed to be equal? At standard temperature and pressure (see chapter 1) the density of oxygen is $1.429\ \mathrm{kg\,m^{-3}}$ which is 10 per cent greater than that of air at $1.293\ \mathrm{kg\,m^{-3}}$. The quadratic equation which results from introducing these values into eqn (2.35) can be readily solved to yield u_1/u_0 and then $\dot{V}_{AIR}/\dot{V}_{FG}$

as functions of a/A. The resulting solution for $\dot{V}_{\mathrm{AIR}}/\dot{V}_{\mathrm{FG}}$ is plotted in Fig. 2.17 alongside the solution for the case $\rho_0 = \rho_1$. The plots lie close together.

In Fig. (2.18) the associated plot for a/A as a function of $F_{\mathrm{IO_2}}$ for $\rho_0 = 1.429 \ \mathrm{kg\,m}^{-3}$ and $\rho_1 = 1.293 \ \mathrm{kg\,m}^{-3}$ lies so close to that for the case $\rho_0 = \rho_1$ that it cannot be distinguished on the form of plot adopted here, and so no attempt has been made to depict the two separate solutions.

A number of commercially available devices adopt a geometry which conforms very closely to the flow depicted in Fig. (2.16). The Ventimask (Vickers Medical) is available for several oxygen fractions, and the corresponding relative jet sizes a/A measured from four masks are plotted in Fig. 2.18. It can be seen that agreement with our uncomplicated one-dimensional flow model is fair, despite the fact that the structural support for the ducting in the Ventimask necessitates a degree of three dimensional flow in the commercial product. The model clearly provides a useful guide to practical engineering design.

Proper function of the HAFOE mask requires there to be no significant elevation of pressure in the face-piece of the mask. We assumed in our derivation of eqn (2.38) that the outlet pressure p_2 of the entrainment duct (Fig. 2.16) was equal to atmospheric pressure. Were the pressure in the face-piece to rise, for example due to obstruction at the expiratory holes (Fig. 2.15), this assumption would become invalid. We now examine the effects of varying p_2.

Solving eqns (2.31–34), this time leaving p_2 as an independent variable, we find

$$\left(p_2 - P_{\mathrm{atm}} + \frac{\rho_1 u_1^2}{2} \right) \left[\frac{A^2}{a(A-a)} \right] = (\rho_1 u_1 - \rho_0 u_0)(u_1 - u_0). \tag{2.40}$$

This equation reduces to eqn (2.35) when $p_2 = P_{\mathrm{atm}}$ as expected. If p_2 were to be progressively raised above P_{atm} we should expect less of the oxygen–air mixture to enter the mask. Assuming u_0 to be constant, this would reveal itself as a rise in $F_{\mathrm{IO_2}}$ as less air is entrained into the mixing duct. At some critical value of p_2 we should get to a condition at which no air is entrained and $F_{\mathrm{IO_2}} = 1$. Further elevation of p_2 would then reverse the sign of u_1 so that gas leaves at the section where air is normally entrained. We term this condition the *stalling* of the mask and it corresponds to $u_1 = 0$. At stalling, eqn (2.40) yields

$$\frac{p_2 - P_{\mathrm{atm}}}{\rho u_0^2} = \frac{a}{A}\left(1 - \frac{a}{A} \right). \tag{2.41}$$

The right-hand side of eqn (2.41) varies between 0 and 0.25 as a/A varies between 0 and 1. The stalling-pressure coefficient on the left-hand side of eqn (2.41) takes its maximum value of 0.25 when $a/A = 0.5$, at which value it is least susceptible to stalling for a given u_0. Masks in common clinical use

(Fig. 2.18) have area ratios well below 0.5 and the corresponding stalling-pressure coefficient is much smaller.

To gain some idea of the size of the stalling-pressure itself, consider the mask designed to generate an F_{IO_2} of 0.35 (Fig. 2.18) for which $a/A = 0.038$, $a = 4.2 \text{ mm}^2$ and an appropriate oxygen flow is $10 \, \text{l min}^{-1}$. Taking ρ to be 1.3 kg m^{-3} we obtain from eqn (2.41)

$$p_2 - P_{atm} = \rho\left(\frac{\dot{V}_{FG}}{a}\right)^2\left(\frac{a}{A}\right)\left(1 - \frac{a}{A}\right)$$

$$= 1.3[10^{-2}/(60 \times 4.2 \times 10^{-6})]^2(0.038 \times 0.962) \qquad (2.42)$$

$$= 75 \text{ N m}^{-2} \, (\text{Pa})$$

$$= 0.075 \text{ kPa},$$

which is a very small pressure difference in comparison with an atmospheric pressure of approximately 100 kPa. This calculation suggests that HAFOE masks may be stalled by very modest increases in pressure in the facepiece. Moreover, if total stalling can be so easily achieved we should expect quite large deviations in F_{IO_2} from design values at back pressures which are smaller, for which u_1 is reduced but not brought equal to zero.

In the next section we examine one way in which the stalling characteristics of an entrainment duct can be improved, even to the extent of permitting the use of such an oxygen–air mixing system to supply a mixture of gas to a T-piece anaesthetic breathing system.

2.5 Venturi breathing systems

The simplicity of the entrainment system examined in the previous section (Fig. 2.16) suggests that such a device may be of value for mixing air with oxygen to supply a mixture with the desired F_{IO_2} to a breathing system such as a T-piece (Fig. 2.19(a)). It is in this kind of application, however, that difficulties are most likely to arise with stalling of the entrainment duct due to back pressure. In this section we examine the effect of small back pressures on the F_{IO_2} of entrainment ducts with and without the addition of a diffuser downstream of the mixing section.

One way in which the stalling properties of an entrainment duct can be minimized can be deduced from eqn (2.42). For a given area ratio a/A and fresh gas (oxygen) flow $\dot{V}_{FG}$, the gauge stalling pressure $(p_2 - P_{atm})$ is inversely proportional to the square of the jet area a. Thus for a given flow a high velocity jet of small area is preferable to a low velocity jet of large area.

A second way in which the stalling properties may be improved is by the introduction of a diffuser (a gradually broadening duct) downstream of the mixing section. In Fig. 2.20 we depict two entrainment systems each designed to generate the same F_{IO_2} from an oxygen jet of fixed flow, area a, and hence

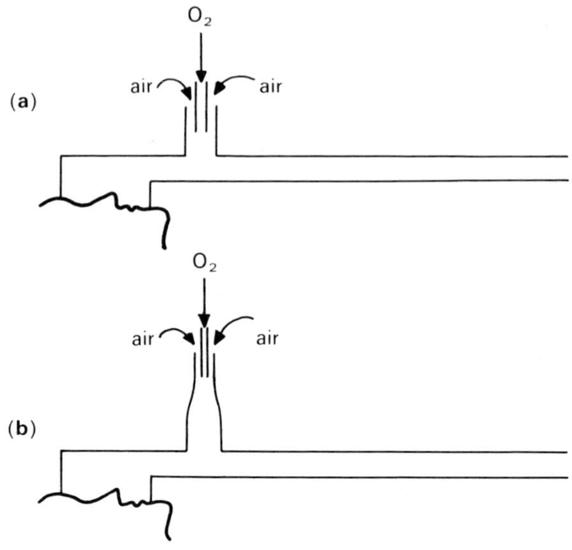

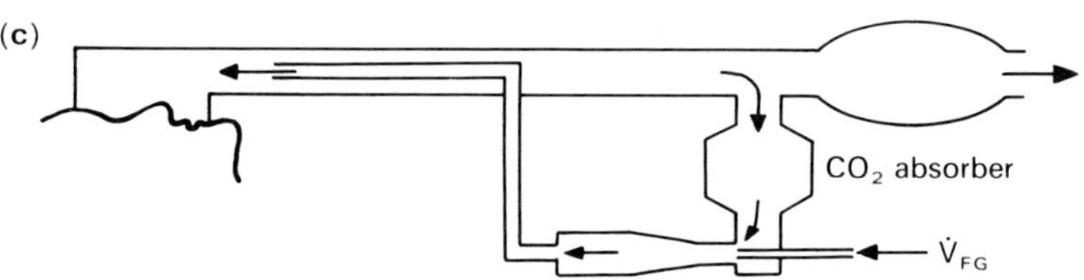

Fig. 2.19. Entrainment systems for supplying T-pieces. (a) Uniform entrainment duct, (b) addition of a diffuser to reduce susceptibility of the system to back pressure, (c) use of a venturi entrainer to recirculate gas in a T-piece. The recirculated gas passes through a CO_2 absorber and is thus depleted of expired CO_2.

velocity u_0. The first system is of the kind we examined in the previous section. We designate the pressure at exit p_e. The second system incorporates a diffuser which increases the duct area from A' to KA' where $K > 1$. It is assumed that the flow along the diffuser conforms to Bernoulli's equation, being steady, incompressible and without energy losses. Inherent in the assumption of zero energy loss is that the rate of increase of area with distance is small enough to avoid boundary layer separation and wake formation at the wall. The divergence angle must be small.

The variable of interest in assessing the susceptibility of the system to changes in F_{IO_2} resulting from small back pressures is $(\partial F_{IO_2}/\partial p_e)$, where the

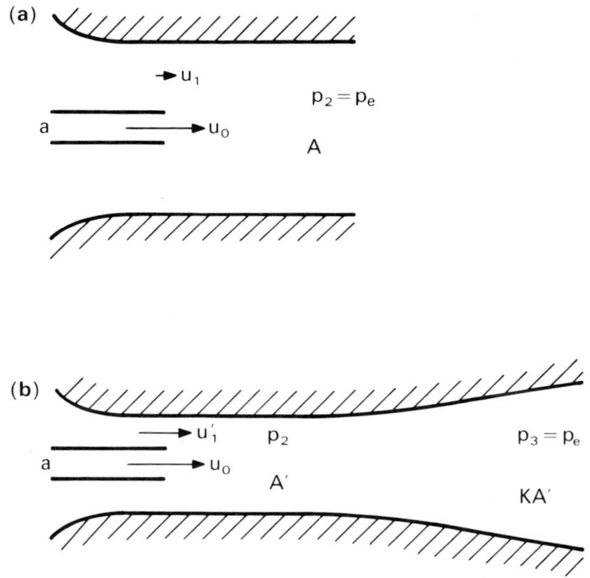

Fig. 2.20. Two entrainment systems each generating the same air–oxygen mixture (and hence F_{IO_2}) from an oxygen jet of fixed area a and velocity u_0. The first system (a) has no diffuser. The addition of a diffuser downstream of the mixing duct yields a true venturi (b), and renders the system more resistant to changes in F_{IO_2} due to back pressure.

partial derivative assumes that u_0, a, A or (A') and K remain constant. For the uniform duct (Figs. 2.16 and 2.20(a)) differentiation of eqn (2.40) (taking $\rho_1 = \rho_0$ and setting $p_2 = p_e$) yields

$$1 + \rho u_1 \frac{\partial u_1}{\partial p_e} = 2\rho \left(\frac{a}{A} \right) \left(1 - \frac{a}{A} \right) (u_1 - u_0) \frac{\partial u_1}{\partial p_e}$$

or

$$\frac{\partial u_1}{\partial p_e} = \left[\frac{1}{2\rho \left(\dfrac{a}{A} \right) \left(1 - \dfrac{a}{A} \right) (u_1 - u_0) - \rho u_1} \right] \tag{2.43}$$

Noting (cf., eqn (2.39)) that

$$F_{IO_2} = \frac{u_0 a + 0.2 u_1 (A - a)}{u_0 a + u_1 (A - a)},$$

$$= 1 - \frac{0.8 u_1 (A - a)}{u_0 a + u_1 (A - a)}, \tag{2.44}$$

we may obtain $\partial F_{IO_2}/\partial u_1$ and then finally obtain $\partial F_{IO_2}/\partial p_e$ from eqn (2.43).

$$\frac{\partial F_{IO_2}}{\partial u_1} = -0.8u_0 \left\{ \frac{\left(\frac{a}{A}\right)\left(1-\frac{a}{A}\right)}{\left[u_0\left(\frac{a}{A}\right)+u_1\left(1-\frac{a}{A}\right)\right]^2} \right\}. \tag{2.45}$$

The result comes from eqns (2.43) and (2.45):

$$\frac{\partial F_{IO_2}}{\partial p_e} = -\frac{1}{\rho u_0^2} \times$$

$$\left\{ \frac{0.8\left(\frac{a}{A}\right)\left(1-\frac{a}{A}\right)}{\left[2\left(\frac{a}{A}\right)\left(1-\frac{a}{A}\right)\left(\frac{u_1}{u_0}-1\right)-\frac{u_1}{u_0}\right]\left[\frac{a}{A}+\frac{u_1}{u_0}\left(1-\frac{a}{A}\right)\right]^2} \right\}. \tag{2.46}$$

In the presence of the diffuser (Fig. 2.20(b)), the pressure p_2 at the end of the uniform section of the mixing duct is related to the exit pressure $p_3 = p_e$ by Bernoulli's equation:

$$\frac{p_2}{\rho} + \frac{[u_0 a + u_1'(A'-a)]^2}{2A'^2} = \frac{p_e}{\rho} + \frac{[u_0 a + u_1'(A'-a)]^2}{2K^2 A'^2}. \tag{2.47}$$

Combine eqns (2.40) and (2.47) to eliminate p_2 (again with $\rho_1 = \rho_0 = \rho$):

$$\left\{ p_e - P_{atm} + \frac{\rho[u_0 a + u_1'(A'-a)]^2}{2A'^2}\left(\frac{1-K^2}{K^2}\right) + \frac{\rho u_1'^2}{2} \right\}$$

$$= \rho\left(\frac{a}{A'}\right)\left(1-\frac{a}{A'}\right)(u_1'-u_0)^2. \tag{2.48}$$

Differentiate to find $\partial u_1/\partial p_e$:

$$1 + \frac{\rho[u_0 a + u_1'(A'-a)](A'-a)}{A'^2}\left(\frac{1-K^2}{K^2}\right)\frac{\partial u_1}{\partial p_e} + \rho u_1 \frac{\partial u_1}{\partial p_e}$$

$$= 2\rho\left(\frac{a}{A}\right)\left(1-\frac{a}{A}\right)(u_1-u_0)\frac{\partial u_1}{\partial p_e},$$

or

$$\frac{\partial u_1}{\partial p_e} = \frac{1}{\rho} \times$$

$$\left\{ \frac{1}{2\left(\frac{a}{A'}\right)\left(1-\frac{a}{A'}\right)(u_1-u_0)-u_1-\left[u_0\frac{a}{A'}+u_1'\left(1-\frac{a}{A'}\right)\right]\left(1-\frac{a}{A'}\right)\left(\frac{1-K^2}{K^2}\right)} \right\}. \tag{2.49}$$

Eqn (2.49) reduces to eqn (2.43) for $K = 1$ as expected. The final result for the system with a diffuser comes from eqns (2.45) and (2.49):

$$\frac{\partial F_{\mathrm{IO}_2}}{\partial p_e} = -\frac{1}{\rho u_0^2}\left\{\frac{0.8\left(\dfrac{a}{A'}\right)\left(1-\dfrac{a}{A'}\right)}{\left[\dfrac{a}{A'}+\dfrac{u_1'}{u_0}\left(1-\dfrac{a}{A'}\right)\right]^2}\right\}\times$$

$$\left\{\frac{1}{2\left(\dfrac{a}{A'}\right)\left(1-\dfrac{a}{A'}\right)\left(\dfrac{u_1'}{u_0}-1\right)-\dfrac{u_1'}{u_0}-\left[\dfrac{a}{A'}+\dfrac{u_1'}{u_0}\left(1-\dfrac{a}{A'}\right)\right]\left(1-\dfrac{a}{A'}\right)\left(\dfrac{1-K^2}{K^2}\right)}\right\}.$$

$$(2.50)$$

Comparison of $(\partial F_{\mathrm{IO}_2}/\partial p_e)$ for the two systems, with and without a diffuser, may be made therefore using eqns (2.46) and (2.50), but the comparison will only be meaningful when both systems generate the same F_{IO_2}. For this to be the case a/A, a/A', u_1/u_0, and u_1'/u_0 will be related according to eqn (2.44) in the following manner:

$$\frac{u_0 a + 0.2u_1(A-a)}{u_0 a + u_1(A-a)} = \frac{u_0 a + 0.2u_1'(A'-a)}{u_0 a + u_1'(A'-a)} \tag{2.51}$$

or since both the numerator and the denominator must be the same on each side of eqn (2.51),

$$\frac{u_1}{u_0}\left(\frac{A}{a}-1\right) = \frac{u_1'}{u_0}\left(\frac{A'}{a}-1\right). \tag{2.52}$$

The following numerical example illustrates the use of eqns (2.46), (2.50), and (2.52). Consider an entrainment duct without a diffuser for which $a/A = 0.03$. For this system eqn (2.37) tells us that $u_1/u_0 = 0.194$ and eqn (2.44) that $F_{\mathrm{IO}_2} = 0.3$. The variability of F_{IO_2} with changes in p_e is thus (eqn (2.46))

$$\frac{\partial F_{\mathrm{IO}_2}}{\partial p_e} = \frac{2.03}{\rho u_0^2}. \tag{2.53}$$

In Fig. (2.21) this point is plotted at $K = 1$ on a graph which gives $\partial F_{\mathrm{IO}_2}/\partial p_e$ as a function of K. Choosing now successively larger values of a/A', the corresponding increasing values of u_1'/u_0 and K may be determined from eqns (2.52) and (2.48) respectively, and the resulting values of $\partial F_{\mathrm{IO}_2}/\partial p_e$ from eqn (2.50).

In Fig. 2.21, $\rho u_0^2 \partial F_{\mathrm{IO}_2}/\partial p_e$ is plotted as a function of K. We can see that as K rises from 1 there is an initial rapid fall in $\partial F_{\mathrm{IO}_2}/\partial p_e$, showing that even a small diffuser can make an entrainment duct substantially more resistant than the uniform duct to changes in F_{IO_2} brought about by small back pressures. However, upon increasing K above about 3 little further improve-

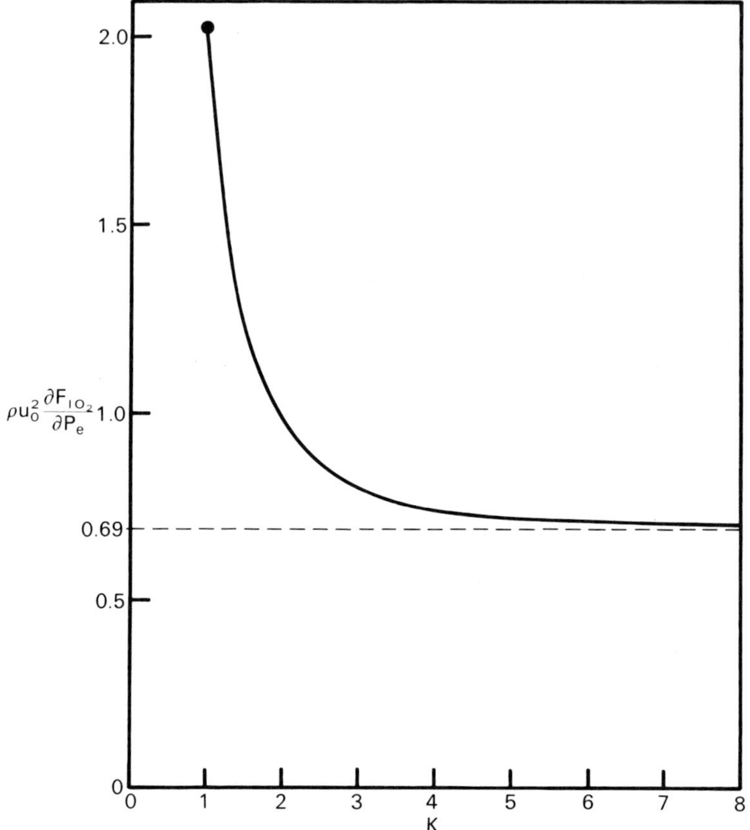

Fig. 2.21. The effect of adding a diffuser with area ratio K to an entrainment duct (Fig. 2.20) on the stalling coefficient $\partial F_{IO_2}/\partial p_e$ (eqn (2.50)). This coefficient measures the extent to which the composition of the air–oxygen mixture generated by the system is varied by back pressure at the diffuser exit. This plot is for the case $F_{IO_2} = 0.31$. The dashed line represents an asymptotic minimum value of $\rho u_0^2 \partial F_{IO_2}/\partial p_e$.

ment can be achieved. Indeed the plot is asymptotic to the line $\rho u_0^2 \partial F_{IO_2}/\partial p_e = 0.69$ which represents the condition $u_1' = u_0$ at which the entrained air velocity equals the velocity of the oxygen jet. The maximum reduction in $\partial F_{IO_2}/\partial p_e$ which can be achieved for this system in which $F_{IO_2} = 0.3$ is thus by a factor of $2.03/0.69 \simeq 3$.

Entrainment systems incorporating a diffuser as in Fig. 2.20(b) may be appropriately called venturi breathing systems because they contain a true venturi: a region in a pipe where the cross-sectional area of the flow first decreases to a minimum value then increases again downstream in what is termed the diffuser. We have already commented on the need to reduce turbulence in the diffuser. To minimize turbulence in the entry region, where the entrained air is converging from an infinite cross-sectional area to the minimum area A, it may also be desirable to introduce a gradually converging duct.

In conclusion, it appears that an entrainment duct may be used to supply a breathing system such as a T-piece with an accurately determined mixture of oxygen and air (Fig. 2.19(a)). The introduction of a diffuser makes the device a true 'venturi' system and reduces the susceptibility of the system to back pressure (Fig. 2.19(b)). Venturi breathing systems are not widely used but continue to be evaluated for various applications. Fig. 2.19(c) is a diagram of a venturi circuit incorporating a CO_2 absorber and using a venturi to recirculate part of the fresh gas flow to a T-piece. The system was described in 1985 by Jorgensen and Hansen (Jorgensen, S. and Hansen, L. K. *Acta Anaesthesiologica Scandinavica*, **29**, 269–72) and evaluated on patients in Denmark. It reduces the fresh gas flow requirement of the T-piece to about 40 per cent of its normal value. The performance of the venturi and its susceptibility to back pressure transmitted along the narrow feed tube have not been examined theoretically. A portable anaesthetic apparatus for use in the Antarctic utilized an air entrainment duct to supply a mixture of oxygen and air to a Magill breathing system. Its analysis forms question 3 in the problem section.

2.6 The Magill and Lack breathing systems

The components of the Magill breathing system (Fig. 2.22(a) and (b)) are virtually identical to those of a T-piece system with a bag (Fig. 2.9(b)) but they perform in a very different manner because the gas entry and exit ports are reversed.

The Magill system is probably the most widely used breathing system among anaesthetists. It was introduced early into modern anaesthesia as an 'attachment' to the Boyle machine which has evolved since 1917 as the dominant style of anaesthetic machine capable of delivering a steady flow of accurately mixed anaesthetic gases and vapours. Legend has it that Ivan Magill* was anaesthetizing in about 1920 using the then current attachment to the Boyle machine which was a tube leading to a three-way stopcock and reservoir bag close to the facemask. The crowding of these pieces around the patient's face apparently limited the surgeon's access and Magill is said to have improvised to improve matters by interposing a piece of tube found in his civilian's gas mask bag between the patient's face and the reservoir bag. Thus was born a breathing system which has dominated anaesthesia for nearly 70 years and which is the least greedy of its kind with respect to fresh

---

* Later Sir Ivan Magill (1888–1986).

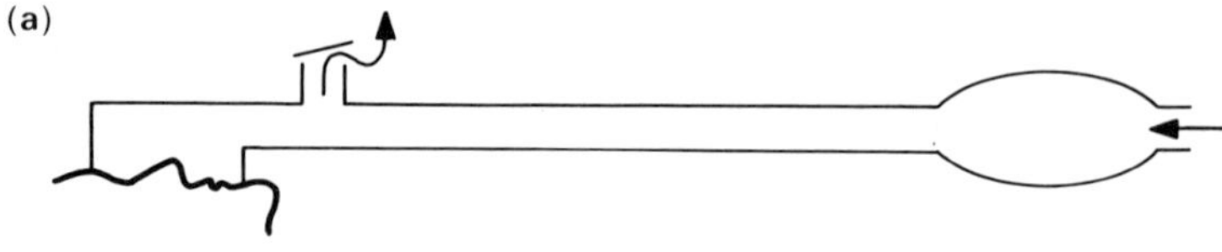

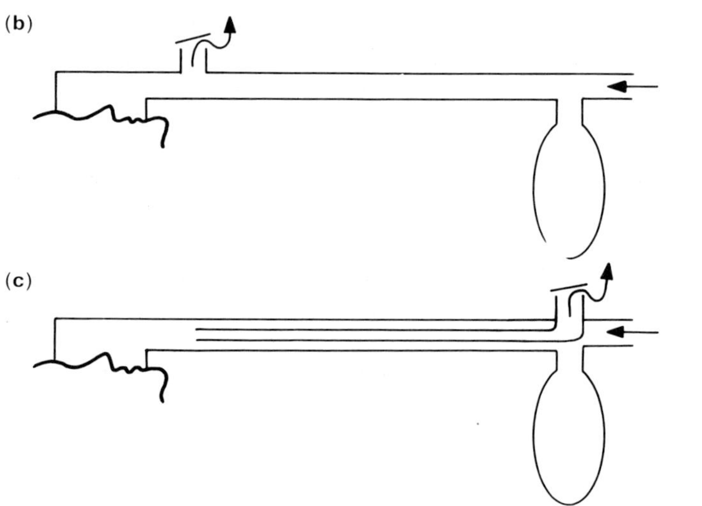

Fig. 2.22. The Magill breathing system has fresh gas delivered through (a) or close to (b), a collapsible reservoir bag separated by a reservoir tube from an expiratory valve. The Lack breathing system (c) is a coaxial form of the Magill system and is functionally identical.

gas flow, but which was never formally described by Magill in the scientific literature.

Fresh gas is delivered through (Fig. 2.22(a)) or close to (Fig. 2.22(b)) a collapsible reservoir bag and thence passes via a reservoir tube to the patient's face mask. The escape of gas from the system is via a one-way valve lying close to the mask. The system differs from the T-piece simply in having an exact reversal of inlet and outlet flows. In the Magill system, fresh gas is inhaled from the reservoir bag and as long as the reservoir tubing interposed between patient and bag is sufficiently large, no CO_2 will find its way to the bag during expiration. We shall now demonstrate that this arrangement allows rebreathing of CO_2 to be minimized at a relatively small fresh gas flow approximately equal to the patient's ventilation, $\dot{V}$.

Consider Fig. 2.23. We again model the patient's breathing by assuming constant inspiratory and expiratory flows (Fig. 2.23(e)). At the moment the

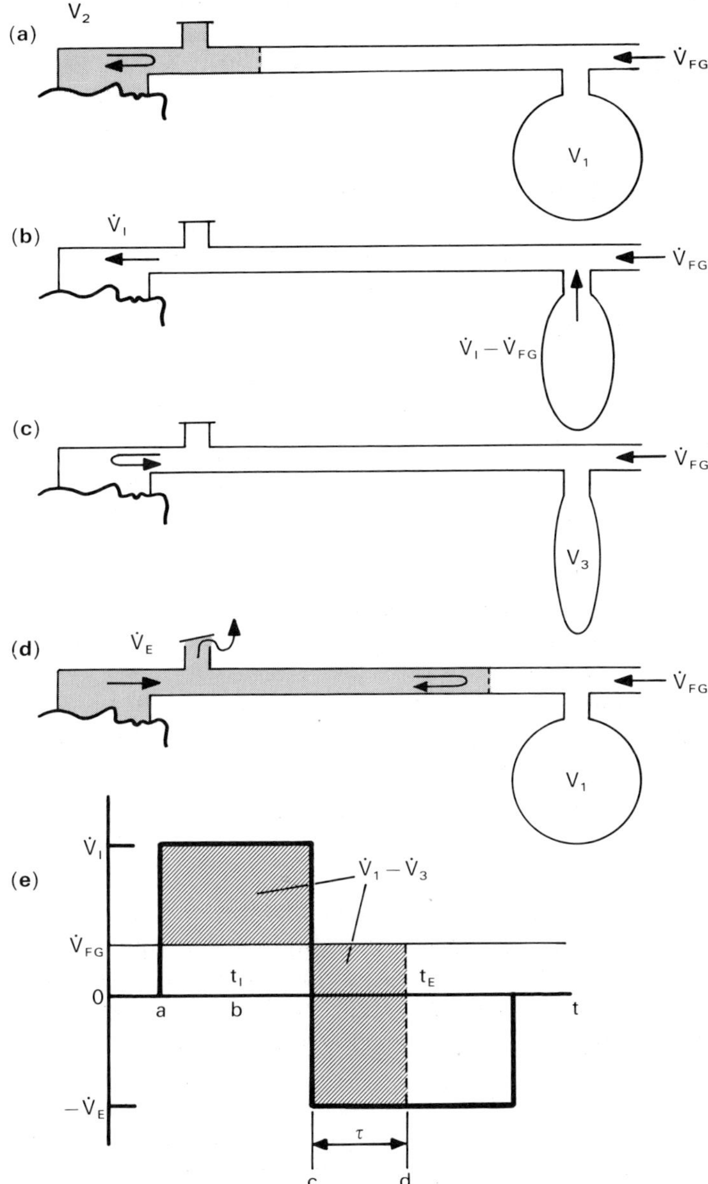

Fig. 2.23. Calculation of the rebreathing properties of the Magill system assuming constant inspiratory and expiratory flows (e). (a) The beginning of inspiration (end of previous expiration); (b) midway through inspiration; (c) end of inspiration (beginning of expiration); (d) at time τ into expiration when the expiratory valve opens.

patient begins to inspire from the system (Fig. 2.23(a)) we shall define the volume of gas in the fully distended reservoir bag to be V_1 and the volume of expired gas remaining at this time in the system (including the dead space) to be V_2. (The reservoir bag must be fully distended at this moment because it has filled during the preceding expiration prior to sufficient pressure being generated in the system to open the expiratory valve.) Note that we assume $V_2 - V_D$ to be smaller than the volume of the reservoir tube lying between the dead space and the reservoir bag, and so no expired gas reaches the bag.

As inspiration continues (Fig. 2.23(b)) the patient rebreathes this volume V_2 of expired gas, followed by a volume $(\dot{V}_1 t_1 - V_2)$ of fresh gas. The fraction of fresh gas inspired is thus

$$F_{IFG} = \frac{\dot{V}_1 t_1 - V_2}{\dot{V}_1 t_1}. \tag{2.54}$$

Throughout inspiration the gas flow from the bag is the difference between the inspiratory flow $\dot{V}_1$ and the fresh gas flow $\dot{V}_{FG}$ (assuming $\dot{V}_{FG} < \dot{V}_1$) and so the volume of the bag at the end of inspiration (Fig. 2.23(c)) must be given by

$$V_1 - V_3 = (\dot{V}_1 - \dot{V}_{FG})t_1. \tag{2.55}$$

In the early stage of expiration the bag volume increases from V_3 to V_1 as gas enters the system from both ends. When the bag is full the expiratory valve opens to permit gases to leave the system. We denote this event as a time τ into expiration (Fig. 2.23(d)). Before the valve opens the gas flow into the system is the sum of $\dot{V}_E$ from the patient and $\dot{V}_{FG}$ from the fresh gas supply and so τ is given by

$$\tau = \frac{V_1 - V_3}{\dot{V}_E + \dot{V}_{FG}}. \tag{2.56}$$

Finally, we relate V_2 to τ. We note that the volume of expired gas remaining in the system at the end of expiration (V_2) equals the volume of expired gas entering the system during the initial τ seconds of expiration $(\dot{V}_E \tau)$ minus the volume of expired gas displaced from the reservoir tube during the remaining $t_E - \tau$ seconds of expiration $[\dot{V}_{FG}(t_E - \tau)]$:

$$V_2 = \dot{V}_E \tau - \dot{V}_{FG}(t_E - \tau). \tag{2.57}$$

$(V_1 - V_3)$ is directly available from eqn 2.55. That leaves three unknowns $(F_{IFG}, V_2$ and $\tau)$ to be found from three equations (2.54, 2.56 and 2.57). The solutions are easily derived:

$$\tau = t_1 \frac{(\dot{V}_1 - \dot{V}_{FG})}{(\dot{V}_E + \dot{V}_{FG})}; \tag{2.58}$$

$$V_2 = \dot{V}_1 t_1 - \dot{V}_{FG}(t_1 + t_E); \tag{2.59}$$

$$F_{IFG} = \frac{\dot{V}_{FG}}{\dot{V}_I} (1 + t_E/t_I) = \frac{\dot{V}_{FG}}{\dot{V}};$$ (2.60)

Recall that the following assumptions have been made in deriving this solution:

(i) $V_3 \geq 0$. (The minimum volume of the reservoir bag must not be required to go below zero.)

(ii) $V_2 \geq 0$. (The rebreathed volume must not appear as negative.)

(iii) $V_{RT} + V_D \geq V_E \tau$, where V_{RT} is the volume of the reservoir tube. (The expired gas does not reach the bag.)

The second assumption is equivalent to saying that $F_{IFG} \leq 1$. If $\dot{V}_{FG}$ exceeds $\dot{V}$ and there is truly no dead space in the system, then V_2 would equal zero and F_{IFG} would remain at 1.

In the presence of a dead space V_D, the minimum value of V_2 which can be achieved is $V_2 = V_D$ and the maximum F_{IFG} becomes less than 1. Equation (2.54) becomes

$$F_{IFG} = 1 - V_D/(\dot{V}_I t_I).$$ (2.61)

To calculate the rebreathing index for the Magill system we need to deduce the expired CO_2 fraction, F_{ECO_2}, which is related to F_{ICO_2} by eqn (2.16)

$$(F_{ECO_2} - F_{ICO_2})\dot{V} = \dot{V}_{CO_2},$$ (2.16)

and also by a relationship involving F_{IFG}:

$$F_{ICO_2} = F_{ECO_2} (1 - F_{IFG}).$$ (2.62)

(Both eqns (2.16) and (2.62) assume that eqn (2.7) holds true, that inspired and expired volumes may be regarded as identical.) Combine eqns (2.16), (2.62) and (2.62) and we get the simple result

$$F_{ECO_2} = \dot{V}_{CO_2}/\dot{V}_{FG}.$$ (2.63)

We thus have the following behaviour from the Magill system. A patient breathing with ventilation $\dot{V}_0$ at high fresh gas flows has a fraction of the inspired breath composed of fresh gas at the minimum value given by eqn (2.61), which with eqn (2.9) yields

$$F_{IFG} = 1 - V_D/[\dot{V}_0(t_I + t_E)]$$

$$= 1 - V_D r/\dot{V}_0$$

$$= 1 - V_D/V_{T0},$$ (2.64)

where r is the respiratory rate and V_{T0} the tidal volume at ventilation $\dot{V}_0$. The minimum fresh gas flow for which this high F_{IFG} is maintained is (eqns (2.60) and (2.64))

$$\dot{V}_{FG} = \dot{V}_0 F_{IFG}$$
$$= \dot{V}_0 - V_D r, \tag{2.65}$$

and the F_{ECO_2} at this fresh gas flow and above is (eqn (2.63))

$$F_{ECO_2} = \dot{V}_{CO_2}/(\dot{V}_0 - V_D r). \tag{2.66}$$

As the fresh gas flow below this critical value the F_{ECO_2} becomes a function of $\dot{V}_{FG}$ alone (eqn (2.63) with $\dot{V}_{CO_2}$ assumed constant). Thus, no amount of hyperventilation will reduce F_{ECO_2} to its value at high fresh gas flows (eqn (2.66)).

It follows that the rebreathing index (Fig. 2.24) for the Magill system takes a value of 1 for all values of $\dot{V}_{FG}/\dot{V}_0$ greater than $1-(V_D/V_{TO})$; it may take any

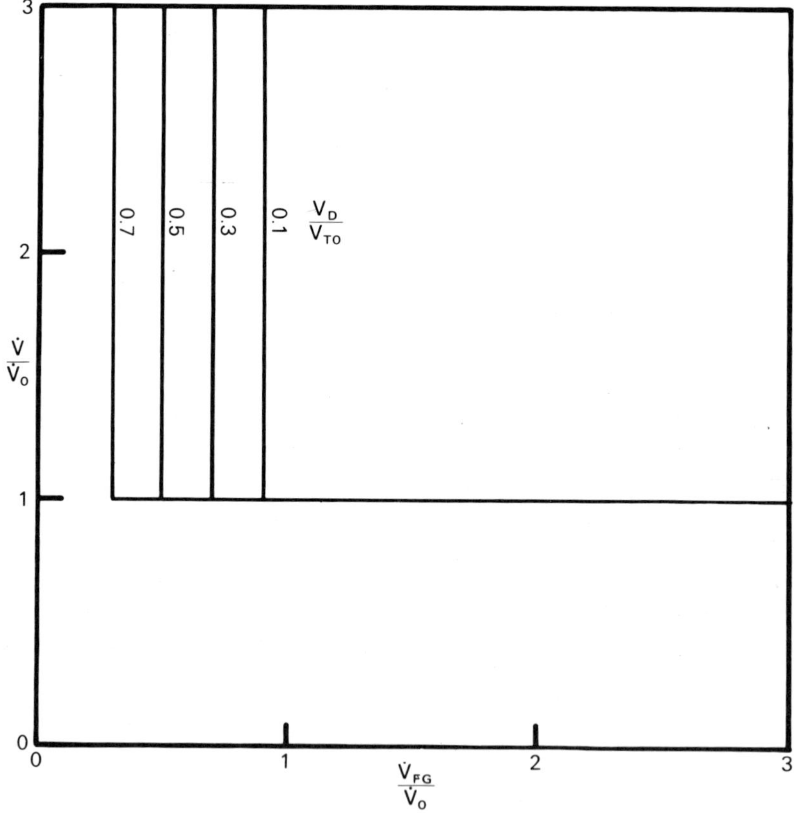

Fig. 2.24. The rebreathing index for the Magill system, plotted for different ratios of the relative dead space V_D/V_{TO}. Constant $\dot{V}_I$ and $\dot{V}_E$ assumed. t_E/t_I may take any value. Respiratory rate constant.

value greater than or equal to 1 at this critical fresh gas flow and is indeterminate at lower fresh gas flows. A comparison of Figs. 2.24 and 2.12 brings out the considerably greater efficiency of the Magill system over the T-piece in generating a low rebreathing index down to relatively low fresh gas flows. Unlike T-piece systems, the Magill system does not permit a subject to maintain normocapnia at low fresh gas flows by increasing ventilation. The F_{ECO_2} rises relentlessly as $\dot{V}_{FG}$ is reduced (eqn (2.63)) regardless of whether $\dot{V}$ is increased or not. The CO_2 retention index for this system becomes a simple result from eqns (2.63) and (2.66)

$$\frac{F'_{ECO_2}}{F_{ECO_2}} = \frac{\dot{V}_0 - V_D r}{\dot{V}_{FG}} = \frac{\dot{V}_0}{\dot{V}_{FG}}\left(1 - \frac{V_D}{V_{TO}}\right), \tag{2.67}$$

and tells us the rise in F_{ECO_2} over its minimum value not only for fixed ventilation $\dot{V}_0$ but for any value of ventilation adopted by the subject in response to the rebreathing to which he is subjected. The CO_2 retention index of eqn (2.67) is consequently a particularly useful result in the clinical setting. We depict the result in Fig. 2.25.

A coaxial form of the Magill system was described by Lack in 1976 (Fig. 2.22(c)). It is analogous to Bain's coaxial form of the T-piece system (Fig. 2.9(d)) but the requirements of the coaxial tubing for the Lack system do differ from the Bain system. In the Lack system the patient has to propel gas along both lumens of the tubing which must therefore both be of a sufficiently large cross-sectional area to minimize resistance to flow. In contrast to this the central lumen of the Bain system is supplied at a constant flow by a high pressure source of gas and need therefore be of only small cross-sectional area.

In both the Magill and Lack systems the reservoir tube plays an important role somewhat independent of the reservoir bag and the reader may find it instructive to calculate the minimum safe tube volume.

2.7 Minimal rebreathing: a graphical approach

Our analysis of the rebreathing characteristics of medical breathing systems has been limited in its precision by the assumption of constant inspiratory and expiratory flows (Fig. 2.4(b) *et seq.*) We noted in Fig. 2.14 one example during anaesthesia of the extent to which this approximation of a 'stepped' respiratory waveform deviates from the observed waveform. We mentioned also the tendency for there to be an 'end-expiratory pause' in the respiratory waveform of patients who are awake rather than anaesthetized. In this section we extend our analysis to the general respiratory waveform and tackle the limited but clinically important problem of determining the minimum fresh gas flow required by different breathing systems to reduce rebreathing to a minimum.

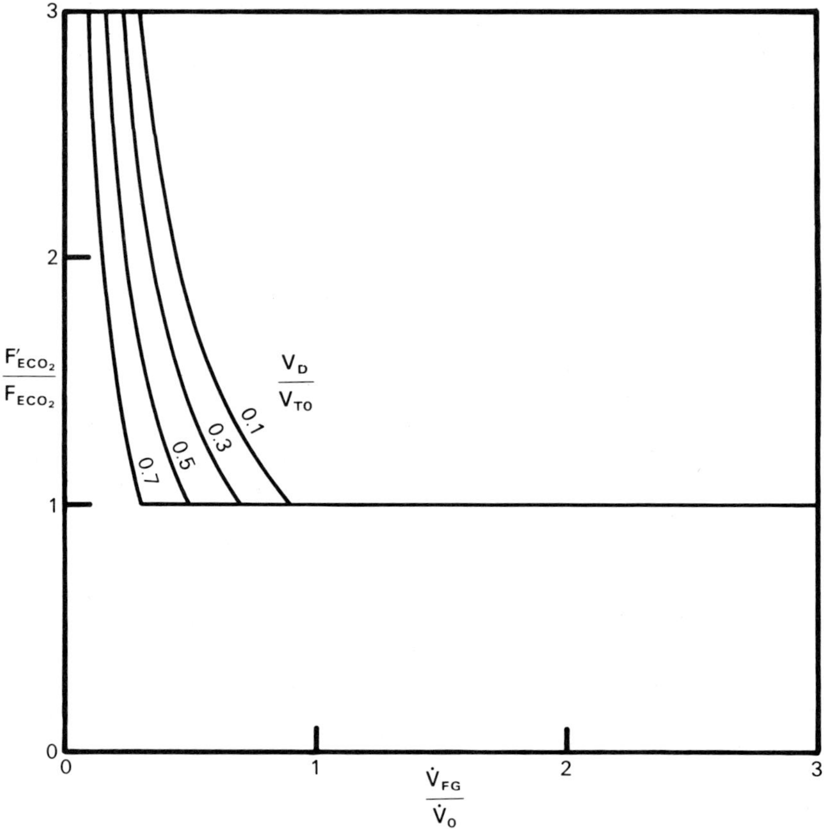

Fig. 2.25. The CO_2 retention index for the Magill system, plotted for different ratios of the relative dead space V_D/V_{TO}. Constant $\dot{V}_I$ and $\dot{V}_E$ assumed. t_E/t_I may take any value.

It is useful here to introduce Mapleson's classification of anaesthetic breathing systems using letters A, B, C, D, E published in 1954 (Fig. 2.26). A sixth system, F, subsequently sneaked into the list. The list of six remains a complete description of all currently used breathing systems having no more than a single one-way valve, in current use by anaesthetists.

The Mapleson A corresponds with the Magill system and its functionally identical counterpart, the Lack (Fig. 2.22). The Mapleson E is the bagless, valveless Ayre T-piece (Fig. 2.9(a)). The Mapleson F is the Jackson Rees modification to the E (Fig. 2.9(b)) and the Mapleson D corresponds with the further addition of a valve yielding a system functionally the same as the Bain (Fig. 2.9(d)).

The Mapleson B and C systems we have not encountered so far in this chapter. In both systems the fresh gas is delivered close to both the expiratory

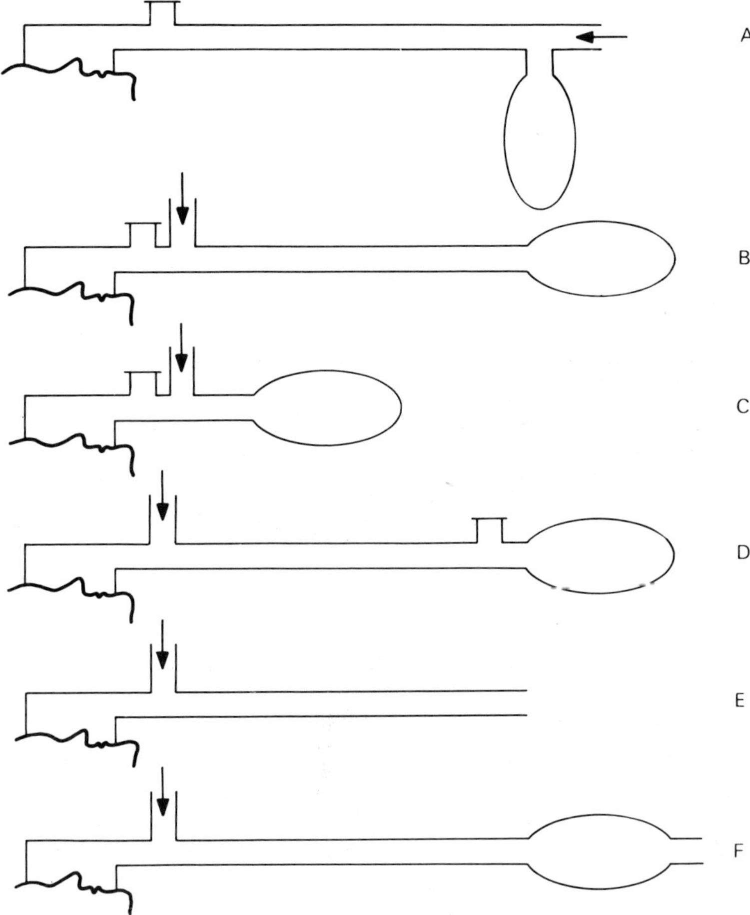

Fig. 2.26. Mapleson's classification of anaesthetic breathing systems, incorporating no more than a single one-way valve. (1954, *British Journal of Anaesthesia* **26**, 323–32. Willis, B. A., Pender, J. W. and Mapleson, W. W. 1975. *British Journal of Anaesthesia* **47**, 1239–45.)

valve and the patient's face. In the C system a collapsible reservoir bag is also attached close to the patient's face; in the B system a reservoir tube is interposed between the bag and the other components. The Mapleson B system is currently unpopular and is rarely used. The C system continues to have its applications. It is often referred to as the 'Waters bag' on account of its similarity with a device described by R. M. Waters in 1926.

In contrast to our earlier depiction of the pattern of breathing as a plot of flow against time (Figs. 2.4 and 2.14, and so on) we now make use of a plot of volume against time of gas passing into and out of the patient. A plot of this

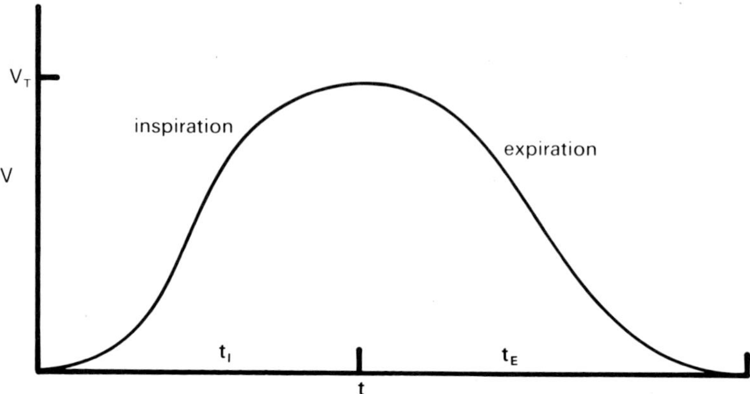

Fig. 2.27. The respiratory waveform depicted as a plot of volume (V) against time (t). V is the volume of gas that passes into or out of the patient and, since the volume of gas expired is usually closely equal to the volume inspired, the plot returns near to the horizontal axis at the end of the cycle. Because physiological gas flows ($\dot{V}$) do not change suddenly, the plot would be expected always to be horizontal at both the beginning and end of the cycle. t_I is the inspiratory time; t_E is the expiratory time.

kind takes the form of the curved line in Fig. 2.27 and represents the integral, with respect to time, of the corresponding $\dot{V}$–t waveform. Time $t = 0$ is taken to be the end of an expiration. In the absence of an end-expiratory pause it is thus the beginning of an inspiration. Volume $V = 0$ is the volume at $t = 0$.

From the origin ($V = 0$, $t = 0$) the plot rises as inspiration proceeds and reaches a maximum volume V_T at the end of inspiration. The plot then falls as expiration occurs. Usually the volume of gas expired is closely equal to the volume inspired, and so the plot meets the horizontal axis at the end of expiration. Small differences between inspired and expired volumes occur due to R differing from one, humidification by the lungs of dry gases, and uptake or elimination of anaesthetic gases. In such cases, the V–t plot will not return exactly to the horizontal axis at the end of expiration. The solution presented in this section will remain precise in such cases.

The fresh gas flow ($\dot{V}_{FG}$) to an anaesthetic breathing system may also be represented on a V–t plot (Fig. 2.28), this time by a line which has a slope equal to $\dot{V}_{FG}$. The position of this line is varied in the following analyses.

The determination of the minimum fresh gas flows needed to eliminate rebreathing, as far as possible, from the anaesthetic systems is achieved simply by superimposing the plot of fresh gas flow (Fig. 2.28) onto the respiratory waveform (Fig. 2.27). The following definitions are adopted. Dead space (V_D) is again the sum of the anatomical dead space and equipment dead space (eqn 2.24). The equipment dead space is taken to be that volume within the breathing system which lies between the patient's anatomical dead space

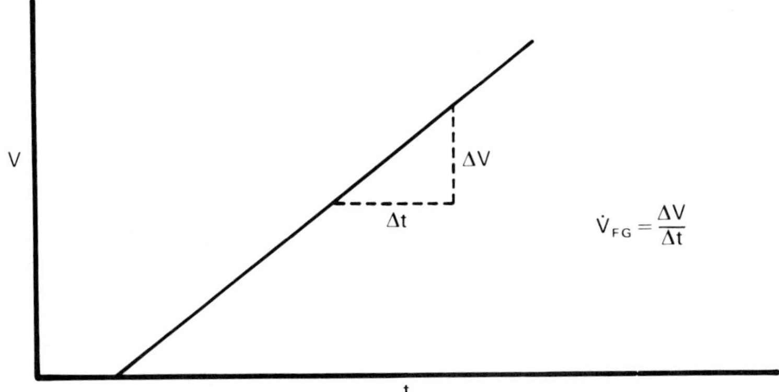

Fig. 2.28. The fresh gas flow $\dot{V}_{FG}$ delivered to a breathing system, depicted as a plot of volume against time. The gradient of the straight line equals $\dot{V}_{FG}$.

and the region within the breathing system flushed by the flow of fresh gas if the patient stops breathing (for example, Fig. 2.11). Minimal rebreathing is the inhalation into the alveoli of a volume of gas containing CO_2 equal only to the gas which is present in the dead space at the time inspiration begins.

Consider firstly the Mapleson A (Magill, Lack) system (Fig. 2.22). We seek the fresh gas flow which before an inspiration begins is just sufficient to displace all alveolar gas from the reservoir tube; only the dead space V_D is left filled with alveolar gas (Fig. 2.23). The gradient of line A in Fig. 2.29 gives the $\dot{V}_{FG}$ which is the solution to this problem.

From the end of expiration ($t = 0$) until point X, where line A becomes a tangent to the respiratory waveform, $\dot{V}_{FG}$ exceeds inspiratory flow and the

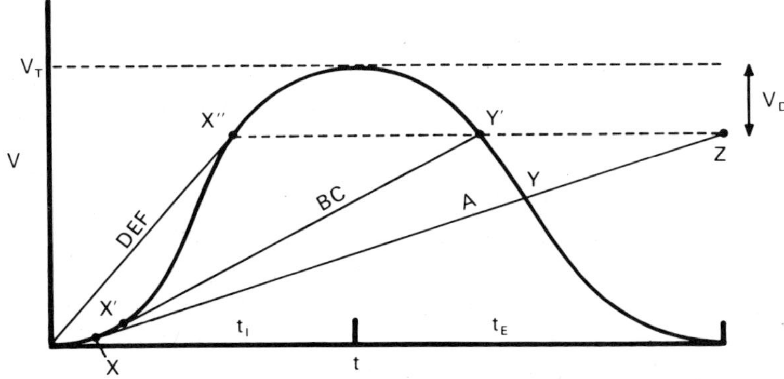

Fig. 2.29. The respiratory wave form with fresh gas flow lines superimposed to obtain minimum flow requirements for anaesthetic breathing systems (Mapleson A/BC/DEF). V_D is the anatomical and equipment dead space volume. (From Dorrington, K. L. and Lehane, J. R. (1987) *Anaesthesia* **42**, 732–7.)

reservoir bag remains full. The expiratory valve remains open at this early stage of inspiration. From point X the valve is closed and the reservoir bag begins to discharge its contents. The loss of volume of the reservoir bag is given by the vertical distance between the line A and the respiratory waveform. The bag starts to fill when the gradient of the V–t curve becomes less than the fresh gas flow. At Y, where the lines cross, the bag is full and the expiratory valve opens. After point Y, the vertical distance between line A and the waveform is a measure of the volume of expired gas that leaves from the valve. At point Z, a volume $V_T - V_D$ of alveolar gas has left the system and the patient has finished breathing out a volume V_T. No gas expired from the alveoli remains in the reservoir tube, and so minimal rebreathing has been achieved. Therefore the gradient of a line which passes through point $Z(t = t_I + t_E, V = V_T - V_D)$ and is also a tangent to the inspiratory waveform (point X) gives the minimum fresh gas flow requirement for the Mapleson A system.

Consider secondly the Mapleson B and C (Waters) systems (Fig. 2.26). These have an identical fresh gas flow requirement. We derive this by noting that no alveolar gas must be permitted to enter the reservoir tube (B system) or bag (C system). The gradient of line BC in Fig. 2.29 gives the $\dot{V}_{FG}$ which is the solution to this problem.

From the end of expiration ($t = 0$) until point X′, where line BC becomes a tangent to the respiratory waveform, $\dot{V}_{FG}$ exceeds inspiratory flow and the reservoir bag remains full. The expiratory valve remains open during this period. From point X′ the valve is closed and the bag discharges gas and then fills again until the expiratory valve opens again at Y′. The vertical distance of point Y′ below the peak volume V_T is a measure of the volume of expired gas which has entered the system at the moment the valve opens. In the B and C systems, as long as this does not exceed V_D no alveolar gas will enter the reservoir tube/bag.

Thus the gradient of a line that passes through Y′ ($V = V_T - V_D$ on expiratory limb of waveform) and is also a tangent to the inspiratory waveform (point X′), gives the minimum fresh gas flow requirement for the Mapleson B and C systems.

Consider thirdly, the Mapleson D, E, and F (Bain, T-piece, Jackson Rees) systems (Fig. 2.9). These have an identical fresh gas flow requirement. We derive this by noting that from the start of inspiration until a volume $V_T - V_D$ has been inspired, no gas that contains CO_2 must be permitted to pass into the equipment dead space from the reservoir tube. The solution is represented by the line DEF in Fig. 2.29.

From the end of expiration ($t = 0$) until the point X″ where the line $V = V_T - V_D$ crosses the inspiratory limb of the $V - t$ curve, the volume of fresh gas delivered at the T-piece exceeds the patient's inspiratory demand. The excess fresh gas is stored at the patient end of the reservoir tube. At X″

the two volumes become equal and gas which contains CO_2 arrives at the T itself. After point X″, gas that contains CO_2 may be inspired into the dead space with no functional significance, since it will never reach the alveoli. Thus the gradient of a line that passes through $V = 0$ at the end of expiration ($t = 0$) and first meets the inspiratory limb of the waveform where $V = V_T - V_D$ gives the minimum fresh gas flow requirement for the Mapleson D, E and F systems.

An important qualification needs to be made for the case in which V_D is so small that a line which joins the origin to the point $V = V_T - V_D$ on the inspiratory limb would cross the limb between these end points. In this case, achievement of minimal rebreathing requires that line DEF should lie tangential to the inspiratory limb. The appropriate X″ which forms the right hand end of the line DEF is then the point at which the line becomes a tangent to (parallel to and just touching) the inspiratory waveform. This situation is unlikely to arise in clinical practice.

It is instructive to derive the solutions for the triangular $V - t$ waveform which corresponds with the 'square wave' $\dot{V}-t$ waveform used extensively earlier in this chapter (Figs. 2.4, 2.11 and 2.23). The graphical constructions applied to this waveform are shown in Fig. 2.30. These can be shown to be in agreement with the earlier analyses using this waveform (Fig. 2.12, 2.13 and 2.24).

The simple graphical technique of deriving fresh gas flow requirements enables us to see at a glance how variations in the pattern of breathing and in the ratio V_D/V_T affect these requirements. The effect of an end-expiratory pause can also readily be seen (Fig. 2.31). Recall that the line DEF originates at the end of expiration, which may differ from the beginning of inspiration in the presence of an end expiratory pause (t_p). Increasing t_p reduces the slope of

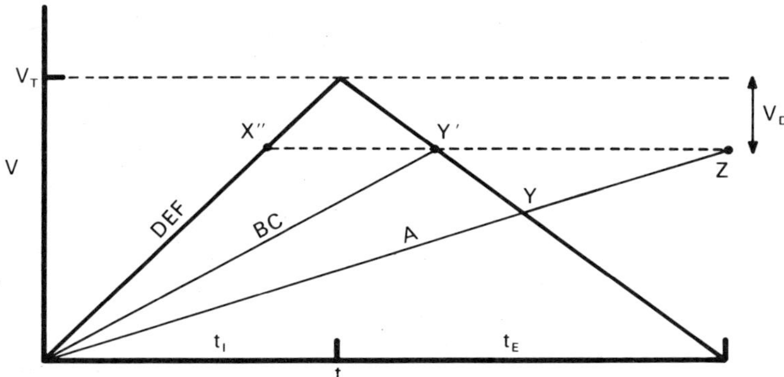

Fig. 2.30. The equivalent construction to Fig. 2.29 for the idealized respiratory waveform that consists of constant inspiratory and expiratory flows. (Source as Fig. 2.29)

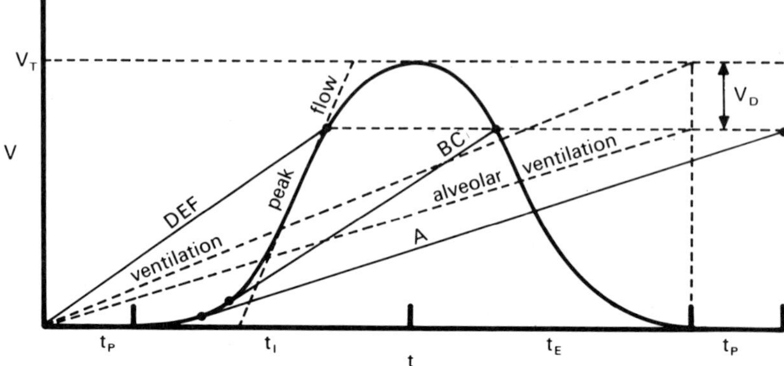

Fig. 2.31. Construction as in Fig. 2.29 but with an end expiratory pause (duration t_p) preceding inspiration. Also included are three sloping dashed lines, the gradients of which equal peak inspiratory flow, ventilation, and alveolar ventilation. The completed construction gives a precise comparison between the minimum fresh gas flow requirements of the Mapleson systems A/BC/DEF and the three flows with which comparisons are often quoted in the research literature. (Source as Fig. 2.29)

line DEF (i.e., reduces the fresh gas flow requirement). However, it can be seen by comparison of the slopes of the fresh gas flow lines that the Mapleson A system is usually more efficient than the other systems. Furthermore, Mapleson B and C systems are more efficient than D, E and F systems except in the presence of a slow respiratory rate (small V_D/V_T) and long t_p, conditions which do not normally prevail during anaesthesia (Fig. 2.14). It should be emphasized that this analysis, like those earlier in this chapter, makes the assumptions of absence of coaxial mixing within the ducts of the breathing system, and that a steady state has been achieved.

Note that fresh gas flow requirements are commonly stated in clinical studies as multiples of either the patient's ventilation (minute volume) or alveolar ventilation (alveolar minute volume). These are given in our construction by the gradients of straight lines that pass through the origin ($t = 0$, $V = 0$) and the respective points $V = V_T$ and $V = V_T - V_D$ at the end of the respiratory cycle ($t = t_p + t_I + t_E$ in Fig. 2.31). A third flow occasionally mentioned in such studies is the peak inspiratory flow which has been erroneously regarded by some as the minimum fresh gas flow requirement of the B and C systems. The peak inspiratory flow, ventilation, and alveolar ventilation are depicted as dashed lines in Fig. 2.31.

The solution shows that the Mapleson A system will be the most efficient of all, and will have a fresh gas flow requirement approximately equal to (but always greater than) the alveolar ventilation. The next most efficient will usually be the B and C systems, with a flow requirement around twice the alveolar ventilation. The D, E, and F systems would only become more efficient than the B and C systems in the presence of a large t_p and small V_D/V_T ratio, which are unlikely to occur during anaesthesia. Of the three families of breathing systems the D, E, F family would appear to have a flow requirement which varies most with the shape of the respiratory waveform. A broad recommendation of a flow approximately equal to 2–3 times the (total) ventilation seems appropriate from Figs. 2.29 and 2.31.

2.8 Minimal rebreathing: use of multiple valves

It may by now be a cause for frustration in the reader that the simplest way of eliminating rebreathing – by the use of valves – has been neglected in favour of less straightforward means. The Mapleson classification of anaesthetic breathing systems (Fig. 2.26) includes only systems with one or no unidirectional valve. The addition of a valve in the fresh gas supply line is shown in Fig. 2.32. During inspiration the valve in the supply line opens (Fig. 2.32(a)) whilst during expiration it closes, preventing the accumulation in the system of expired gas other than that filling the dead space (Fig. 2.32(b)).

In this system problems still arise in accommodating a constant flow of fresh gas to the rhythmic inspiratory and expiratory demand at the patient end. If $\dot{V}_{FG}$ exceeds the patient's ventilation the addition of a reservoir bag (Fig. 2.32(c)) is sufficient to overcome the problem. With this arrangement, however, a fall in $\dot{V}_{FG}$ to below the ventilation will lead to collapse of the reservoir bag and unrewarded inspiratory efforts.

One of the most satisfactory arrangements for the use of a 'non-rebreathing' double valve system is the addition of an open reservoir tube (Fig. 2.32(d)) at the point of entry of the fresh gas supply. In this mode an excess of gas leaves from the tube, whilst a deficit of fresh gas can be made up for by entrainment of air along the tube in the opposite direction. The dilution of anaesthetic gases by air may lead to a lightening of anaesthesia but at least provides a safe source of oxygen. A system of this kind is much used for anaesthesia in difficult circumstances, such as by the military or in remote areas (Fig. 2.32(e)). Oxygen is used economically at a flow of around $1\,l\,min^{-1}$ to enrich to around 30 per cent the greater flow of air entrained down the reservoir tube. Only after the air–oxygen mixture is formed are one or more anaesthetic vapours added to the gas, by one or more vaporizers which lie between the oxygen 'T' and the inspiratory valve.

Finally, Fig. 2.32(f) depicts a system which eliminates rebreathing of CO_2 by the use of two one-way valves but permits the economy of rebreathing of anaesthetic gases. This 'circle system' incorporates a CO_2 absorption canister containing soda lime, the cost of which partially offsets the economy of the system. During the maintenance of anaesthesia when little anaesthetic is being taken up by the patient, the fresh gas flow to this circle system can be reduced to a theoretical and safe practical minimum of around $250\,ml\,min^{-1}$

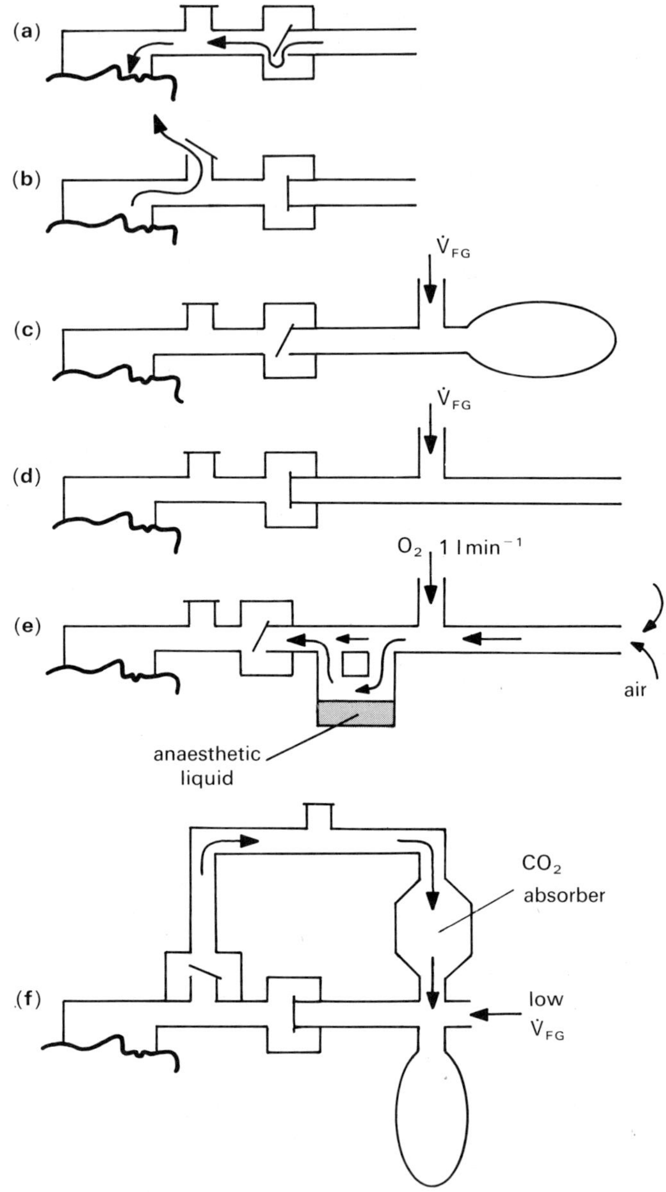

Fig. 2.32. Non-rebreathing systems. The presence of two valves prevents rebreathing of expired CO_2 from other than the dead space. (a) Valve on inspiratory limb opens during inspiration and closes (b) during expiration. (c) A reservoir bag is adequate only if $\dot{V}_{FG}$ exceeds the patient's ventilation. (d) A reservoir tube permits escape of excess fresh gas and entrainment of air. (e) The 'Triservice' system for economical use of oxygen to enrich air. (f) The circle system for rebreathing of anaesthetic gases but not CO_2.

of oxygen, i.e., the patient's oxygen consumption alone. This circle system shares some similarity with that shown in Fig. 2.19(c) in which circulation through the CO_2 absorber is maintained by a jet entrainment system rather than by valves. Circle systems are popular for anaesthetic use in the USA but less widely used in this country.

Problems

2.1 Small babies do not readily tolerate an oxygen mask. An alternative way of controlling the composition of their inspired gas is to nurse them inside an oxygen tent supplied with a flow $\dot{V}_{FG}$ of the appropriate mixture of gas (Fig. 2.33).

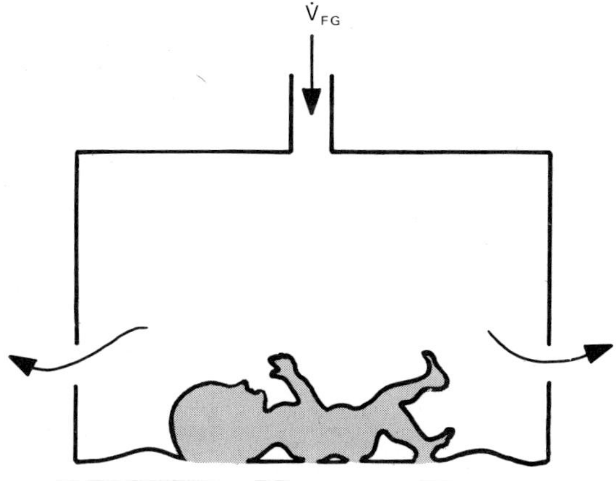

Fig. 2.33

By modelling a baby's breathing as a steady flow of oxygen out of the tent and a steady flow of CO_2 into the tent, and by assuming perfect mixing of gas within the tent, show that the rebreathing index of the system may be given by the approximate relation

$$\frac{\dot{V}}{\dot{V}_0} \simeq \frac{\dot{V}_{FG}/\dot{V}_0}{(\dot{V}_{FG}/\dot{V}_0 - 1)},$$

where $\dot{V}$ is the ventilation and $\dot{V}_0$ is the ventilation in the absence of rebreathing. Under what conditions does this solution become inaccurate? Estimate the minimum safe fresh gas flow required for a baby with a normal P_{aCO_2} of 5 kPa consuming 50 ml min^{-1} of oxygen if it is intended to avoid a rebreathing index of higher than 1.2.

Fig. 2.34 is a plot of this solution. Compare this with Fig. 2.7 and explain in general terms why T-piece systems (Figs. 2.5(b) and 2.9) generate a smaller rebreathing index than the oxygen tent.

2.2 Explain the meaning of the term High Air Flow with Oxygen Enrichment (HAFOE) as applied to one form of oxygen mask.

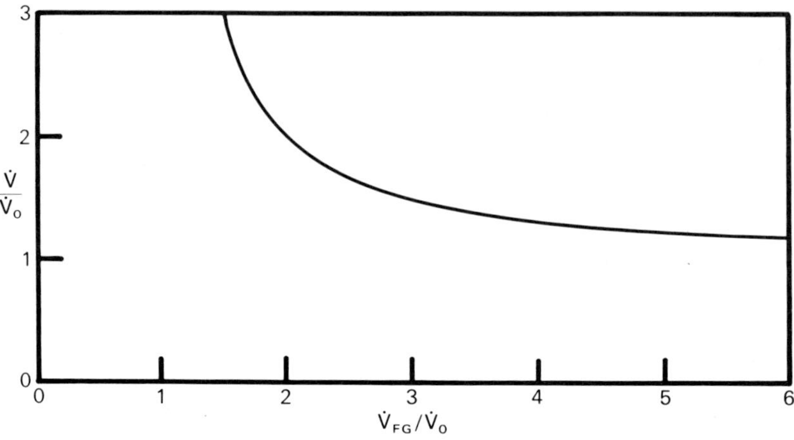

Fig. 2.34

A HAFOE mask is designed in such a way that a variable oxygen concentration is provided by sliding a screen across the air entry region close to where the oxygen jet enters the mixing duct (Fig. 2.35). The area of the oxygen jet is a and the total area of the duct is A. ϕ is the manually variable fraction of the area available to air flow $(A - a)$ which remains not occluded by the screen.

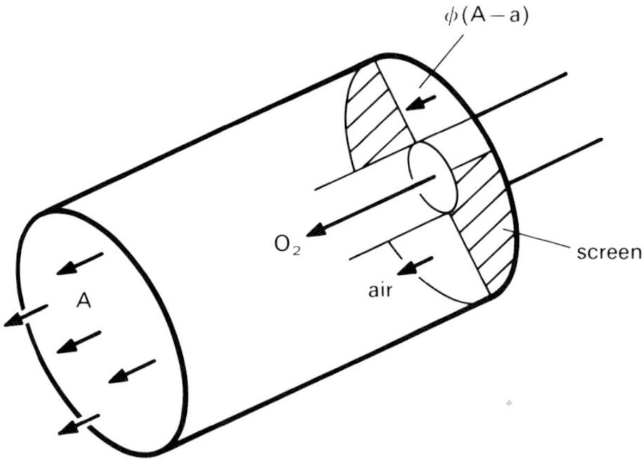

Fig. 2.35

Assuming that the air–oxygen mixture leaves the duct with uniform velocity across the outlet and at atmospheric pressure, show that the inlet velocity of the oxygen u_0 and inlet velocity of the entrained air u_1 are related by the quadratic equation

$$u_1^2 \left\{ \frac{A^2}{2} + (A - a)[\phi^2(A - a) - \phi A] \right\} + u_0 u_1 [2a(A - a)\phi] + u_0^2 a(a - A) = 0.$$

You may assume that the density of air is the same as that of oxygen.

Use this equation to calculate the oxygen fraction of gas delivered to the mask when $a/A = 0.019$ and $\phi = 0.3$.

2.3   A portable anaesthetic apparatus for use in the Antarctic utilizes an oxygen driven air entrainment duct to supply a mixture of oxygen and air to a Magill breathing system (Nunn, J. F. (1961). *British Medical Journal*, **i**, 1139–43). The device incorporates a uniform entrainment duct, of the form depicted in Fig. 2.20(a), driven by an oxygen jet with constant flow of $1\,l\,min^{-1}$. It is designed to produce an air–oxygen mixture containing approximately 30 per cent oxygen when the back pressure on the entrainer is 1 cm H_2O. During an assessment of the entrainer Nunn measured the total flow delivered at eight different back pressures between 0 and 6 cm H_2O (Fig. 2.36, data points).

Show using eqn (2.40), with equal values of density assumed for air and oxygen, that the relationship between the back pressure Δp and the total flow through the device

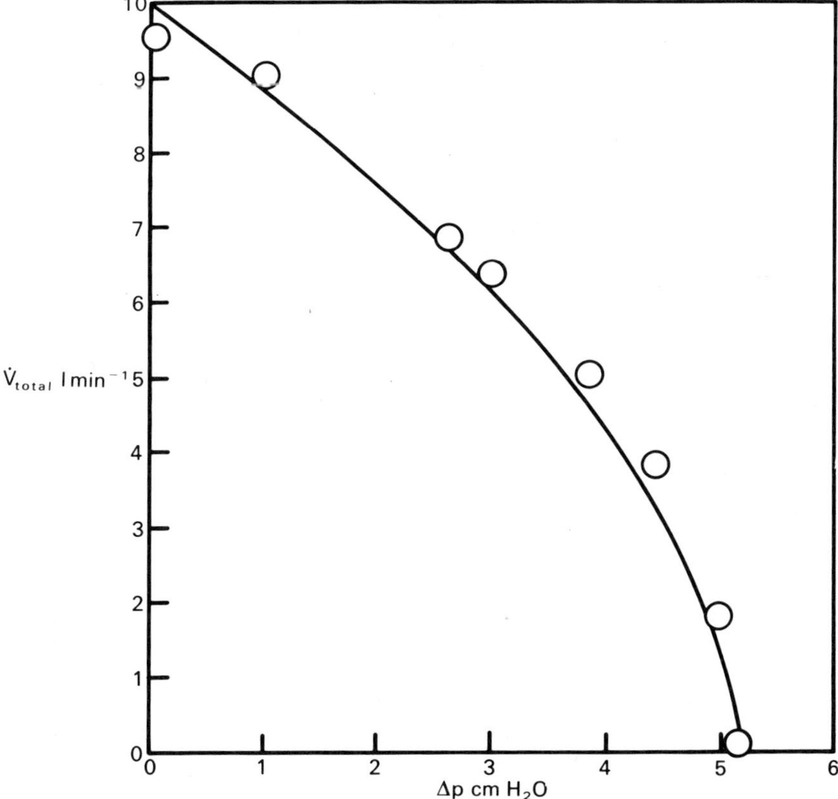

Fig. **2.36.**

V_{total} is expected to be of the form

$$\Delta p = q + r V_{total} + s V_{total}^2,$$

where q, r, and s are constants.

Assuming $\Delta p = 5.2$ cm H_2O when $V_{total} = 0$, and $V_{total} = 10\,l\,min^{-1}$ when $\Delta p = 0$, estimate the area A of the entrainment duct, the jet to duct area ratio a/A, and the values of the constants q, r, and s. Take $\rho = 1.3$ kg m^{-3} throughout. (The solution to this problem is depicted by the continuous line in Fig. 2.36.)

2.4   A patient breathes through a system of the Mapleson C type with a pattern of breathing represented by the equation

$$V = (V_T/2)[1 - \cos(2\pi t/\tau)],$$

where V_T is the tidal volume and τ is the duration of each breath.

Find the theoretical minimum fresh gas flow requirement if the dead space V_D equals 150 ml, $V_T = 500$ ml, and $\tau = 5$ s. What error would be incurred in the calculation if we made the simplification of assuming X′ in Fig. 2.29 to lie exactly at the origin?

Further reading

Ayre, P. (1937). Anaesthesia for intracranial operation. A new technique. *Lancet* **i,** 561–3. (Description of a T-piece).

Bain, J. A. and Spoerel, W. E. (1972). A streamlined anaesthetic system. *Canadian Anaesthetists Society Journal* **19,** 426–35.

Campbell, E. J. M. (1960). A method of controlled oxygen administration which reduces the risk of carbon dioxide retention. *Lancet* **ii,** 12–14.

Dorrington, K. L. and Lehane, J. R. (1987). Minimum fresh gas flow requirements of anaesthetic breathing systems during spontaneous ventilation: a graphical approach. *Anaesthesia* **42,** 732–7.

Eger, E. I. and Ethans, C. T. (1968). The effects of inflow overflow and valve placement on economy of the circle system. *Anesthesiology* **29,** 93–100.

Jackson Rees, G. (1950). Anaesthesia in the newborn. *British Medical Journal* **2,** 1419–22. (Addition of a bag to the system of Ayre.)

Jonsson, L. O. and Zetterström, H. (1987). Influence of the respiratory flow pattern on rebreathing in Mapleson A and D circuits. *Acta Anaesthesiologica Scandinavica* **31,** 174–8.

Lack, J. A. (1976). Theatre pollution control. *Anaesthesia* **31,** 259–62. (Description of the 'Lack' breathing system.)

Mapleson, W. W. (1958). Theoretical considerations of the effects of rebreathing in two semi-closed anaesthetic systems. *British Medical Bulletin* **14,** 64–8.

Scacci, R. (1979). Air entrainment masks: jet mixing is how they work; the Bernoulli and Venturi principles are how they don't. *Respiratory Care* **10,** 928–31.

Waters, R. M. (1926). Advantages and technique of carbon dioxide filtration with inhalation anesthesia. *Anesthesia and Analgesia* **15,** 160–2.

Watt, O. M. (1968). The evolution of the Boyle apparatus 1917–67. *Anaesthesia* **23,** 103–18.

3 Anaesthetic vaporizers

3.1 Introduction

Most surgical operations would be impossible without anaesthesia. Less than 150 years ago, surgeons were largely limited to performing amputations, setting fractures, and repairing superficial wounds. The primary characteristic of a good surgeon was speed: a leg could be amputated in as little as 25 s. No satisfactory way of reducing the agony of the unfortunate patient was available, and surgical treatment of diseases within the abdomen, the chest, or the skull was considered virtually impossible.

The earliest anaesthetics and the agents which form the mainstay of anaesthesia today are all gases or vapours which are administered to a patient by inhalation. Ether was first used for anaesthesia in the 1840s and is still arguably the safest all-purpose anaesthetic. Its use in surgery was first formally demonstrated at the Massachusetts General Hospital on 16 October 1846, when William Morton administered ether during the painless excision of a tumour from the jaw of one Gilbert Abbott.

The inhalational agents which have subsequently been used as anaesthetics form a motley collection of molecules with widely varying properties and chemical structure. Figure 3.1 depicts features of nine prominent anaesthetics, all of which still find some clinical use with the exception of chloroform (the merits of which are regarded now as outweighed by its dangers, despite the enhancement of its popularity by its administration to Queen Victoria in 1853). A measure of potency called the minimal alveolar concentration (MAC) is plotted on the vertical logarithmic scale against a measure on the horizontal logarithmic scale of the relative oil solubility of the agents.

The MAC of an anaesthetic agent is the concentration of the agent required in alveolar gas to eliminate a reflex movement in 50 per cent of subjects when a knife incision is made in the skin. It is expressed here as a partial pressure in a percentage of atmospheric pressure in a wide range from 0.16 per cent for methoxyflurane to approximately 100 per cent for nitrous oxide. Potent anaesthetics have a low MAC and weak anaesthetics have a high MAC. When using the concept of MAC it is important to remember this inverse relation to potency. The oil/gas partition coefficient is a dimensionless ratio of the relative molar concentrations of an agent, with respect to volume, in oil and gas, when the oil and gas are in equilibrium.

The striking inverse relationship seen in Fig. 3.1 between the MAC ($\simeq 1/\text{potency}$) of the inhalational anaesthetics and their relative solubility in oils (and fats) implies that the anaesthetic action of these agents in the fatty

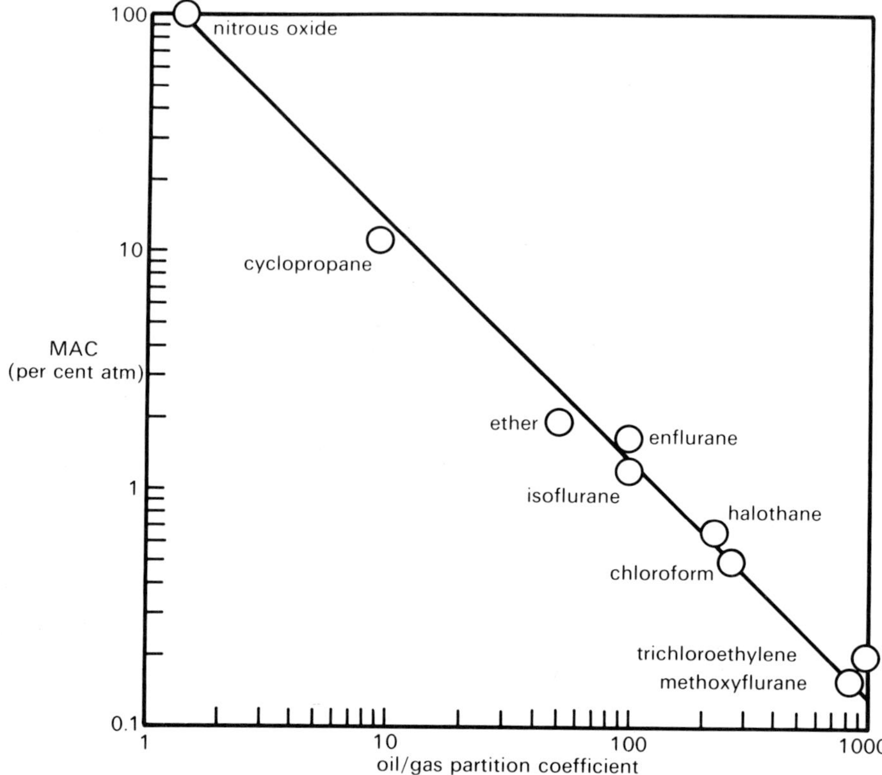

Fig. 3.1. The close relationship between potency and relative solubility in oil for nine prominent inhalational anaesthetics. Minimal alveolar concentration (MAC) is plotted against the oil/gas partition coefficient. Data are from Table 3.1. The solid line has slope −1. Note the wide range over three decades in potency ($\simeq 1/\text{MAC}$) of these agents.

cell membranes of the brain occurs in almost exact proportion to the numbers of molecules dissolved in the brain, regardless of the chemical structure of the agent. This can be seen from the fact that all points joined by a line of gradient −1 in Fig. 3.1 will satisfy the equation

$$\text{MAC} \times \frac{\text{oil molar concentration per ml}}{\text{gas molar concentration per ml}} = \text{const.} \tag{3.1}$$

Since MAC is a gas concentration in percentages of atmospheric pressure, to the extent that Avogadro's law holds it will also be a percentage gas molar concentration. For alveolar gas in equilibrium with the fatty cell membranes of brain, eqn (3.1) therefore yields the result that the brain molar concentration per ml is a constant for all agents lying along the prescribed line. This concept of 'isonarcosis' being equivalent to equal numbers of molecules in the brain (per ml of tissue) was first established as long ago as 1920. It seems therefore that anaesthesia is mediated by a physical rather than chemical action of the agents, but the detailed mechanism of this process remains a mystery.

Two of the anaesthetic agents in Fig. 3.1, nitrous oxide and cyclopropane, exist at ambient temperature and pressure only as gases. Their critical temperatures are respectively 36.5 °C and 125 °C and it is therefore possible for both agents to be stored at room temperature as liquids under pressure. The saturated liquid/vapour pressures at 20 °C of nitrous oxide and cyclopropane are 50.5 bar and 5.6 bar (50 atm and 5.5 atm). The problems of storage and delivery of these anaesthetics are consequently related to the use of high pressure cylinders, reducing valves, and in the case of cyclopropane, avoidance of explosions. We shall not discuss further the supply of high pressure gases; the interested reader is referred to the bibliography at the end of this chapter.

The remaining seven of the anaesthetic agents in Fig. 3.1 exist at ambient temperature and pressure as saturated liquid–vapour mixtures. Since only the vapour component can be safely delivered for inhalation, it has been necessary to devise equipment in which the vapour can be extracted from its mixture with liquid and introduced to carrier gases (always including oxygen) to be delivered to the patient via breathing systems such as those discussed in Chapter 2. Moreover, for all anaesthetic vapours the difference between an adequate concentration for keeping the surgical patient asleep and a dangerous concentration may be small. The amount of vapour delivered must be both known and controllable to a fair degree of accuracy over a wide range of concentrations. The history of inhalational anaesthesia is one of increasing ingenuity in tackling this apparently straightforward, but in practice taxing, engineering problem.

3.2   Saturated vapour pressures of inhalational anaesthetics

The *saturated vapour pressure* of an anaesthetic agent is the pressure at which pure vapour will exist in equilibrium with its liquid in a sealed container. This pressure depends heavily on temperature, and the *critical temperature* is the highest temperature at which such a vapour–liquid mixture can exist. *Boiling* of a liquid occurs in an unsealed container when the pressure of its vapour becomes equal to the ambient atmospheric pressure.

The ease with which an anaesthetic vapour can be 'creamed off' its corresponding liquid is directly proportional to its saturated vapour pressure. Data for our seven examples are plotted in Fig. 3.2. There is a striking temperature-dependence in the vapour pressures and a wide variation in behaviour among the anaesthetics. The more *volatile* agents are those with

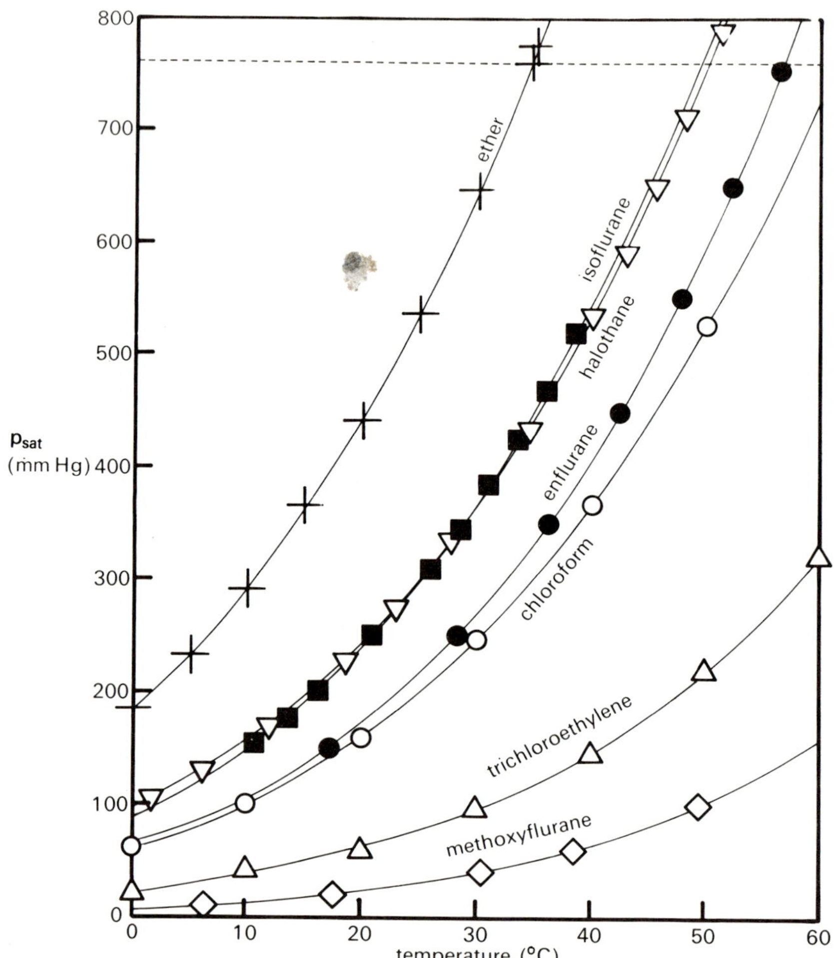

Fig. 3.2. Saturated vapour pressures (mmHg) as a function of temperature (°C) for seven prominent inhalational anaesthetics that exist as a liquid at ambient conditions of temperature and pressure. Sources: ether, chloroform, and trichloroethylene, Jordan, T. E. (1954). *Vapor Pressure of Organic Compounds*, pp. 47, 48, 104. Interscience Publishers; halothane, Bottomley, G. A. and Seiflow, G. J. (1963). *Applied Chemistry* **13**, 339–402; isoflurane, Nahrwold, M. L., Archer, P. G., and Cohen, P. J. (1973). *Anesthesiology* **39**, 444–6; enflurane, Rogers, R. C. and Hill, G. E. (1978). *British Journal of Anaesthesia* **50**, 415–24 (incorrectly labelled 'isoflurane' on p420); methoxyflurane, Nahrwold, M. L., Archer, P., and Cohen, P. J. (1973). *Anesthesia and Analgesia* **52**, 866–7. The horizontal dashed line represents a pressure of 1 atmosphere (760 mmHg, 101.3 kPa). The normal boiling points of the liquids lie at the intercepts on this line.

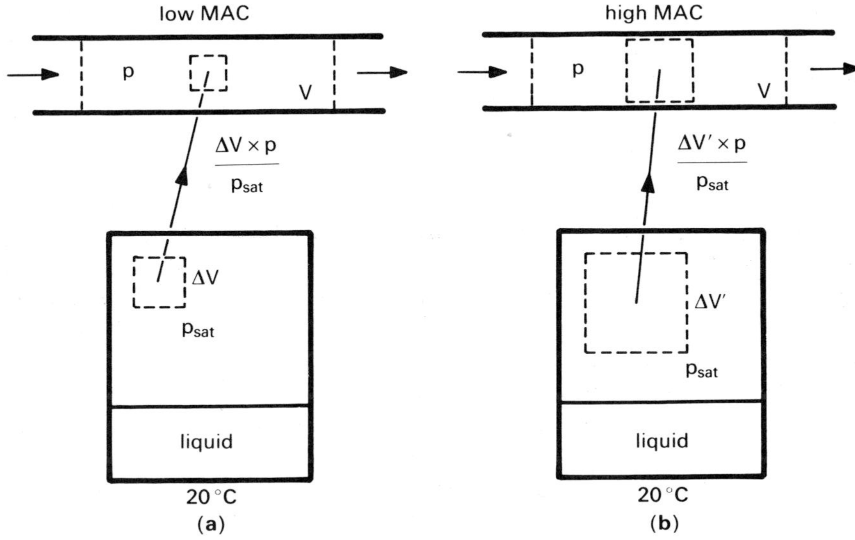

Fig. 3.3. The ease with which an anaesthetic agent may be vaporized and delivered to a carrier gas depends upon the minimal alveolar concentration (MAC) and the saturated vapour pressure (p_{sat}). See text.

higher saturated vapour pressures at any given temperature. The curves for these therefore lie towards the top left hand corner of Fig. 3.2.

In what way then is the ease with which a vapour may be generated related to the saturated vapour pressure of an anaesthetic? Consider a container (Fig. 3.3(a)) holding pure liquid and vapour of an anaesthetic agent at room temperature, say 20 °C. The saturated vapour pressure is p_{sat}. We remove a volume ΔV of vapour under these conditions and introduce it into the main gas flow running to the patient's breathing system. This *carrier gas* would typically consist of a minimum of 30 per cent oxygen in a mixture with nitrous oxide or nitrogen. Pure oxygen is sometimes preferred.

p is the pipeline pressure at which a volume of carrier gas is mixed with the bolus ΔV from the vapour chamber, to form a mixture of total volume V. We can deduce the partial pressure p_{anaes} of the anaesthetic in the final mixture by assuming that the dispersed vapour molecules conform to our kinetic model of gases (eqn (1.4)), and therefore that the vapour satisfies Boyle's law (eqn (1.6)):

$$p_{\text{sat}}\Delta V = p_{\text{anaes}} V. \tag{3.2}$$

The fraction by which the anaesthetic vapour contributes to the total pressure of the mixture is

$$\frac{p_{\text{anaes}}}{p} = \frac{p_{\text{sat}}}{p}\left(\frac{\Delta V}{V}\right). \tag{3.3}$$

If Avogadro's Law is satisfied (see chapter 1), the fraction by numbers of molecules F_{anaes} of the anaesthetic vapour in the final mixture will be equal to the pressure ratio of eqn (3.3):

$$F_{\text{anaes}} = \frac{p_{\text{sat}}}{p}\left(\frac{\Delta V}{V}\right). \tag{3.4}$$

Equation (3.4) is a justification of the earlier claim that the ease with which an anaesthetic vapour can be 'creamed off' its corresponding liquid is directly proportional to p_{sat}. We can see now that this statement must be qualified by saying that we envisage a constant pipeline pressure p and some kind of device which is limited in the ratio of the volume ΔV of saturated vapour it can supply to a given volume V of the mixture generated at the pressure p.

Clearly, anaesthetics with low saturated vapour pressures, such as methoxyflurane and trichloroethylene, are more difficult to vaporize than anaesthetics with high p_{sat}, such as ether, in the sense that a relatively greater volume of vapour ΔV has to be extracted for the less volatile agents to achieve a similar F_{anaes} in the final mixture of volume V. However, the anaesthetic agents are not all required at the same molar fraction F_{anaes} because they vary greatly in their potencies. A glance at the progression from methoxyflurane at the bottom right hand corner of Fig. 3.1 to ether near the centre of the diagram shows some correlation with the line-up of agents in Fig. 3.2, with the saturated vapour pressure curve for methoxyflurane lying bottom right and that for ether lying top left.

It is convenient that the less volatile agents, having a relatively low p_{sat} at any given temperature, also tend to be the more potent agents, having a lower MAC. The correlation is, however, by no means exact. In Fig. 3.4 are plotted the MAC values for our seven agents (Table 3.1) against their saturated vapour pressures at $20\,^{\circ}\text{C}$, a representative ambient temperature (data from Fig. 3.2). These data clearly do not lie on a single straight line.

Figure 3.3(b) depicts the vaporization of an agent having a high MAC in contrast to the one having a low MAC shown in Fig. 3.3(a). According to eqn (3.2), the value of $\Delta V/V$ when an agent is delivered at the Minimum Alveolar Concentration is given by

$$\left(\frac{\Delta V}{V}\right)_{\text{MAC}} = \left(\frac{p_{\text{anaes}}}{p_{\text{sat}}}\right)_{\text{MAC}} = \left(\frac{\text{MAC}}{p_{\text{sat}}}\right)\left(\frac{p_{\text{atm}}}{100}\right), \tag{3.5}$$

where p_{atm} is atmospheric pressure. It follows that the gradient of a line in Fig. 3.4 joining the origin to a data point for an agent gives a measure of $(\Delta V/V)_{\text{MAC}}$, itself an indicator of the difficulty of generating a vapour mixture of a given clinical potency. These lines in Fig. 3.4 fan out from the origin in the shaded region. The most easily vaporized agents are trichloroethylene, chloroform, and halothane, which lie almost exactly on the same line. Ether, isoflurane, and methoxyflurane take intermediate values of respectively in-

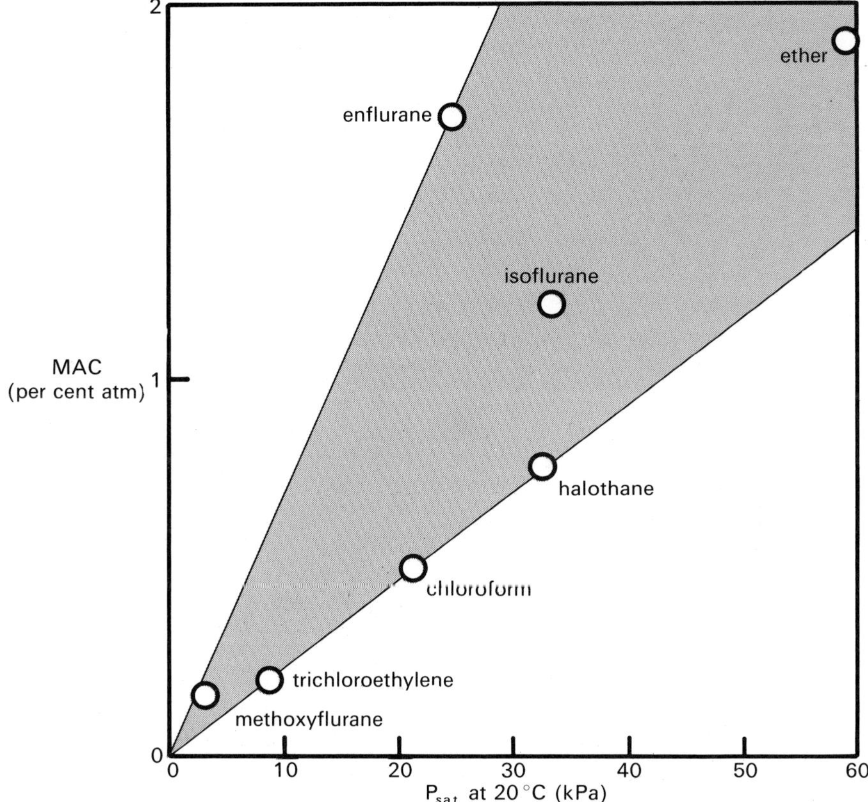

Fig. 3.4. With regard to vapour volume, the difficulty with which anaesthetic agents can be delivered, for maintenance of a common degree of anaesthetic effect, is given by the relative gradients joining the origin to data points on a plot of minimal alveolar concentration (MAC) against saturated vapour pressure (p_{sat}) at ambient temperature (here taken to be 20 °C). We shall see later that in the chapter that thermodynamic considerations change the assessment of difficulty of vaporization.

creasing $(\Delta V/V)_{MAC}$. Enflurane is the extreme case, with a value of $(\Delta V/V)_{MAC}$ almost three times its value for halothane.

We have seen that MAC is a clinically useful measure of the potency of an inhalational anaesthetic agent. We have seen too that the ease with which any given vapour fraction can be generated is proportional to p_{sat}. Since we do not require the same fraction of vapour for all the different agents, the quotient MAC/p_{sat} gives a more informative measure of the difficulty of vaporizing an agent than either of its two components alone. This is not, however, the end of the story.

We shall find that the need to supply heat for the process of vaporization gives rise to a further important difference between anaesthetic agents. The

Table 3.1. *Minimal alveolar concentrations and oil/gas partition coefficients of nine inhalational anaesthetics.*

Agent	MAC (per cent atm)	oil/gas partition
nitrous oxide	101	1.4
cyclopropane	9.2	11
ether	1.9	50
enflurane	1.7	98
isoflurane	1.2	99
halothane	0.77	224
chloroform	0.5	265
trichloroethylene	0.2	960
methoxyflurane	0.16	825

Data from Grant, W. J. (1978). *Medical Gases. Their Properties and Uses.* HM & M Publishers; Hill, D. W. (1980). *Physics Applied to Anaesthesia* (4th edn). Butterworths, London; Atkinson, R. S., Rushman, G. B., and Lee, J. A. (1987). *A Synopsis of Anaesthesia* (10th edn). IOP Publishing Ltd, Bristol. There is considerable variability in the published data for MAC and oil/gas partition coefficients because of differences between subjects and oils studied. The above values should be regarded as typical but not precise. The data are plotted in Fig. 3.1.

ease with which a given volume ΔV of anaesthetic vapour can be generated is not the same for thermodynamic reasons. The way in which this further consideration affects the league table of agents based on ease of vaporization will be discussed later in this chapter.

3.3   The laws of thermodynamics and the Clausius–Clapeyron equation

The dependence of saturated vapour pressure on temperature (Fig. 3.2) is so striking, and of such importance to the design and use of anaesthetic vaporizers, that we devote space to its theoretical description by the Clausius–Clapeyron equation. This equation derives from the first and second laws of thermodynamics, which we here review.

The first law of thermodynamics is a statement about the way in which *heat*, Q, and *work*, W, may be regarded as equivalent. It leads to the concept of *internal energy*, U, an invisible store of energy within a thermodynamic system of which heat and work are the two visible manifestations whereby it may be either replenished or depleted.

The first law states that when any closed* thermodynamic system under-

---

* A closed system is one across the boundary of which no mass can be transferred but heat and work can be transferred.

goes a cyclic process[†], the sum of all increments of heat, dQ, delivered to the system must equal the sum of all increments of work, dW, done by the system:

$$\oint dQ = \oint dW \qquad (3.6)$$

The modified integral sign simply denotes summation for a cyclic process. Equation (3.6) can be written

$$\oint dQ - \oint dW = 0, \qquad (3.7)$$

or

$$\boxed{\oint (dQ - dW) = 0} \quad . \qquad (3.8)$$

It is a general principle that something which always sums to zero round any cyclic path will always sum to the same non-zero total along a non-cyclic path regardless of the path taken between the two fixed endpoints. We denote these two endpoints by 1 and 2, and the non-zero total by $U_2 - U_1$ and write

$$\boxed{\int_1^2 (dQ - dW) = U_2 - U_1} \quad . \qquad (3.9)$$

An analogy of this principle derives from mountain walking. Let dA and dD be the number of metres of ascent or descent respectively mastered during each step taken whilst climbing Snowdon. At the end of the day, on returning to the place of your departure, the sum of $(dA - dD)$ will be zero regardless of the route taken, and whether or not you retraced your exact steps of the ascent during the walk down:

$$\oint (dA - dD) = 0. \qquad (3.10)$$

Considering now just the ascent from the Pen-y-Pass Youth Hostel (356 m), point 1, to the summit (1085 m), point 2, the sum of $(dA - dD)$ between these end points will always be the same, regardless of whether we ascend via Crib-

---

[†] During a process, changes occur in the parameters such as pressure, temperature, and volume, which define the state of a system. If a process is cyclic, these parameters return at the end of the process to the values they had before it started.

goch, the Pig Track, or the Miners' Track:

$$\int_1^2 (\mathrm{d}A - \mathrm{d}D) = 729 \text{ m.} \tag{3.11}$$

Note that this remains true despite the fact that the sums $\int_1^2 \mathrm{d}A$ and $\int_{1^\bullet}^2 \mathrm{d}D$ may differ markedly for the different routes. The up and down clamber over the boulders of Crib-goch will lead to large sums of $\int_1^2 \mathrm{d}A$ and $\int_1^2 \mathrm{d}D$, in contrast to a more continuous gentle ascent of a track which tends towards the extreme case $\int_1^2 \mathrm{d}A = 729$ m, $\int_1^2 \mathrm{d}D = 0$. Thus $\int_1^2 \mathrm{d}A$ and $\int_1^2 \mathrm{d}D$ vary greatly among different routes between points 1 and 2, but their difference is independent of the route taken and we may write

$$\int_1^2 (\mathrm{d}A - \mathrm{d}D) = H_2 - H_1, \tag{3.12}$$

where H_1 and H_2 are the altitudes above sea level of points 1 and 2. H may be regarded as a function of position, not a function of how one gets to the position. In terms of differentials

$$\mathrm{d}A - \mathrm{d}D = \mathrm{d}H. \tag{3.13}$$

The corresponding equation of differentials for the first law of thermodynamics is

$$\mathrm{d}Q - \mathrm{d}W = \mathrm{d}U. \tag{3.14}$$

U is perceived as a function of the state of a thermodynamic system, not a function of how that state was reached. The heat taken up ($\int_1^2 \mathrm{d}Q$) and the work expended ($\int_1^2 \mathrm{d}W$) during a process taking a system from state 1 to state 2 will depend upon the route chosen between these endpoints. Their difference (eqn (3.9)) does not. U is called the *internal energy* of the system.

The second law of thermodynamics is a statement about the way in which heat and work may be regarded as different from each other. It leads to the concept of *entropy*: something which can pass into or out of a thermodynamic system when heat enters or leaves the system, but not when work is done on or by the system.

The second law states that when any closed thermodynamic system undergoes a cyclic process, it is impossible for all the heat delivered to the system to be expended by the system as work. Of the heat delivered to the system during such a process, a fraction must also leave the system. It cannot all, therefore, be 'converted' to work; an outcome which would not in itself violate the first law.

It is a corollary of the second law that heat flow under near-equilibrium conditions may be related to the temperature of the system at the time the heat is being exchanged. If the system undergoes a cyclic process and exchanges heat with reservoirs at only two temperatures, some heat, $\mathrm{d}Q_1$, whilst it is at temperature 1, and some time later some heat, dQ_2, whilst at temperature 2, then it can be demonstrated from simple principles that

$$\frac{dQ_2}{dQ_1} = f(\text{temperature 1, temperature 2}), \tag{3.15}$$

where the right hand side of eqn (3.15) denotes 'some function of temperature 1 and temperature 2'. This relationship enables us to define absolutely some scale of temperature, and the simplest and most widely used is the Kelvin temperature scale in which temperature is denoted by T and the function of eqn (3.15) chosen to be*

$$\frac{dQ_2}{dQ_1} = -\frac{T_2}{T_1}, \tag{3.16}$$

or

$$\frac{dQ_1}{T_1} + \frac{dQ_2}{T_2} = 0. \tag{3.17}$$

For a thermodynamic system undergoing a cyclic process in which it exchanges increments of heat dQ over a whole range of temperatures T, the extension of eqn (3.17) can be shown to be

$$\boxed{\oint \frac{dQ_{eq}}{T} = 0} \,, \tag{3.18}$$

where the subscript 'eq' has been appended to remind us that the equation is valid only for processes in which the system is in near equilibrium conditions throughout.[†]

Equation (3.18) summarizes the second law. It has the same structure as eqn (3.8) which summarized the first law. Consequently the deductions which led us to the concept of internal energy (eqn (3.9)) lead identically to the concept of entropy:

$$\boxed{\int_1^2 \frac{dQ_{eq}}{T} = S_2 - S_1} \,. \tag{3.19}$$

---

* the definition is complete only if we include the internationally agreed definition that $T = 273.16$ K at the triple point of water.
† A system which is always very nearly in *equilibrium* is one without large differences within it of temperature, pressure, and so on between one part of the system and another.

The corresponding equation of differentials for the second law of thermo-dynamics is

$$dQ_{eq} = T dS. \tag{3.20}$$

Equation (3.20) confirms our earlier claim that entropy may be regarded as something which can pass into or out of a thermodynamic system (changing its entropy by dS) when heat enters or leaves the system (dQ_{eq}) but not when work is done on or by the system.

The first and second laws can be combined in differential form by substituting eqn (3.20) into eqn (3.14), remembering to specify for the latter that a near-equilibrium process is envisaged

$$T dS - dW_{eq} = dU. \tag{3.21}$$

For the systems of liquids and vapours we are examining, work is only performed by a closed system by the movement of the system boundary against some pressure p through incremental volume changes dV:

$$dW_{eq} = p dV. \tag{3.22}$$

Substituting from eqn (3.22) into (3.21) we generate the result

$$\boxed{T dS - p dV = dU} \quad , \tag{3.23}$$

which is the root equation of classical thermodynamics.

Our aim in this section is to make use of the first and second laws of thermodynamics to derive a relationship for anaesthetic agents between their saturated vapour pressure p_{sat} and temperature T so that the performance of anaesthetic vaporizers at different temperatures can be both understood and predicted.

The distinctive feature of a phase transition, such as that from liquid to vapour, is that it may occur at constant pressure and temperature. A kilogram of liquid with a volume v_f may be expanded to a kilogram of vapour with a volume v_g^* by the addition of heat, whilst p and T remain constant. During such a process dp and dT are both zero. It follows that, if we could find a relationship like that expressed in eqn (3.23) but with dp and dT appearing on the left-hand side instead of dS and dV, then the resulting differential on the right-hand side of such an equation would be zero. We should then have discovered a third function of the state of a system (in addition to p and T) which remains constant during the change from liquid to vapour.

---

* It has become a convention to denote liquid and vapour by subscripts f and g respectively.

This function can easily be confirmed to be given by

$$U + pV - TS \equiv G \qquad (3.24)$$

because

$$dU + pdV + Vdp - TdS - SdT = dG, \qquad (3.25)$$

and substitution for dU from eqn (3.23) in eqn (3.25) yields a relationship of the kind we require:

$$(TdS - pdV) + pdV + Vdp - TdS - SdT = dG, \qquad (3.26)$$

or

$$VdP - SdT = dG. \qquad (3.27)$$

Equation (3.27) tells us that during the conversion of an anaesthetic liquid to its vapour at constant pressure and temperature there will be no change in the property of state G. G is known as the Gibbs function.*

Consider now a single kilogram of saturated liquid (volume v_f, entropy s_f and Gibbs function g_f) experiencing changes dp and dT. The corresponding change in Gibbs function will be

$$v_f dp - s_f dT = dg_f \qquad (3.28)$$

Consider also a kilogram of saturated vapour experiencing the same changes in pressure and temperature:

$$v_g dp - s_g dT = dg_g. \qquad (3.29)$$

We have already concluded that the Gibbs function for a given mass of liquid and vapour at fixed p and T is identical and consequently the changes dg_f and dg_g must be the same for similar changes dp and dT in both liquid and vapour:

$$dg_f = dg_g. \qquad (3.30)$$

Substitution from eqns (3.28) and (3.29) into (3.30) therefore generates the result we have been aiming for:

$$v_f dp - s_f dT = v_g dp - s_g dT \qquad (3.31)$$

or

$$\frac{dp_{sat}}{dT} = \frac{(s_g - s_f)}{(v_g - v_f)}, \qquad (3.32)$$

which is known as the Clapeyron[†] equation.

The numerator on the right-hand side of eqn (3.32) equals the change in entropy occurring when a kilogram of liquid becomes a kilogram of vapour

---

* Josiah Willard Gibbs (1839–1903), American physicist.
† Benoit Pierre Emile Clapeyron (1799–1864), French civil engineer.

at constant temperature and pressure. For a near-equilibrium (reversible) process of this kind eqn (3.20) tells us that this numerator must be given by

$$s_g - s_f = \frac{q_{eq}}{T} ,$$
(3.33)

where q_{eq} is the heat needed to generate the change of phase, and is known variously as the *latent heat of vaporization* or the *enthalpy of vaporization*, h_{fg}.

$$s_g - s_f = \frac{h_{fg}}{T} .$$
(3.34)

Substituting from eqn (3.34) into eqn (3.32) we obtain an alternative form of the Clapeyron equation

$$\boxed{\frac{\mathrm{d}p_{sat}}{\mathrm{d}T} = \frac{h_{fg}}{T(v_g - v_f)}} .$$
(3.35)

Equation (3.35) is exact but of limited practical value as it stands because it retains three variables v_g, v_f and h_{fg} which are in general unknown. Useful approximate forms of eqn (3.35) can be derived on the basis of assumptions about these variables. Firstly, the vapour specific* volume v_g is usually very much greater than the liquid specific volume v_f by several orders of magnitude. This being the case we may set $(v_g - v_f) \simeq v_g$. Secondly, we may assume that the vapour conforms to our kinetic model of a gas (chapter 1) and consequently obeys Boyle's law

$$pV = \text{constant} \Big|_{\text{temp. const.}}$$
(1.6)

which applied here yields

$$pv_g = \text{constant} \Big|_{\text{temp. const.}}$$
(3.36)

To extend the theory set out in chapter 1 we now associate the specific internal energy u of our model gas with the sum of all the mean kinetic energies $\overline{mc^2}/2$ of the molecules contained within one kilogram of the gas, plus any energy associated with spinning motion of molecules made up of more than one atom bound together. According to the Principle of Equipartion of Energy[†], the energy associated with rotation of molecules equals an

---

* the term 'specific' refers to a single kilogram.
† The justification of this principle lies within the realms of statistical thermodynamics rather than classical mechanics. The reader will find a discussion of the subject in Atkins, P. W. (1986). *Physical Chemistry* (3rd edn) Chapter 22 Oxford University Press.

exact multiple of the kinetic energy associated with translational motion in a single direction. Since the translational motion in three directions has a mean kinetic energy $m\overline{c^2}/2$, this 'unit' of molecular energy is $m\overline{c^2}/6$ and most molecules at body temperature are found to have total energies given by $v(m\overline{c^2}/6)$ where v is an integer. v tends to equal 3 for monatomic gases like argon, to equal 5 for diatomic gases like oxygen (with spin about 2 axes) and to equal 6 for gases made up of more than two atoms (with rotation about 3 axes). These include CO_2 and all the anaesthetic agents of Fig. 3.1. We previously defined n to be the number of molecules per cubic metre of gas, and since v is the volume occupied by 1 kg, it follows that nv equals the number of molecules in 1 kg. We therefore write

$$u = (nv)v\tfrac{1}{6}\,m\overline{c2}. \tag{3.37}$$

Recalling from eqn (1.4) that $p = nm\overline{c^2}/3$, eqn (3.37) yields the result

$$u = (v/2)(pv). \tag{3.38}$$

Equation (3.38) tells us that u, like pv (eqn (3.36)) is constant when temperature is constant and is thus a function only of temperature. This observation can be combined with eqn (3.23) to show* that u (and hence pv) for our model gas is proportional to Kelvin temperature T,

$$u = (v/2)(R_{kg}T), \tag{3.39}$$

$$pv = R_{kg}T, \tag{3.40}$$

where R_{kg} is the constant of proportionality between pv and T, and is called the *gas constant per kilogram*. Equation (3.40) will be recognized as the equation of an *ideal gas*. Substituting $v_g = R_{kg}T/p_{sat}$ from eqn (3.40) as applied to a vapour, into eqn (3.35), we get

$$\frac{\mathrm{d}p_{sat}}{\mathrm{d}T} = \frac{h_{fg}p_{sat}}{R_{kg}T^2}, \tag{3.41}$$

which is known as the Clausius–Clapeyron[†] equation.

Our third unknown variable in the Clapeyron eqn (3.35), the enthalpy of vaporization, still remains in eqn (3.41). As a first approximation we may assume h_{fg} to be a constant and integrate:

$$\int \frac{\mathrm{d}p_{sat}}{p_{sat}} = \frac{h_{fg}}{R_{kg}} \int \frac{\mathrm{d}T}{T^2}, \tag{3.42}$$

---

* Since u is a function only of temperature $(\partial u/\partial v)_T = 0$. From eqn (3.23) we may deduce $(\partial u/\partial v)_T = T(\partial s/\partial v)_T - p = T(\partial p/\partial T)_v - p$. Hence, $(\partial p/\partial T)_v = p/T$ and so $pv \propto T$, or $pv = R_{kg}T$.
[†] Rudolf Clausius (1822–1888), German physicist.

or

$$p_{\text{sat}} = p_0 \exp\left(-\frac{h_{\text{fg}}}{R_{\text{kg}}T}\right). \tag{3.43}$$

Figure 3.5 assesses the validity of the last two assumptions we have made in deriving eqn (3.43) for the case of ether. Measured values of v_{g} and h_{fg} are

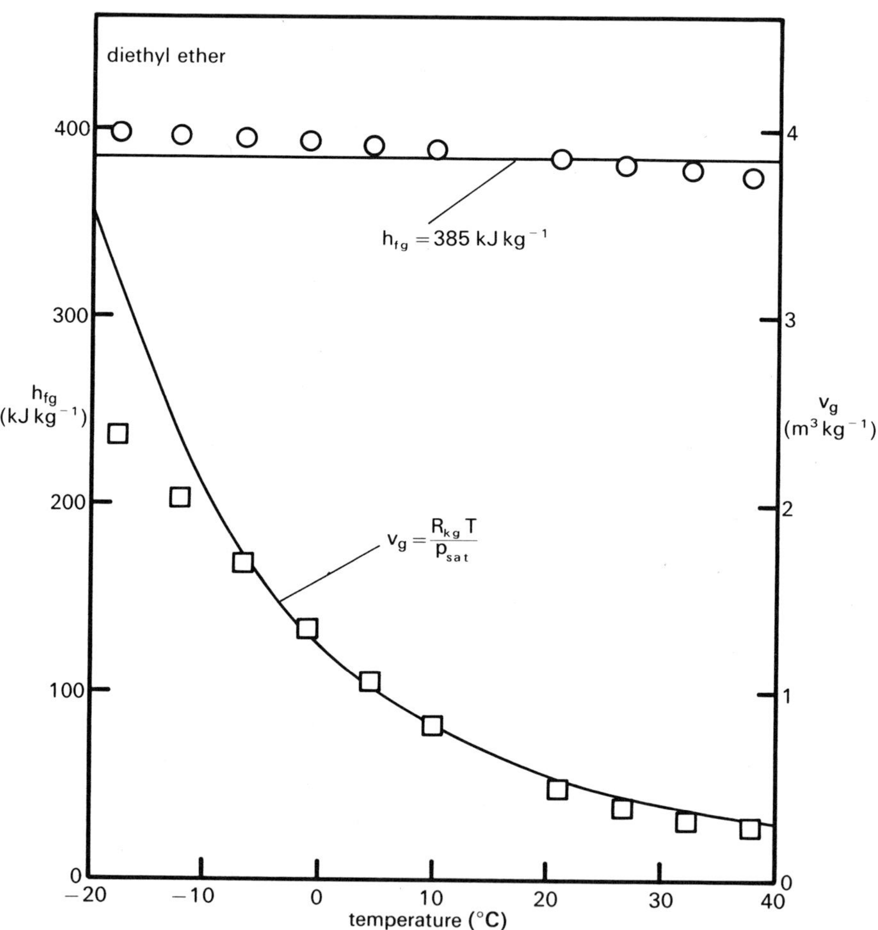

Fig. 3.5. Graphical assessment of two theoretical assumptions made in the derivation of eqn (3.43) for the case of ether. The enthalpy of vaporization h_{fg} ($\bigcirc$) and the vapour specific volume v_{g} ($\square$) are plotted against temperature (Weast, R. C. (ed.) (1975). *Handbook of Chemistry and Physics* (56th edn). CRC Press, Ohio). The theoretical lines plotted are as follows: $h_{\text{fg}} = 385\ \text{kJ kg}^{-1}$ (constant), the measured value at 20 °C; $v_{\text{g}} = R_{\text{kg}}T/p_{\text{sat}}$ (the ideal gas equation), taking measured values for p_{sat} from the same source (see Fig. 3.6). R_{kg} for ether is $0.1121\ \text{kJ kg}^{-1}\,\text{K}^{-1}$.

plotted against temperature in the range of clinical interest. The data for v_g agree well with the ideal gas equation except for temperatures below $-10\,^\circ\mathrm{C}$; h_{fg} is approximately constant.

Equation (3.43) is plotted in Fig. 3.6 for comparison with measurements of p_{sat} for ether at different temperatures. h_{fg} is chosen to be equal to the

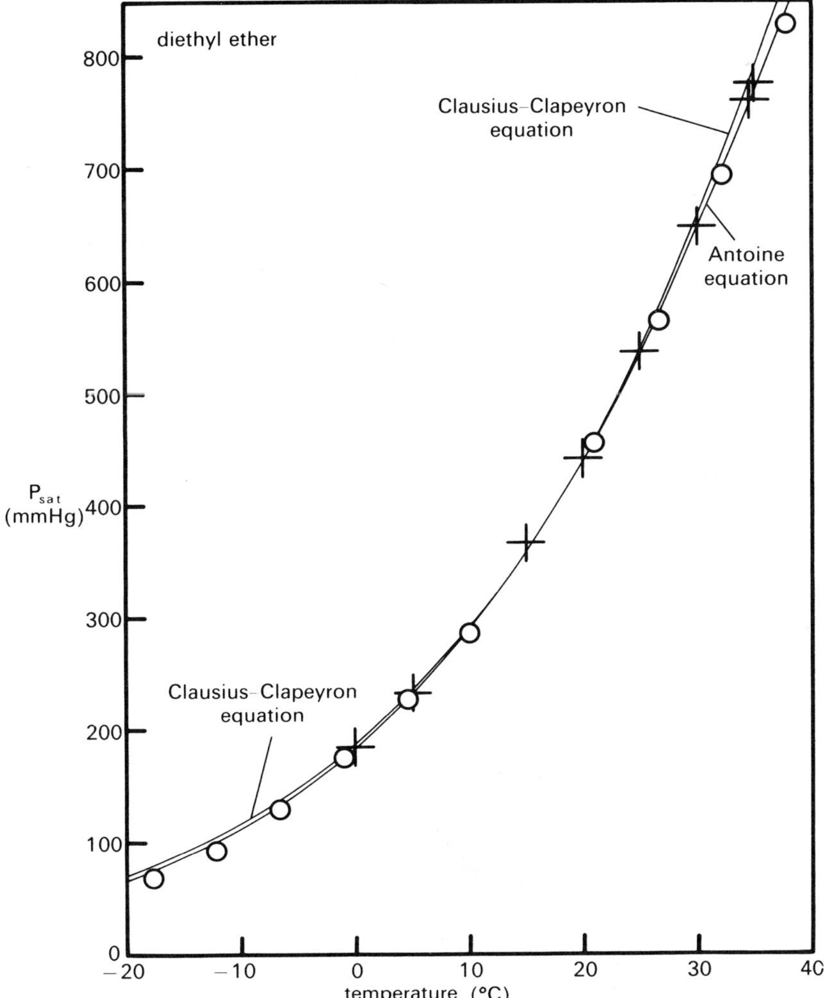

Fig. 3.6. Saturated vapour pressure as a function of temperature for ether: comparison of experimental data with theory. $+$ as Fig. 3.2; $\bigcirc$ Weast, R. C. (ed.) (1975). *Handbook of Chemistry and Physics*, (56th edn). CRC Press, Ohio (converted from $\mathrm{lb\,in}^{-2}$). The Clausius–Clapeyron eqn (3.43) is plotted taking $h_{fg} = 385\ \mathrm{kJ\,kg}^{-1}$ (the measured value at $20\,^\circ\mathrm{C}$, see Fig. 3.5). $R_{kg} = 0.1121$ $\mathrm{kJ\,kg}^{-1}\,\mathrm{K}^{-1}$. In p_0 (17.8059) is chosen to give coincidence of data and theory at $20\,^\circ\mathrm{C}$. The Antoine equation (eqn 3.46) is plotted using the empirical constants given in Table 3.2.

measured value at 20 °C (385 kJ kg^{-1}) and p_0 chosen to give coincidence of theory and data similarly at 20 °C. Equation (3.43) clearly describes the data to a fair degree of accuracy in addition to having a credible theoretical foundation. There has, however, been a vogue amongst anaesthetists for making use of an even more precise but empirical equation for the description of p_{sat}. We turn to this in the next section.

3.4   The Antoine equation

The Clausius–Clapeyron eqn (3.43) can be written in the form

$$\ln p_{sat} = \ln p_0 - \frac{h_{fg}}{R_{kg}T},\tag{3.44}$$

or

$$\log_{10} p_{sat} = A - \frac{B}{T},\tag{3.45}$$

where A and B are constants which take different values for the different anaesthetic agents. When fitting eqn (3.45) empirically to experimental data there are only two constants A and B with which a good fit can be obtained. A useful modification to eqn (3.45) is a relation first published by Antoine in 1888, incorporating three constants:

$$\log_{10} p_{sat} = A - \frac{B}{(T+C)}.\tag{3.46}$$

Using a method of least squares, Rogers and Hill (Rogers, R. C. and Hill, G. E. (1978). *British Journal of Anaesthesia* **50**, 415–24.) have calculated A, B, and C for most anaesthetic agents, and were able to limit deviations of the theoretical expressions from the measured values of p_{sat} they consulted to

Table 3.2. *Constants computed for the Antoine equation by least squares regression by Rogers and Hill (see text).*

Agent	A (log$_{10}$mmHg)	A (log$_{10}$kPa)	B	C (K)	C (°C)
ether	7.02683	6.15068	1109.577	−39.995	233.155
enflurane	6.98840	6.11225	1107.839	−60.087	213.063
isoflurane	5.69778	4.82163	536.4589	−132.159	140.991
halothane	6.76799	5.89184	1043.697	−54.888	218.262
chloroform	6.85426	5.97811	1125.046	−51.136	222.014
trichloroethylene	6.83695	5.96080	1198.477	−56.714	216.436
methoxyflurane	7.08219	6.20604	1336.580	−59.670	213.480

only about 1 per cent. Their results are presented in Table 3.2 for the seven agents we have already considered.

The resulting Antoine equation for ether is plotted in Fig. 3.6 for comparison with the Clausius–Clapeyron eqn (3.43). The Antoine relation clearly represents an improvement in fitting the data, giving a curve which is less concave to the vertical axis. (There is deviation of considerably more than 1 per cent at low temperatures from the data of Weast, but this data was not used by Rogers and Hill for their regression analysis on ether.) The Antoine equation, loaded with the empirical constants determined from fitting data, is a useful empirical reference for the saturated vapour pressures encountered in the design of anaesthetic vaporizers.

3.5 The plenum vaporizer

The earliest method of delivering anaesthetic vapours was to pour the liquid drop by drop on to a napkin held over the patient's face. This technique is still used in some remote hospitals in the third world. A development of this method involved the use of a wire frame, known as the Schimmelbusch mask, to support a variable number of layers of gauze around the nose and mouth, according to which agent was in use. Most modern devices for delivering anaesthetic vapours take the form of the *plenum* vaporizer (Fig. 3.7(a)) in

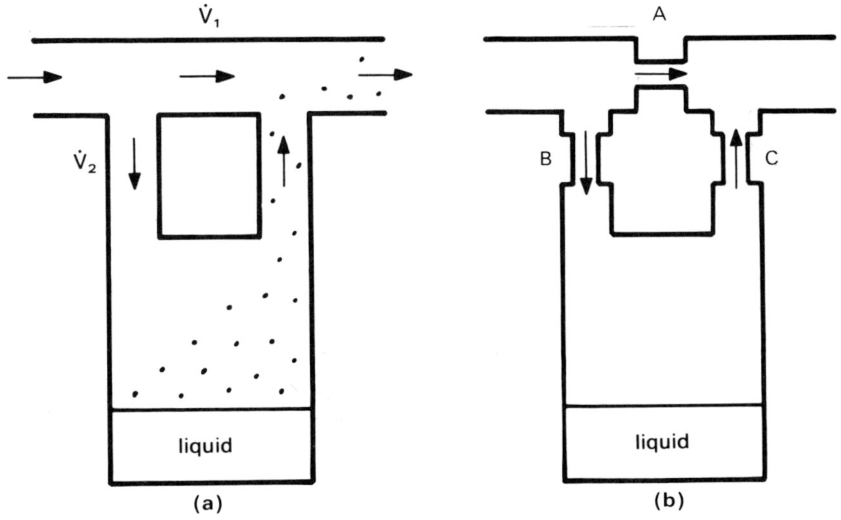

Fig. 3.7. The plenum vaporizer contains anaesthetic liquid in a closed chamber. (a) The ratio of bypass flow $\dot{V}_1$ to chamber flow $\dot{V}_2$ is known as the splitting ratio, (b) control of the splitting ratio is achieved by varying flow resistances at one or more of the sites A, B and C.

Table 3.3. *Control of splitting ratio in different designs of anaesthetic vaporizer (see Fig. 3.7).*

Model	Site of manual flow control	Site of flow control of temperature compensator
Halothane 4	A	B
Tec Mark 2	A	C
Boyle's Bottle	A and B	none
Copper Kettle	A and B	none
Ohio calibrated	A and B	A
Tec Mark 4	A and B	A
Goldman	A, B and C	none
Oxford Miniature	A, B and C	none
Abingdon	A and C	B
E.M.O.	A and C	C
Blease Universal	B and C	C
Penlon Plenum	C	A
Vapor 19.n	C	A
Tec Mark 3	C	A
Fluomatic	C	C

which the liquid is held in a closed chamber to which all or part of a flow of carrier gas is given access via inlet and outlet connections*.

Plenum vaporizers are usually designed to ensure that all gas which passes through the vaporization chamber becomes highly saturated with anaesthetic vapour. Consequently the final concentration of anaesthetic in the gas leaving the vaporizer depends upon the relative magnitudes of the volume flow $\dot{V}_2$ through the vaporization chamber and the bypass volume flow $\dot{V}_1$ (Fig. 3.7(a)). The ratio $\dot{V}_1/\dot{V}_2$ is known as the *splitting ratio*.

Control of the vaporizer output depends upon control of the splitting ratio. The splitting ratio may be varied by changing the relative resistances of the alternative gas paths through the device, which in turn can be achieved by changing the relative resistances of the bypass, chamber inlet, and chamber outlet, respectively labelled A, B, and C in Fig. 3.7(b). To illustrate the variety of control modes selected by the various manufacturers of vaporizers we have listed in Table 3.3 which one, or more, of the sites A, B and C have been used for manual adjustment of the splitting ratio. In fact six out of the seven possible combinations of the three sites can be found in the table: A, C, A and B, B and C, A and C, and A with B and C. Site B alone has not been used.

* the word 'plenum' is derived from the Latin *plenus*, meaning 'full'. It tends, however, to be used to describe containers holding variable amounts of matter, usually in a fluid form.

We calculate the vaporizer output, expressing a volume fraction of anaesthetic vapour as a function of the splitting ratio. Whatever value is taken by the total pressure p_c in the vaporizing chamber, the partial pressure of the anaesthetic vapour in the chamber cannot exceed the saturation vapour pressure p_{sat}. In terms of the kinetic theory outlined in chapter 1, this is because the vapour molecules are indifferent to the carrier gas molecules in the chamber with which they rarely collide. The density of the vapour molecules and their contribution to the pressure of their container are thus independent of the densities and partial pressures of other gases in the chamber.

If full saturation with anaesthetic vapour occurs of the gas in the chamber, the volume fraction of anaesthetic in the chamber will be given by

$$F_{c,\,max} = \frac{p_{sat}}{p_c}.\tag{3.47}$$

The extent to which full saturation is achieved is likely, however, to fall short of the ideal. We define an efficiency of vaporization η_{vap} such that the actual anaesthetic volume fraction of gas leaving the chamber is given by

$$F_c = \frac{\eta_{vap} p_{sat}}{p_c}.\tag{3.48}$$

Engineering techniques for maximizing η_{vap} involve the use of large surface areas of anaesthetic liquid, in part generated by wicks, and the design of chambers in which the carrier gas is directed towards the liquid surface. In a few vaporizers the carrier gases are actually bubbled through the liquid.

If a flow $\dot{V}_2$ enters the chamber, then the flow leaving will equal $\dot{V}_2/(1-F_c)$ and upon mixing with the bypass flow $\dot{V}_1$ a total flow will be generated of $\dot{V}_1 + \dot{V}_2/(1-F_c)$. The final volume fraction of anaesthetic vapour is thus

$$F_{anaes} = \frac{F_c \dot{V}_2/(1-F_c)}{\dot{V}_1 + \dot{V}_2/(1-F_c)}$$

$$= \frac{\eta_{vap}(p_{sat}/p_c)}{[1 - \eta_{vap}(p_{sat}/p_c)]\,\dot{V}_1/\dot{V}_2 + 1}.\tag{3.49}$$

It is important to be clear about the exact meaning of $\dot{V}$ in these equations. We defined $\dot{V}_1$ and $\dot{V}_2$ earlier to be volume flows of gas, but now add the qualification that they are volume flows referred to the same standard temperature and pressure (STP). The need to add this qualification arises because the volume flow corresponding to a fixed mass flow of a gas will vary from one part of a pipe to another if the temperature and pressure change between those sites. Thus, for example, the mass flow of gas at entry to the pipe constriction at A in Fig. 3.7(b) is identical to the mass flow at exit from the constriction. However, the true volume flows of gas at entry to and exit from the constriction will not be exactly identical because of changes in pressure, and possibly temperature, across the constriction. It is only when the gas volumes are referred to identical temperatures and pressures that the volume flow will remain a constant like the mass flow. The splitting ratio $\dot{V}_1/\dot{V}_2$ of volume flows defined in this way is then identical to the ratio $\dot{m}_1/\dot{m}_2$ of mass flows in the alternative paths through the vaporizer.

Equation (3.49) shows how the fractional concentration of an anaesthetic vapour is related to the size of the splitting ratio $\dot{V}_1/\dot{V}_2$. It also shows that this F_{anaes} is a function of the ratio p_{sat}/p_c. Equation (3.49) is plotted in Fig. 3.8, with F_{anaes} shown as a function of p_{sat}/p_c for different values of splitting ratio in the range of clinical interest. η_{vap} is taken to be 1. Clearly

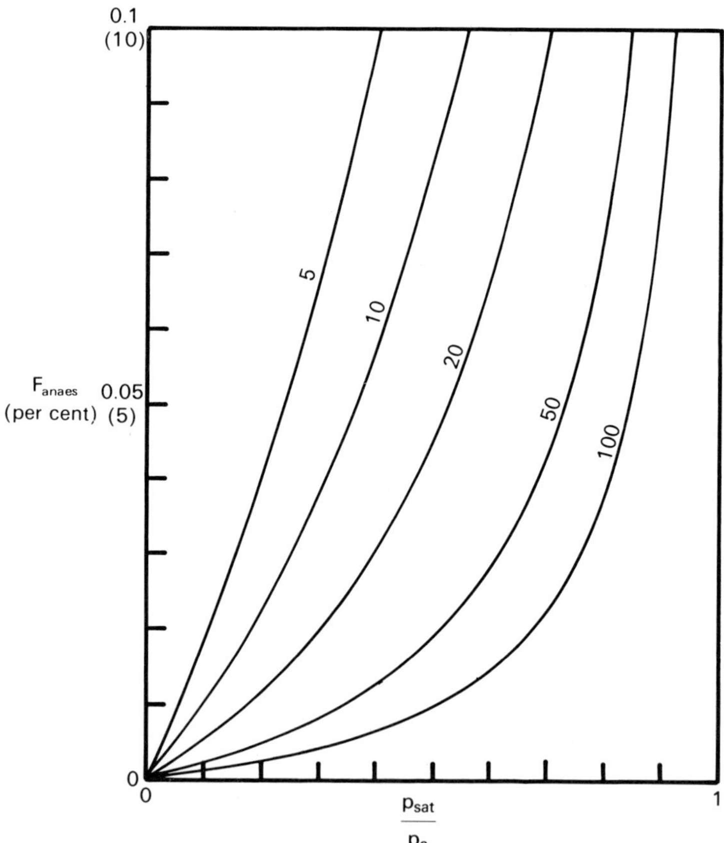

Fig. 3.8. Fractional concentration F_{anaes} of anaesthetic vapour delivered by a plenum vaporizer, plotted according to eqn (3.49). p_{sat}/p_c is the ratio of saturated vapour pressure to chamber pressure. Five values of splitting ratio between 5 and 100 are represented. In parentheses are percentages of anaesthetic vapour. $\eta_{\text{vap}} = 1$.

changes in p_{sat}/p_c may have profound effects on the output of a vaporizer in addition to the effects of changes in the splitting ratio. In the following sections we consider the practical importance of the relationship depicted in Fig. 3.8.

3.6   The effect of temperature on the output from plenum vaporizers

It was shown in Fig. 3.2 that p_{sat} is highly temperature-dependent for all anaesthetic agents. It follows that the output of a plenum vaporizer should be expected also to be highly dependent on the ambient temperature. The behaviour with regard to temperature is further complicated by the marked cooling which can occur of the anaesthetic liquid as evaporation takes place, which reduces the internal energy of the liquid available to provide the enthalpy (latent heat) for evaporation.

The relationship between F_{anaes} and p_{sat} can be predicted by combining eqn (3.43) and (3.49):

$$F_{anaes} = \frac{\eta_{vap}(p_0/p_c)\exp[-h_{fg}/(R_{kg}T)]}{\{1-\eta_{vap}(p_0/p_c)\exp[-h_{fg}/(R_{kg}T)]\}\,\dot{V}_1/\dot{V}_2+1} \qquad (3.50)$$

An alternative, slightly more accurate expression can similarly be derived by combining the empirical Antoine eqn (3.46) with eqn (3.49):

$$F_{anaes} = \frac{(\eta_{vap}/p_c)\,10^{(A-B/(T+C))}}{(1-(\eta_{vap}/p_c)\,10^{(A-B/(T+C))})\,\dot{V}_1/\dot{V}_2+1}. \qquad (3.51)$$

Figure. 3.9 is a plot of eqn (3.51) for halothane over the range in temperature 0–40 °C. The MAC of halothane being 0.77, anaesthetists usually deliver halothane at a percentage concentration in the range 0.5–4.0, which at 20 °C is shown by the figure to correspond with splitting ratios in the range 10–100. The variability of output with changes in temperature at a set splitting ratio is clearly large. Whilst delivering approximately 1 per cent halothane at 20 °C ($\dot{V}_1/\dot{V}_2=50$), for example, a fall in temperature of 5 °C reduces the output concentration by 26 per cent, and a rise in temperature of 5 °C increases the concentration by 37 per cent.

Ambient temperatures in modern operating theatres rarely extend over a range of more than 10 °C. However, even in surroundings held at a constant temperature, the liquid anaesthetic in a plenum vaporizer may cool to a low temperature because of the process of evaporation. A particularly striking example of this was offered by Macintosh, Mushin and Epstein for the case of a Boyle's bottle in which the whole of a carrier gas flow of oxygen equal to 8 l min^{-1} was bubbled through liquid ether to observe the effects on vaporizer temperature and output of the evaporative cooling. The result is shown in Fig. 3.10.

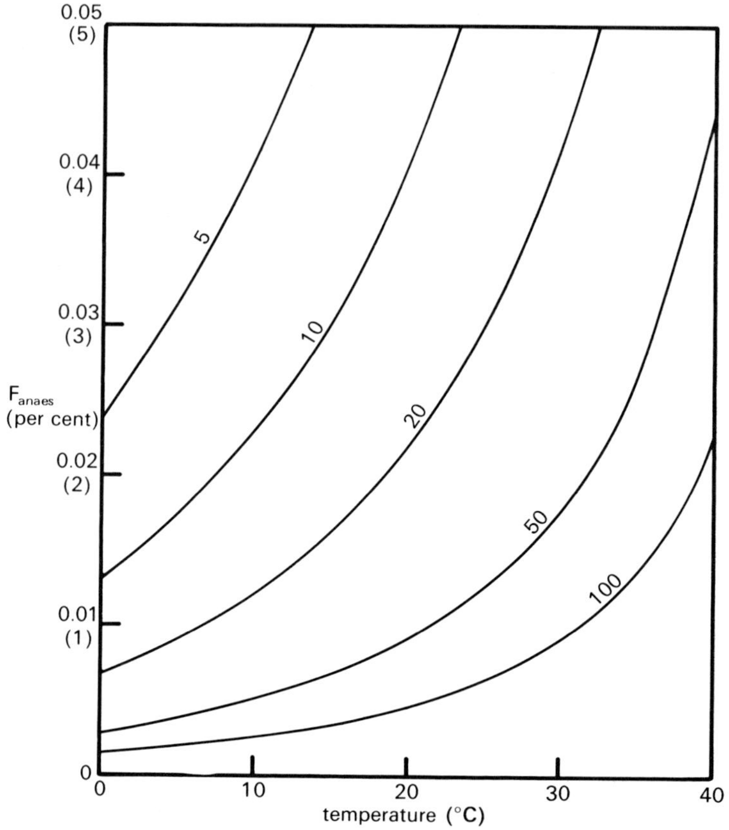

Fig. 3.9. Fractional concentration F_{anaes} of halothane delivered by a plenum vaporizer, plotted as a function of temperature for five values of the splitting ratio $\dot{V}_1/\dot{V}_2$. This theoretical estimation is from eqn (3.51) with $\eta_{vap} = 1$ and $p_c = 101.3\ \text{kPa}$. In parentheses are percentages of halothane.

We now examine the thermodynamics of this evaporative cooling. To apply the first law of thermodynamics to estimate the cooling of liquid anaesthetic in the plenum chamber, we define a closed system (Fig. 3.11) undergoing a non-steady flow process lasting unit time (for example 1 second) in which a mass of carrier gas m_1 enters the chamber, which initially contains a mass m of anaesthetic liquid at temperature T. By the end of the process a total mass m_2 of gas and anaesthetic vapour has left the chamber, which finally contains a mass $m - \Delta m$ of liquid at temperature $T - \Delta T$. Let p_1 be the pressure of the carrier gas upstream of the plenum chamber. Let p_2 be the pressure of the gas–vapour mixture downstream of the chamber. Let v_1, u_1, v_2 and u_2 be respectively the specific volumes and internal energies in these

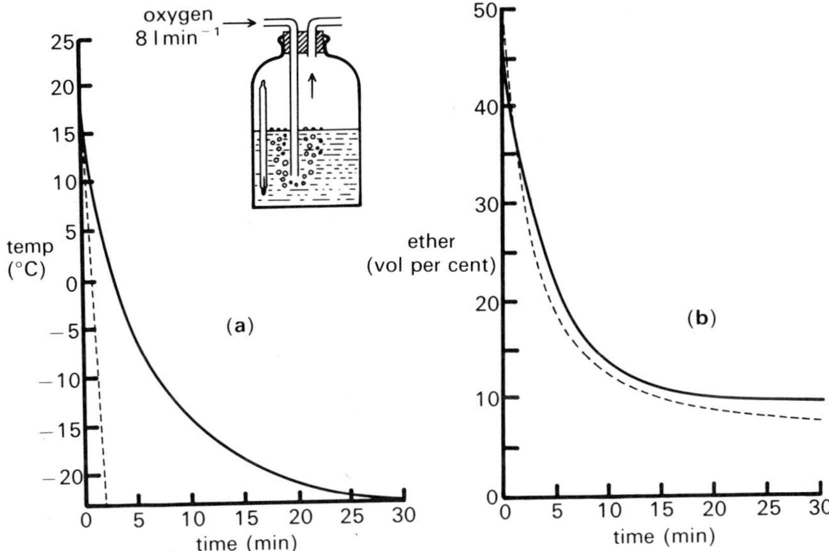

Fig. 3.10. The effect of evaporative cooling on the temperature (a) and the output (b) of a Boyle's bottle containing ether. The whole of a carrier gas flow of $8\,l\,min^{-1}$ of oxygen was bubbled through the liquid ether (the splitting ratio was zero). The dashed line in (b) represents the expected vaporizer output calculated according to the Antoine equation for ether (Table 3.2) based on the temperature in (a). The initial volume of liquid ether present was 285 ml. The volume decreased to half this value at 30 min. The dashed line (a) represents the initial rate of fall in temperature calculated according to eqn (3.65). From Macintosh, Mushin and Epstein (1987). *Physics for the Anaesthetist* (4th edn) p. 143. Blackwell Scientific Publications, Oxford.

upstream and downstream flows. We apply eqn (3.9) to the process,

$$U_2 - U_1 = \int_1^2 \mathrm{d}Q - \int_1^2 \mathrm{d}W, \tag{3.9}$$

where subscripts 1 and 2 here refer to the initial and final states of the whole closed system.

Note firstly that the only work expended by the closed system is due to the displacement of an upstream boundary through a diminishing volume $m_1 v_1$, and a downstream boundary through an increasing volume $m_2 v_2$. Assuming near equilibrium (reversible) conditions at these boundaries we may utilize eqn (3.22) to obtain

$$\int_1^2 \mathrm{d}W = m_2 p_2 v_2 - m_1 p_1 v_1. \tag{3.52}$$

We allow for possible heat flow into the plenum chamber from a surrounding atmosphere or other components of the equipment by assuming the source temperature to be constant at T_0 and the flow of heat in unit time to be

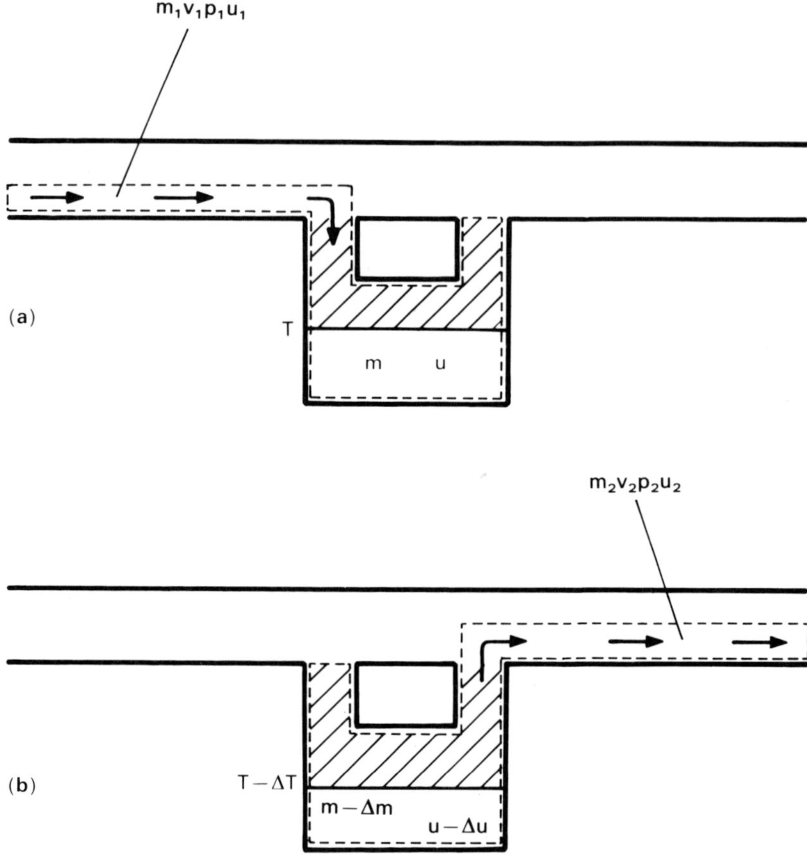

Fig. 3.11. Evaporative cooling in a plenum vaporizer. A fixed mass of gas, vapour, and liquid (a) before and (b) after the passage of unit time, during which the liquid temperature falls by ΔT. For other parameters see text.

proportional to $T_0 - T$:

$$\int_1^2 \mathrm{d}Q = K(T_0 - T), \tag{3.53}$$

where K is the heat transfer coefficient for this process.

The left-hand side of eqn (3.9) involves the internal energy change of all components within the closed system: pipeline gases and vapour, plenum-chamber liquid, and plenum-chamber gas and vapour. We simplify our analysis by neglecting the change of internal energy of the region within the chamber (shaded in Fig. 3.11) occupied by gas and vapour alone. This can be justified for our purposes by reference to the hugely greater density of liquid to that of the gas–vapour mixture lying above it. Taking u to be the specific internal energy of the anaesthetic liquid at temperature T, and Δu to be its decrease with the fall in temperature ΔT, we find

$$U_2 - U_1 = [m_2 u_2 + (m - \Delta m)(u - \Delta u)] - (m_1 u_1 + mu).$$

$$= m_2 u_2 - m_1 u_1 - m\Delta u - \Delta mu + \Delta m \Delta u. \tag{3.54}$$

We neglect the final term of eqn (3.54) as of second order smallness, and combine eqns (3.52), (53) and (54) to obtain

$$m_2 u_2 - m_1 u_1 - m\Delta u - \Delta mu = K(T_0 - T) - m_2 p_2 v_2 + m_1 p_1 v_1$$

or

$$m_2(u_2 + p_2 v_2) - m_1(u_1 + p_1 v_1) - m\Delta u - \Delta mu = K(T_0 - T). \tag{3.55}$$

Readers familiar with thermodynamics will recognize the assemblies of terms in brackets on the left-hand side of eqn (3.55) as enthalpies: $h_1 = u_1 + p_1 v_1$, $h_2 = u_2 + p_2 v_2$. It is precisely because this collection of terms so frequently arises in applications of the first law of thermodynamics to flow problems that enthalpy may usefully be regarded as a separate entity. Equation (3.55) can then be written more succinctly as

$$m_2 h_2 - m_1 h_1 - m\Delta u - \Delta mu = K(T_0 - T). \tag{3.56}$$

We now note that to a high degree of accuracy the difference between the mass of gas and vapour leaving the chamber (m_2) and the mass of carrier gas entering the chamber (m_1) equals the reduction in mass of the anaesthetic liquid:

$$\Delta m = m_2 - m_1. \tag{3.57}$$

This relation is not exact because of the small change during the process in the mass of gas–vapour mixture lying above the liquid in the chamber. Substitution of eqn (3.57) into (3.56) gives

$$m_2 h_2 - m_1 h_1 - (m_2 - m_1)u - m\Delta u = K(T_0 - T). \tag{3.58}$$

Equation (3.58) summarizes the process of evaporative cooling. The following discussion evaluates the relative magnitudes of the five terms in this equation and yields a solution for the way temperature T varies with time as the cooling takes place.

Consider first the relative magnitudes of m_1 and m_2. In the presence of full saturation $(\eta_{\text{vap}} = 1$, eqn (3.48)) the fraction by volume and by molecular number of anaesthetic vapour in the gas–vapour mixture leaving the chamber equals p_{sat}/p_c. The ratio of the mass of vapour leaving to the mass of gas arriving will then be given by

$$\frac{m_2 - m_1}{m_1} = \frac{M_{\text{vap}}(p_{\text{sat}}/p_c)}{M_{\text{car}}(1 - p_{\text{sat}}/p_c)}. \tag{3.59}$$

Table 3.4. *Molecular weights (M_w) of oxygen, nitrogen, and nine inhalational anaesthetics.*

Gas/vapour	M_w (g mol^{-1})
oxygen	32.0
nitrogen	28.0
nitrous oxide	44.0
cyclopropane	42.1
ether	74.1
enflurane	184.5
isoflurane	184.5
halothane	197.4
chloroform	119.4
trichloroethylene	131.4
methoxyflurane	165.0

Data from Grant, W. J. (1978). *Medical Gases. Their Properties and Uses.* HM & M Publishers.

where M_{vap} is the molecular weight of the vapour molecules, and M_{car} the mean molecular weight of the carrier gas*. It follows that

$$\frac{m_2}{m_1} = 1 + \frac{M_{vap}(p_{sat}/p_c)}{M_{car}(1 - p_{sat}/p_c)}. \tag{3.60}$$

Table 3.4 lists the molecular weights of the major carrier gases oxygen, nitrogen and nitrous oxide, and the anaesthetic agents considered earlier. Note that there is up to a sevenfold variation. Table 3.5 lists calculated values of m_2/m_1 for seven vapours saturating three typical carrier gases: pure oxygen, a 30 per cent mixture of oxygen in nitrogen (for example, oxygen-enriched air), and a 30 per cent mixture of oxygen in nitrous oxide. The data are calculated according to eqn (3.60) with values of p_{sat}/p_c taken at 20 °C. We see that the relative mass flows range from 1.13 for methoxyflurane in the O_2/N_2O mixture to 4.48 for ether in the O_2/N_2 mixture.

The interpretation of the left-hand side of eqn (3.58) in terms of published thermodynamic data requires the recognition that the enthalpy $m_2 h_2$ associated with a mixture (mass m_2) of gas plus vapour equals the sum of the individual enthalpies of the two components taken at the same temperature. This will be true insofar as the kinetic gas model holds true, since eqns (3.39)

* Molecular 'weights' are conventionally given as the *mass*, not of an individual molecule m, but of N_{Av} molecules, where $N_{Av} = 6.022 \times 10^{23}$ and is known as Avogadro's number. The reason for this is that N_{Av} molecules of ^{12}C (the commonest carbon isotope) have a mass of exactly 12 g. Any collection of N_{Av} particles is known as one mole (strictly one gram mole).

Table 3.5. *Ratio m_2/m_1 of the mass of a gas–vapour mixture leaving a plenum chamber (m_2) to the mass of carrier gas entering the chamber (m_1) according to eqn (3.60) for three different carrier gases at 20°C. (p_{sat}/p_c according to eqn (3.46), Table 3.2., with $p_c = 101.3\,kPa$ (760 mm Hg) is in parentheses below the name of each vapour.)*

Carrier gas: $(\bar{M}_w\,\mathrm{g\,mol^{-1}})$	O_2 (32)	30 per cent O_2/ 70 per cent N_2 (29.2)	30 per cent O_2/ 70 per cent N_2O (40.4)
Ether (0.578)	4.17	4.48	3.51
Enflurane (0.266)	2.68	2.84	2.33
Isoflurane (0.305)	3.53	3.77	3.00
Halothane (0.320)	3.90	4.18	3.30
Chloroform (0.211)	2.00	2.09	1.79
Trichloroethylene (0.077)	1.34	1.38	1.27
Methoxyflurane (0.030)	1.16	1.17	1.13

and (3.40) for this model predict that for each component

$$h = u + pv = \frac{v}{2}R_{kg}T + R_{kg}T = \left(\frac{v}{2} + 1\right)R_{kg}T. \tag{3.61}$$

This suggests that enthalpy, like internal energy (cf., eqns (3.37) and (3.38)) is the sum of contributions from individual molecules which depend only on the temperature of a mixture. We rewrite eqn (3.58) in the following form

$$(m_2 - m_1)h_{fg} + m_1 c_p(T - T_0) - mc\Delta T = K(T_0 - T), \tag{3.62}$$

where $c_p \equiv (\partial h/\partial T)_p^*$ is the specific heat capacity at constant pressure of the carrier gas mixture which enters the chamber at temperature T_0 and leaves at temperature T; c is the liquid specific heat capacity ($\Delta u/\Delta T \simeq (\partial h/\partial T)_p$ for a liquid); and h_{fg} is the latent heat (enthalpy) of vaporization of the anaesthetic agent. Strictly the introduction of h_{fg} in eqn (3.62) represents the replacement

---

* For the model gas we have from eqn (3.61) $c_p = \left(\dfrac{v}{2} + 1\right)R_{kg}$. On the basis of the model R_{kg} can be shown to equal R_{mol}/M_w, where R_{mol} is the gas constant associated with one mole and equals $8.31\,\mathrm{J\,mol^{-1}\,K^{-1}}$ universally.

Table 3.6. *Latent heat (enthalpy) of vaporization* h_{fg}, *liquid specific heat capacity c, and liquid specific volume v of anaesthetic agents. Where available, the temperature at which measurements were made is stated in parenthesis.*

Agent	h_{fg} (kJ kg^{-1})	c (kJ kg^{-1} K^{-1})	v (l kg^{-1})
ether	385	2.3	1.4
	(20°C)	(20°C)	(0°C)
enflurane[1]	176	—	0.66
isoflurane[1]	153	—	0.67
halothane	147	0.80	0.54
		(20°C)	(0°C)
chloroform	247	0.97	0.67
		(25°C)	(0°C)
trichloroethylene	239	1.05	0.68
		(20°C)	(0°C)
methoxyflurane	205	1.21	0.70
		(20°C)	(0°C)

[1] It is not the policy of the Ohmeda company to give details of specific heat capacity of liquid enflurane and isoflurane.

Data from West, R. C. (ed.) (1975). *Handbook of Chemistry and Physics* (56th edn). E32. CRC Press, Cleveland, Ohio; Schreiber, P. (1972). *Anaesthesia Equipment*, p. 37. Springer-Verlag, Berlin (Conversions from kcal kg^{-1} to kJ kg^{-1} on multiplication by 4.19); Abbott Laboratories Ltd, Queenborough, Kent; Macintosh, Mushin, and Epstein. (1987). *Physics for the Anaesthetist* (4th edn). pp. 598–9. Blackwell Scientific Publications, Oxford.

Table 3.7. *Specific heat capacity* c_p *for the major carrier gases.*

Gas	c_p (kJ kg^{-1} K^{-1})
Oxygen	0.915
	(STP)
Nitrogen	1.039
	(STP)
Nitrous oxide	0.88
	(20°C)

Data from Howatson, A. M., Lund, P. G., and Todd, J. D. (1972). *Engineering tables and data,* p. 69. Chapman and Hall, London; Macintosh, Mushin and Epstein (1987). *Physics for the Anaesthetist,* (4th edn). pp. 598–9. Blackwell Scientific Publications, Oxford.

of u in eqn (3.58) with $u + p_c v$, the liquid specific *enthalpy*, but since $u \gg p_c v$ for a liquid this error is negligible in relation to the accuracy we are seeking here.

Finally substitution from eqn (3.59) into eqn (3.62) brings the result

$$m_1 \left[\frac{h_{fg} M_{vap}(p_{sat}/p_c)}{M_{car}(1 - p_{sat}/p_c)} + c_p(T - T_0) \right] - mc\Delta T = K(T_0 - T). \qquad (3.63)$$

We saw in Fig. 3.5 that h_{fg} for ether was a gradually varying function of temperature over the range of practical interest to us. It is unfortunate that most sources fail to state the temperature at which h_{fg} measurements were made. Table 3.6 lists the available h_{fg} as well as liquid specific volumes v. The latter allow calculation of m from plenum chamber liquid volumes.

Table 3.7 lists values of c_p for the major carrier gases. In accordance with our concept that enthalpy contributions in a mixture of gases will vary in proportion to the masses of the components (eqn(3.61)), the relevant values of c_p for mixtures of two of these carrier gases will be given by

$$c_p = \frac{M_{w1} p_1 c_{p1} + M_{w2} p_2 c_{p2}}{M_{w1} p_1 + M_{w2} p_2}, \qquad (3.64)$$

where M_{w1} and M_{w2} are molecular weights, c_{p1} and c_{p2} specific heat capacities, and p_1 and p_2 the partial pressure of the constituent gases. This for air we obtain approximately* to be

$$c_p = \frac{(32 \times 21 \times 0.915) + (28 \times 79 \times 1.039)}{(32 \times 21) + (28 \times 79)}$$

$$= 1.010 \text{ kJ kg}^{-1} \text{ K}^{-1}.$$

For 30 per cent oxygen in nitrous oxide the corresponding result is

$$c_p = \frac{(32 \times 30 \times 0.915) + (44 \times 70 \times 0.88)}{(32 \times 30) + (44 \times 70)}$$

$$= 0.888 \text{ kJ kg}^{-1} \text{ K}^{-1}.$$

For the experiment of Fig. 3.10 eqn (3.63) predicts the initial rate of fall of liquid temperature to be

$$\frac{dT}{dt} = -\frac{m_1 h_{fg} M_{vap}(p_{sat}/p_c)}{mc M_{car}(1 - p_{sat}/p_c)}$$

$$\doteq -\frac{p_1 \dot{V}_1 h_{fg} M_{vap} p_{sat}/p_c}{R_{mol} T_0 mc(1 - p_{sat}/p_c)}, \qquad (3.65)$$

where $\dot{V}_1$ is the oxygen flow. Terms in $T_0 - T$ are zero at the beginning of the

---

* A more precise calculation taking into account components other than oxygen and nitrogen yields $c_p = 1.004 \text{ kJ kg}^{-1} \text{ K}^{-1}$ at STP.

experiment, when $T = T_0$. Noting that the initial volume of liquid ether is 285 ml, that $v = 1.41\,\mathrm{kg}^{-1}$ (Table 3.6), and setting $p_1 = p_c = 100\,\mathrm{kPa}$, $T_0 = 16\,°\mathrm{C}$, eqn (3.65) predicts

$$\frac{\mathrm{d}T}{\mathrm{d}t} = -\frac{8 \times 10^{-3}(\mathrm{m^3\,min^{-1}}) \times 385\,(\mathrm{kJ\,kg^{-1}}) \times 74.1 \times 10^{-3}(\mathrm{kg\,mol^{-1}})}{8.31 \times 10^{-3}(\mathrm{kJ\,mol^{-1}\,K^{-1}}) \times 289(\mathrm{K}) \times 2.3\,(\mathrm{kJ\,kg^{-1}\,K^{-1}})}$$

$$\times \frac{50\,(\mathrm{kPa}) \times 1.4\,(\mathrm{kg\,l^{-1}})}{0.285(\mathrm{l}) \times (1 - 0.5)}.$$

$$= -20\,°\mathrm{C\,min}^{-1}$$

$$\equiv -0.33\,°\mathrm{C\,s}^{-1}.$$

The steep dashed line in Fig. 3.10(a) represents this result and shows fair agreement with the experimental line. It is unfortunate, however, that the authors of the experiment do not depict data points to give us some idea of the accuracy of the temperature–time plot at this early stage of the experiment.

Equation (3.63) also permits us to make an estimate of K for the experiment of Macintosh, Mushin and Epstein. This can be most easily achieved by considering the near steady-state conditions of output and temperature achieved towards the end of the 30 min experimental period. We set $\Delta T = 0$, $T = -23\,°\mathrm{C}$, $m_1 = p_1 V_1 M_{\mathrm{car}}/(R_{\mathrm{mol}} T_0)$, and $p_{\mathrm{sat}}/p_c = 0.095$ (corresponding to their measured volume percentage) and obtain

$$K = \frac{p_1 V_1 M_{\mathrm{car}}}{R_{\mathrm{mol}} T_0}\left[\frac{h_{\mathrm{fg}} M_{\mathrm{vap}} p_{\mathrm{sat}}/p_c}{M_{\mathrm{car}}(1 - p_{\mathrm{sat}}/p_c)(T_0 - T)} + c_{\mathrm{p}}\right]$$

$$= \frac{8 \times 10^{-3} \times 385 \times 74.1 \times 10^{-3} \times 9.5}{8.31 \times 10^{-3} \times 289 \times 0.905 \times 39}$$

$$+ \frac{100 \times 8 \times 10^{-3} \times 32 \times 10^{-3} \times 0.915}{8.31 \times 10^{-3} \times 289}$$

$$= 0.0256 + 0.0097$$

$$= 0.035\,\mathrm{kJ\,min^{-1}\,K^{-1}}.$$

Note that the term involving h_{fg} dominates this result, showing that the term representing the enthalpy change of the carrier gas alone is of secondary importance ($\simeq 30$ per cent). The computed value of K is appropriate to the end of the 30 min experiment, at which time the volume of ether remaining in the Boyle's bottle was, according to the authors, half the starting volume. K is likely to vary with the volume of liquid present and probably took a value nearer $0.05\,\mathrm{kJ\,min^{-1}\,K^{-1}}$ at the beginning of the experiment.

An experiment similar to that of Fig. 3.10 has been conducted by Palayiwa, Hahn and Sugg using halothane rather than ether. A flow of $600\,\mathrm{ml\,min^{-1}}$ of

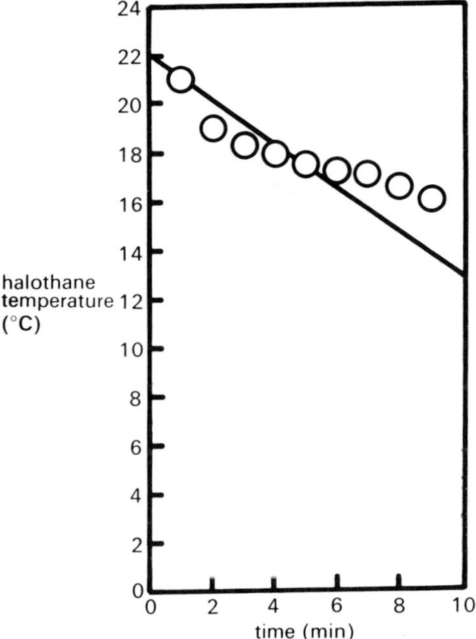

Fig. **3.12.** Variation of halothane temperature with time as oxygen is bubbled at a flow 600 ml min^{-1} through a bottle initially containing 250 ml. The solid line depicts the predicted decline in temperature according to eqn (3.65), with $T_0 = 20\,^{\circ}$C, $p_1 = 101$ kPa, $p_{\mathrm{sat}}/p_{\mathrm{c}} = 0.320$, and data for halothane from relevant preceding tables. Data (1985) from *Anaesthesia* **40**, 415–19.

oxygen was bubbled through a bottle initially containing 250 ml of halothane, and the temperature was recorded over a 10-min period. Figure 3.12 shows that the results of this experiment are in fair agreement with the prediction of eqn (3.65) for the rate of change of temperature in the early stages of evaporative cooling.

The preceding calculations have related to a rather gross evaporative cooling of ether in a relatively well insulated plenum chamber. We have assumed uniformity of temperature within the anaesthetic liquid despite the transfer to the liquid of heat from its surroundings. In modern vaporizers temperature control is achieved in part by surrounding the liquid with metal (for example, brass) or liquid (for example, water) of high heat capacity with which the anaesthetic liquid has close thermal contact. The associated effect of markedly increasing K in eqn (3.63) can be expected to introduce a greater variability in temperature from one part of the liquid to another. Within the approximate model we have set up this will best be represented as an increase in the term mc which will no longer represent the total heat capacity (kJ K^{-1}) of the liquid, but of the liquid plus the surrounding thermal reservoir. In short, such measures increase both K and mc in eqn (3.63). The two effects can be separated experimentally by studying the initial and steady state regions of the evaporation temperature profile.

3.7   Automatic temperature compensation in plenum vaporizers

It is clear from our examination of the effect of temperature changes on the output of plenum vaporizers, that attempts at maintaining constant vaporizer output in the face of changing temperature will benefit the anaesthetist. The provision of a heat sink and its influence on K and mc in eqn (3.63) have already been mentioned. This is now a feature of all modern vaporizers, even to the extent with some models that they are too heavy to carry around easily by hand.

The more definitive approach to maintaining a constant output in the presence of evaporative cooling and changes in ambient temperature involves variation of flow resistances at one of the sites A, B and C in Fig. 3.7(b). The manoeuvre consists of changing $\dot{V}_1/\dot{V}_2$ in eqn (3.49) to compensate for changes in $p_{\mathrm{sat}}/p_{\mathrm{c}}$ and thereby maintain both sides of the equation constant. Table 3.3 shows that each one of the three sites has been selected for this role in two or more designs of vaporizer. Design engineers of the most modern vaporizers have invariably adopted site A in the bypass carrier flow for automatic temperature compensation. We illustrate the design concept in detail for the Penlon Plenum Vaporizer (PPV) shown in cross section in Fig. 3.13.

The PPV incorporates a bellows made from brass which is only 0.1 mm thick and which is surrounded by liquid ether. The mechanism lies in close thermal contact with the anaesthetic liquid in the plenum chamber. The bellows expands and contracts with heating and cooling and displaces a vertical metal rod by 0.23 mm per °C change in its temperature. On the upper end of this rod lies a conical needle machined to a half taper of 2 °C. This needle lies centrally in a short orifice which has a minimum diameter 3.5 mm and through which all bypass carrier gas flows. As the temperature of the anaesthetic liquid changes, the vertical movement of the tapered needle changes the orific area available for the bypass flow and thereby changes the bypass resistance.

The nature of the flow through this orifice can be deduced from a plot of pressure drop against gas flow at fixed temperature. Figure 3.14 shows the result of an experiment in which the pressure drop across the bypass resistance was measured at 20 °C for flows of air in the range 0–10 l min^{-1}. The near parabolic form of the relationship demonstrates that the flow is highly *turbulent* in contrast to the linear relationship which would be expected for *laminar* flow.

To demonstrate the validity of this claim and to examine theoretically the

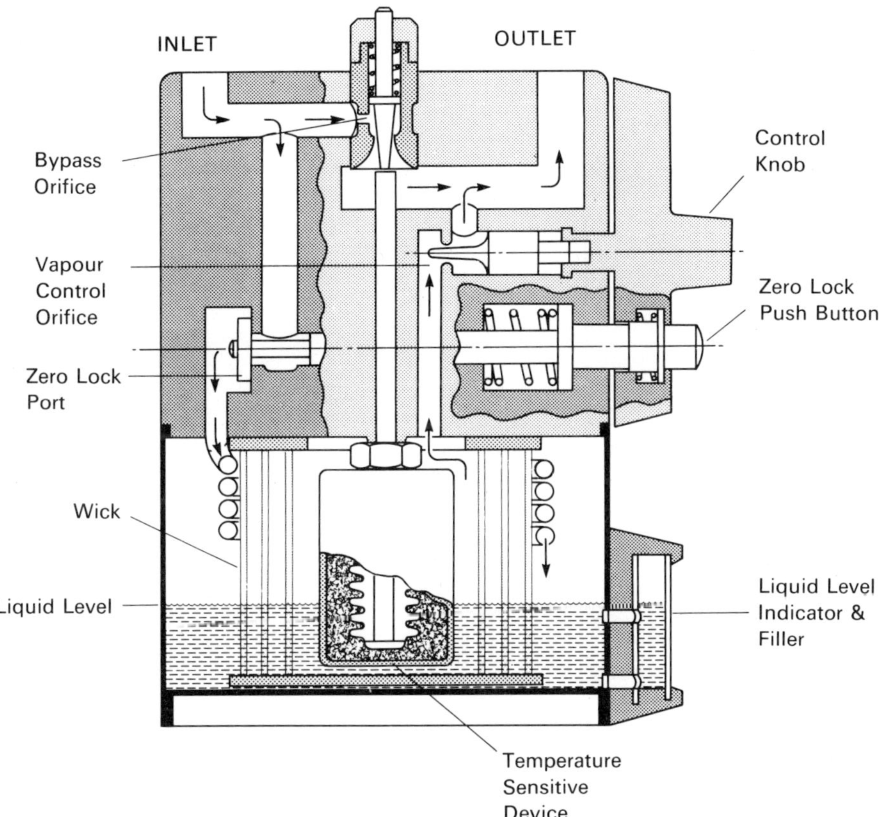

Fig. 3.13. Cross sectional view of the Penlon Plenum Vaporizer (PPV) available for use with halothane, enflurane and isoflurane. Arrows indicate the direction of flow of bypass gas and plenum chamber gas. The manual vapour control orifice lies in the outflow from the chamber (position C in Fig. 3.7(b)); the automatic temperature compensator controls an orifice in the bypass flow (position A in Fig. 3.7(b)). (Courtesy of Penlon, Abingdon, UK)

temperature dependence of the pressure drop across the orifice, we model the orifice choosing a one dimensional flow in which a high velocity stream of cross-sectional area A_1 enters a duct of much larger cross-sectional area A_2 adjacent to a turbulent wake. Figure 3.15 shows the orifice and needle in section, and Fig. 3.16 depicts our assumptions.

If there were no sudden change in area of the flow, with its associated turbulence, the relationship between the hypothetical downstream pressure p_2' and the pressure p_1 at the orifice would be given by Bernoulli's equation:

$$\frac{p_1}{\rho} + \frac{u_1^2}{2} = \frac{p_2'}{\rho} + \frac{u_2^2}{2}. \tag{3.66}$$

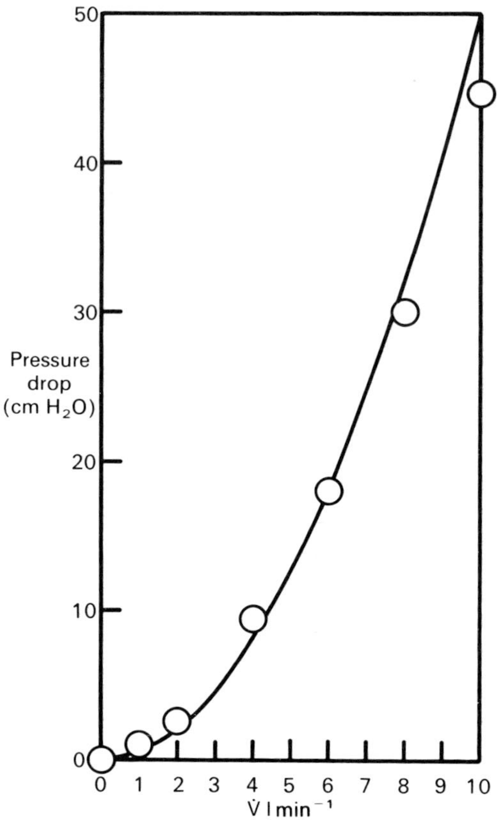

Fig. 3.14. Measurements of pressure drop (in cm H_2O) across the bypass of a Penlon Plenum Vaporizer supplied with a steady flow of air. The experiment was conducted at $20°$ C. The solid line represents the quadratic relationship $\Delta p = a\dot{V}^2$ where $a = 0.5$ cm H_2O min^2 l^{-2}. The near quadratic relationship between measured pressure drop and flow suggests that the flow is turbulent. (Data courtesy of Penlon, Abingdon, UK)

Since continuity of flow requires $u_1 A_1 = u_2 A_2$, eqn (3.66) can be written

$$\frac{p_1 - p_2'}{\rho \dot{V}^2} = \frac{1}{2}\left(\frac{1}{A_2^2} - \frac{1}{A_1^2}\right),\tag{3.67}$$

where $\dot{V}$ is the volume flow of gas. The presence of the wake, however, causes a pressure approximately equal to p_1 to act over the whole of the upstream (left-hand) end of the dashed control volume in Fig. 3.16, resulting in the following momentum equation applied to the control volume*

$$(p_1 - p_2)A_2 = \rho u_2^2 A_2 - \rho u_1^2 A_1,\tag{3.68}$$

* for a similar application of the momentum equation see Fig. 2.16 and eqn (2.31).

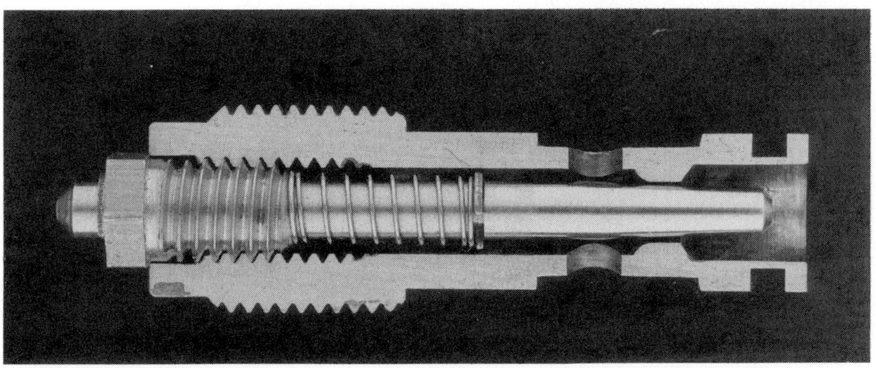

Fig. 3.15. Automatic temperature-compensation orifice of the Penlon Plenum Vaporizer, shown in section.

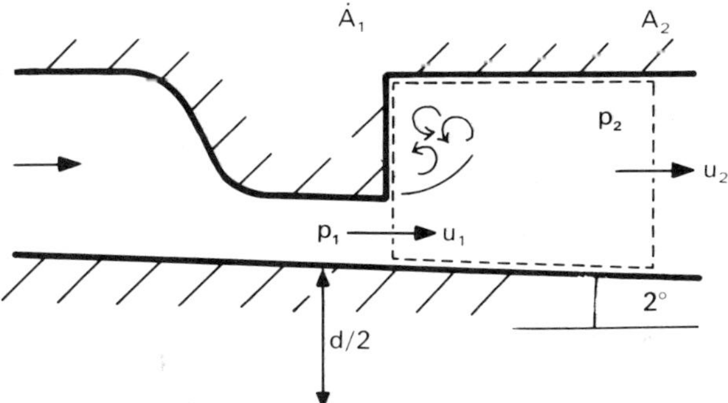

Fig. 3.16. Turbulent flow bypass orifice of the PPV (see Fig. 3.15). The dashed stationary (open) control volume sits at exit from the narrowest portion of the orifice and lies between the sliding tapered needle, depicted as the lower surface in the diagram, and the stationary upper wall of the component. For other variables see text.

or

$$\frac{p_1 - p_2}{\rho \dot{V}^2} = \left(\frac{1}{A_2^2} - \frac{1}{A_1 A_2} \right). \tag{3.69}$$

It follows from eqns (3.67) and (3.69) that the loss of pressure $p_2' - p_2$ arising from the turbulence generated by the orifice is given by

$$\frac{p_2' - p_2}{\rho \dot{V}^2} = \frac{1}{2} \left(\frac{1}{A_2} - \frac{1}{A_1} \right)^2. \tag{3.70}$$

Since A_2 greatly exceeds A_1 (Fig. 3.15) we may approximate the pressure loss using

$$p'_2 - p_2 = \left(\frac{\rho \dot{V}^2}{2A_1^2} \right) \tag{3.71}$$

which is consistent with the parabolic relationship between pressure drop and flow as found in Fig. 3.14.

As the needle valve moves with temperature the flow area A_1 at the orifice varies from some value a_0 at temperature T_0 according to

$$A_1(T) = a_0 - \alpha(T - T_0), \tag{3.72}$$

where $\alpha = 2\Pi \times (3.5/2) \times 4 \times (\Pi/180) \times 0.23 = 0.177 \text{ mm}^2 \text{ K}^{-1}$. The pressure drop across the orifice is given as a function of temperature by substitut-

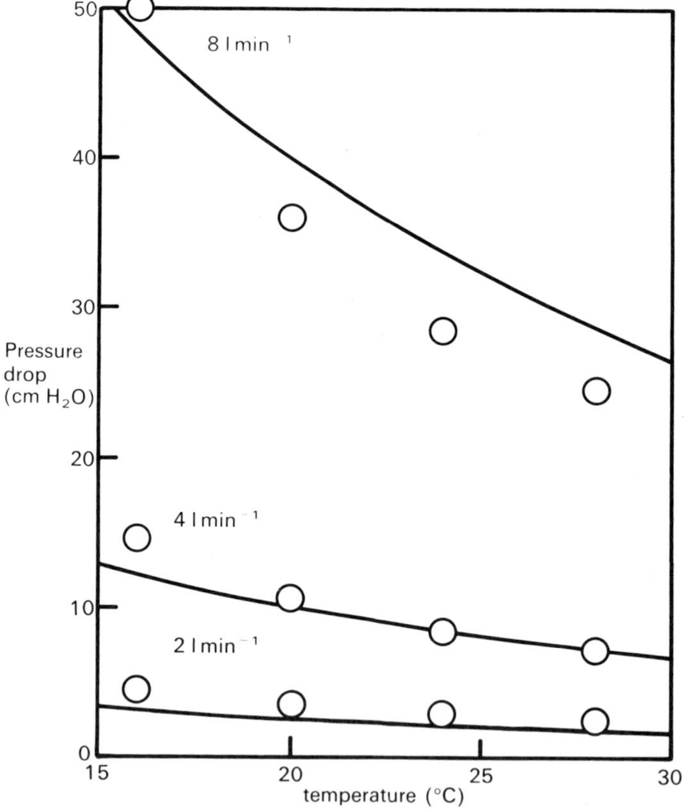

Fig. 3.17. Performance of the bypass orifice in the Penlon Plenum Vaporizer. Measurements of pressure drop at three flows of air in the temperature range 15–30 °C are compared with eqn (3.73) (solid lines); $a_0 = 1.65 \text{ mm}^2$, $\alpha = 0.177 \text{ mm}^2 \text{ K}^{-1}$ (from 2 degree needle half taper). (Data courtesy of Penlon, Abingdon UK.)

ing eqn (3.72) into (3.71):

$$p'_2 - p_2 = \frac{\rho \dot{V}^2}{2[a_0 - \alpha(T - T_0)]}.$$ (3.73)

Equation (3.73) is compared with measurements in Fig. 3.17 for three flows in the temperature range 15–30 °C. $a_0 (= 1.65 \text{ mm}^2)$ has been estimated from the manufacturer's design specification of a pressure drop of 10 cm H_2O at 20 °C when the flow is 4 l min^{-1}. The simple one dimensional flow theory generates a fair approximation to the observed performance.

As temperature increases the resistance to flow in the bypass to the plenum chamber decreases. This results in less carrier gas entering the chamber. The higher vapour saturation pressure at higher temperatures (Fig. 3.2) is thereby compensated for, at least partly, by a reduction in the flow which picks up the anaesthetic vapour (eqn (3.49)).

The degree of independence from temperature which is achieved by this automatic temperature compensation is shown in Fig. 3.18 for halothane and enflurane models of the PPV. The isoflurane model has a virtually identical performance to the halothane model. The contrast between variations in halothane output expected in the absence of temperature compensation (Fig. 3.9) and those seen in Fig. 3.18(a) are striking. Similarly, good temperature compensation is achieved in other modern vaporizers such as the Ohmeda Tec 4 and Dräger Vapor though design features differ considerably between manufacturers (see below).

3.8 The effect of flow on the output from plenum vaporizers

The flow required by an anaesthetist from a plenum vaporizer may vary widely in the approximate range 1–10 l min^{-1}. A low flow may be all that is required, for example, to supply a breathing system incorporating a CO_2 absorber such as that shown in Fig. 2.32(f). Conversely, a high flow is commonly required to supply a T-piece system for a spontaneously ventilating patient (Fig. 2.9 and 2.31). A desirable feature of anaesthetic vaporizers is therefore an ability to deliver a defined vapour concentration over a wide range of flows.

It might at first be thought that a vaporizer which shows little variation in output with changes in temperature would show correspondingly little variation in output with changes in flow. Figure 3.19 shows this not to be the case, even in one of the most modern vaporizers, the Ohmeda Tec Mk 4 (Fig. 3.20). The reason for this kind of behaviour is that the bypass and plenum chamber flows may differ in the degree to which they are either turbulent or laminar. Areas of resistance to flow (Fig. 3.7(b)) exhibit behaviour with respect to changes in flow which differs according to whether the flow through them is turbulent or laminar. In fact there are three types (or

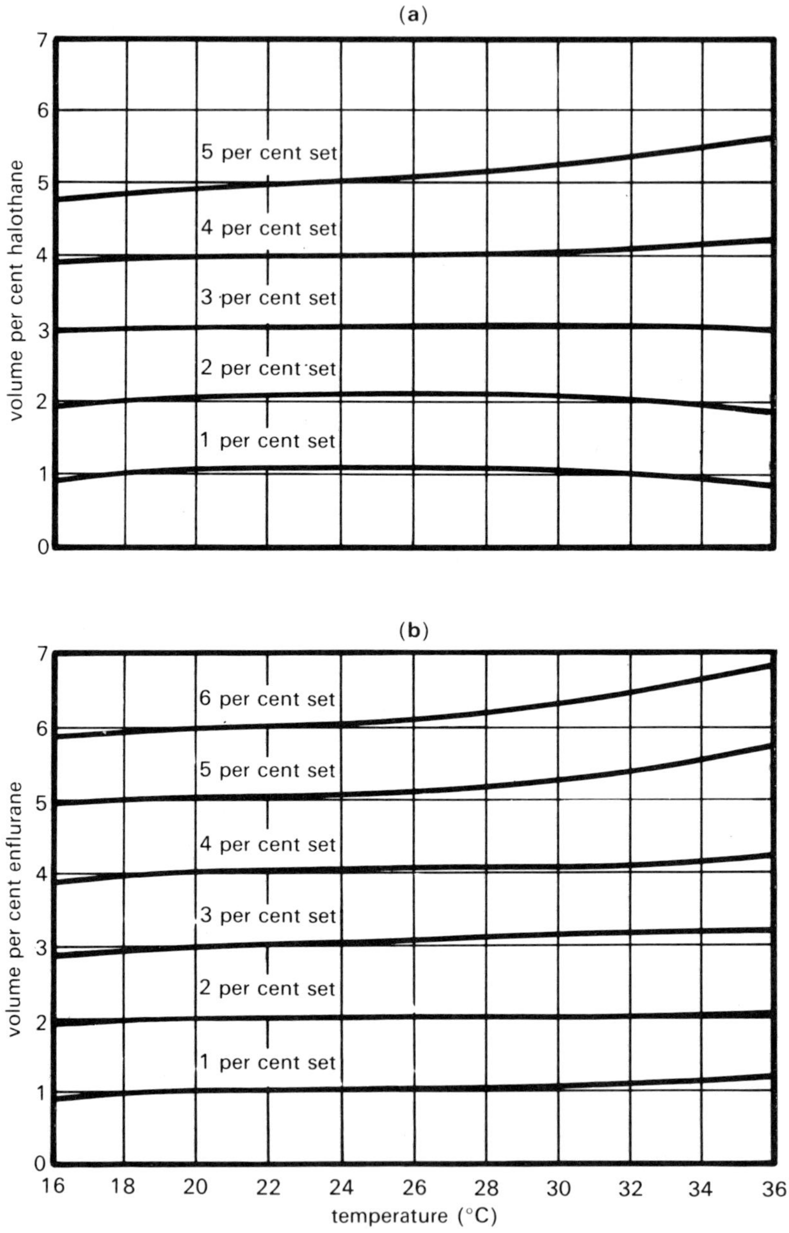

Fig. 3.18. Variation of PPV output with temperature at gas flow $4\,l\,min^{-1}$: (a) halothane model, (b) enflurane model. Data as provided by manufacturer. Gas not specified.

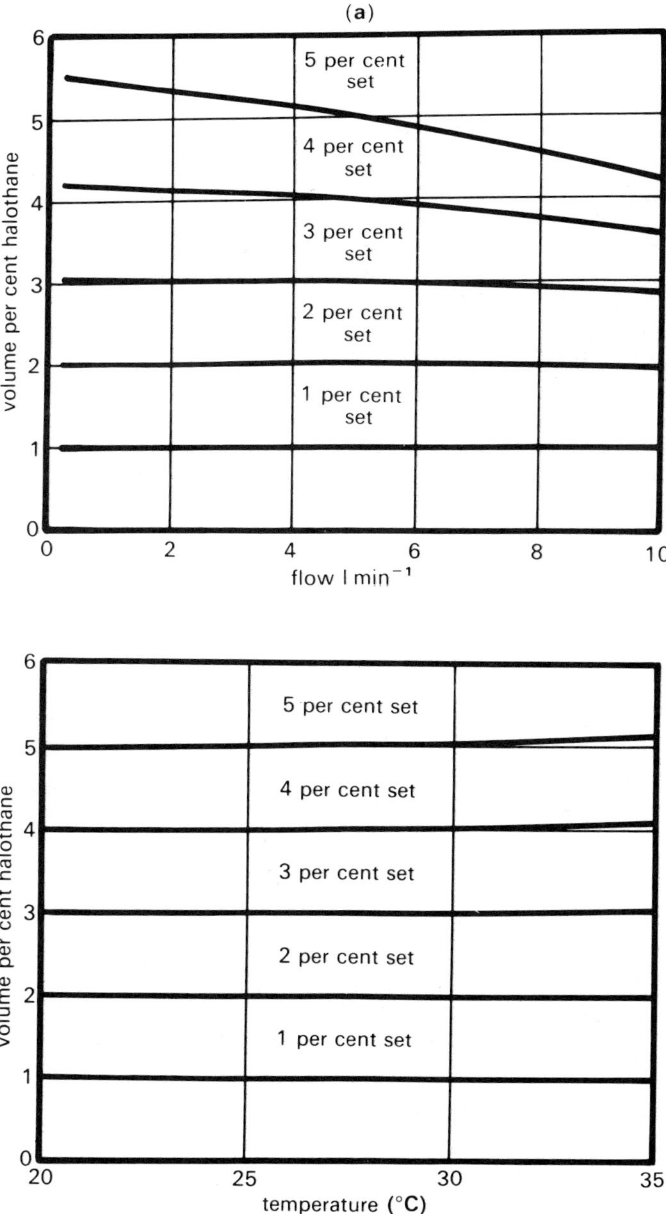

Fig. 3.19. Effect of (a) flow (at 22 °C) and (b) temperature (at flow 5 l min⁻¹) on the output of a Tec 4 vaporizer delivering halothane (Fluotec 4). Data as provided by the manufacturer. Oxygen used throughout. Note that excellent temperature stability coexists with moderate changes of output with flow at high settings. The performance of the isoflurane model (Fig. 3.20) is very similar to that shown here.

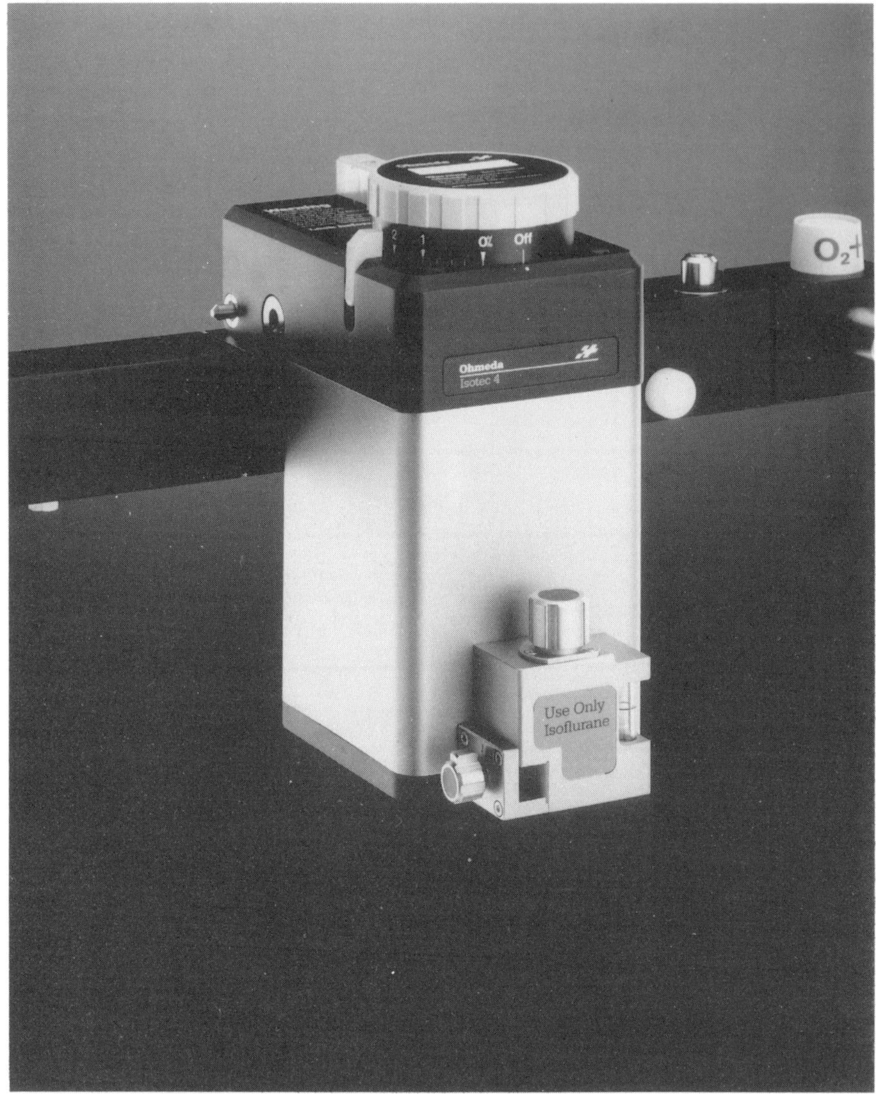

Fig. 3.20. The Ohmeda Tec Mk 4 vaporizer (isoflurane model).

'regimes') of flow which we need to consider in order to understand this problem. They are *turbulent flow in rough piping* (or past obstructions such as orifices), *turbulent flow in smooth piping*, and *laminar flow*.

Recall that we are dealing with gas flows which may be regarded as steady (not varying with time) and incompressible (of constant density). We saw earlier in relation to eqn (2.33) that the assumption of incompressibility was equivalent to saying that flow velocities remain well below the velocity of sound. We define the *resistance* of any flow path to be the ratio of the pressure drop Δp across the path to the volume flow $\dot{V}$ through it:

$$r = \frac{\Delta p}{\dot{V}}. \tag{3.74}$$

Turbulent flow* in rough piping or past obstructions such as orifices is characterized by having a flow resistance which is proportional to both density and flow:

$$r \propto \rho \dot{V}. \tag{3.75}$$

We have met an example of this in the bypass orifice of the PPV (Fig. 3.14) for which eqn (3.73) can be written in the form of eqn (3.75).

Turbulent flow in smooth piping is characterized by a flow resistance which varies less markedly with $\rho \dot{V}$ than that of eqn (3.75). To a fair approximation this kind of flow can be represented by[†]

$$r \propto (\rho \dot{V})^{\frac{4}{5}}. \tag{3.76}$$

For many purposes eqn (3.76) may be regarded as only a slight deviation from eqn (3.75) and this latter equation used as a single representative of all turbulent flows.

Laminar flows are dominated by viscous friction and are characterized by

$$r = \text{constant (for a given gas).} \tag{3.77}$$

Cases of uniform laminar flow will be examined in some detail in Chapter 5 as typical of the flow of blood through membrane lungs.

The dependence of the splitting ratio $(\dot{V}_1/\dot{V}_2)$ on ρ and total gas flow $(\dot{V}_1 + \dot{V}_2)$ can be predicted from the requirement that the pressure drop across two parallel paths must be equal:

$$\Delta p_1 = \Delta p_2 \tag{3.78}$$

or

$$\frac{\dot{V}_1}{\dot{V}_2} = \frac{r_2}{r_1}. \tag{3.79}$$

For example, consider a vaporizer in which the bypass flow is predominantly laminar and the flow through the vaporizing chamber is dominated by a

---

* The terms 'turbulent' and 'laminar' are used here without elaboration. Readers unfamiliar with them will find further explanation in any basic fluid mechanics text.
† This result is obtained by adopting the fifth root approximation to the Moody diagram. See, for example, Howatson, A. M., Lund, P. G. and Todd, J. D. (1972). *Engineering tables and data*, p. 106. Chapman and Hall.

turbulent-flow orifice. This would yield

$$\frac{\dot{V}_1}{\dot{V}_2} \propto \rho \dot{V}_2$$

or

$$\frac{\dot{V}_1}{\dot{V}_2} \propto (\rho \dot{V}_1)^{\frac{1}{2}}. \tag{3.80}$$

Since the total gas flow into the vaporizer $\dot{V}$ equals $\dot{V}_1 + \dot{V}_2$ and since $\dot{V}_1 \gg \dot{V}_2$ in most situations (see Fig. 3.8) the splitting ratio is given approximately by

$$\frac{\dot{V}_1}{\dot{V}_2} \propto (\rho \dot{V})^{\frac{1}{2}}. \tag{3.81}$$

Reduction in total gas flow $\dot{V}$ would then lead to a fall in splitting ratio with a consequent enrichment with vapour. This appears to be the explanation for the performance seen at intermediate flows and high dial settings in the old Fuotec 2 vaporizer (Fig. 3.21(a)) which incorporates a turbulent flow orifice at the outflow from the plenum chamber (position C in Fig. 3.7(b)). The dimensions of this orifice vary with the deflection of a bimetallic strip, which acts as the automatic temperature compensator in this device (see Table 3.3). It has been suggested that the fall in output of this vaporizer at very low flows and at very low settings arises from poor mixing of gas and vapour in the plenum chamber (i.e., low η_{vap} in eqn (3.49)).

Consider secondly a vaporizer in which the bypass flow is dominated by a turbulent flow orifice and the flow through the vaporizing chamber is predominantly laminar. Equation (3.79) would yield

$$\frac{\dot{V}_1}{\dot{V}_2} \propto (\rho \dot{V}_1)^{-\frac{1}{2}} \tag{3.82}$$

Again, since $\dot{V} = \dot{V}_1 + \dot{V}_2 \simeq \dot{V}_1$ in most situations the spilitting ratio is given approximately by ·

$$\frac{\dot{V}_1}{\dot{V}_2} \propto (\rho \dot{V})^{-\frac{1}{2}}. \tag{3.83}$$

Reduction in total gas flow $\dot{V}$ would in this case lead to a rise in splitting ratio with a consequent weakening of the mixture. This appears to be the explanation for the performance seen at low and intermediate flows in the old MIE Halothane 4 vaporizer (Fig. 3.21(b)) which incorporates a turbulent flow butterfly valve in the bypass flow (position A in Fig. 3.7(b)) and a long thin tube at outlet from the plenum chamber.

In general, it follows from eqns (3.75) to (3.79) that where the parallel flows through a vaporizer conform to different flow regimes, a relationship will

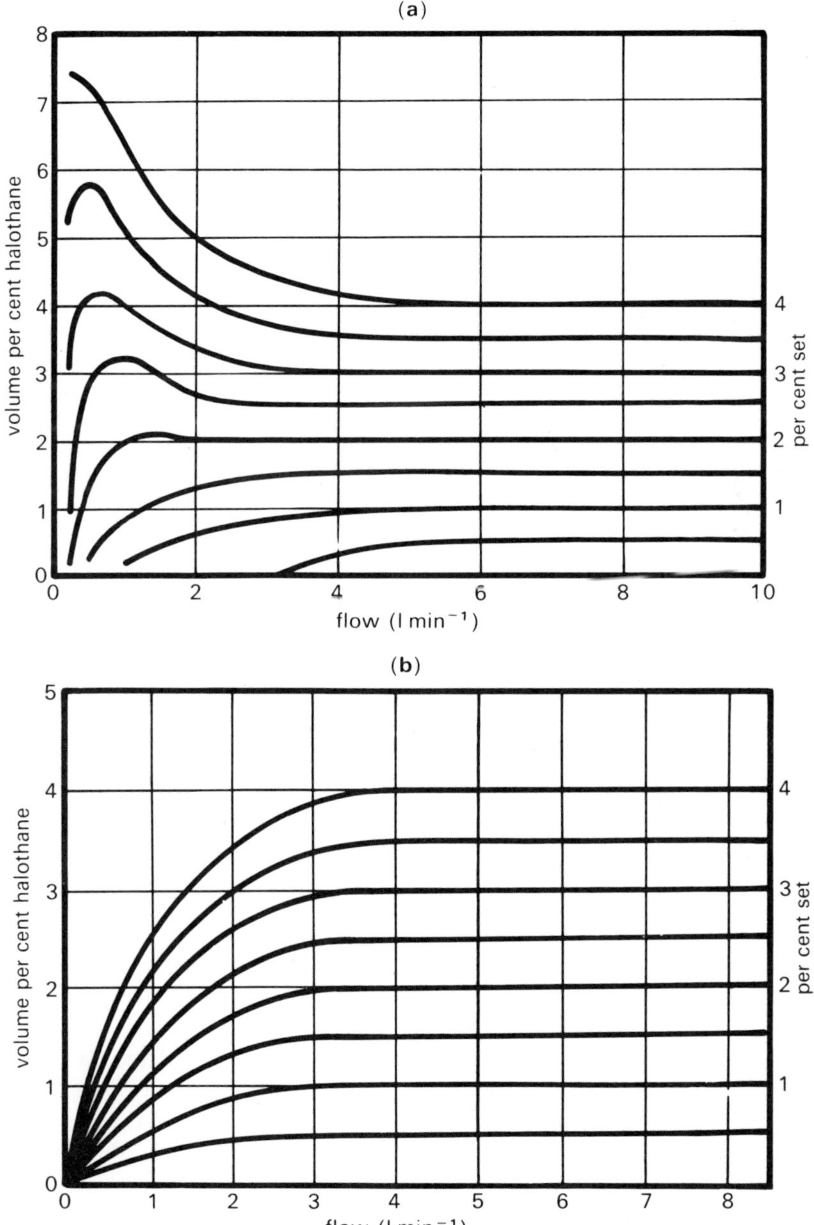

Fig. 3.21. Variation of output with flow for two halothane vaporizers (a) Cyprane Fluotec 2 (b) MIE Halothane 4. At intermediate and low flows these vaporizers display a deviation from the output setting which can be explained by reference to eqns (3.81) and (83). Data as provided by manufacturers with each unit. Temperature and gas not specified.

exist of the form

$$\frac{\dot{V_1}}{\dot{V_2}} = f(\rho \dot{V_1}), \qquad (3.84)$$

where f expresses a general functional dependence of the splitting ratio on the product of ρ and $\dot{V_1}$. This gives the approximate result

$$\frac{\dot{V_1}}{\dot{V_2}} \simeq f(\rho \dot{V}). \qquad (3.85)$$

$f(\rho \dot{V})$ will only be a constant if both parallel paths conform to the same flow regime.

In the Penlon Plenum Vaporizer (Fig. 3.13) this aim is to a large extent achieved by causing both paths to be dominated by turbulent flow orifices. In the bypass we have already examined that in some detail (Fig. 3.15). The orifice dominating the flow through the plenum chamber lies at the outlet from the chamber (site C in Fig. 3.7(b)) and is the site for manual control of vaporizer output The needle valve at this site has a more complex shape than that of the bypass needle valve, being machined to a radius in two dimensions rather than to a simple taper. The resulting output–flow curves for this design are shown in Fig. 3.22(a) for the halothane model and Fig. 3.22(b) for the enflurane model. As for Fig. 3.18, the performance of the isoflurane model is virtually identical to the halothane model.

Another way of achieving similar flow regimes in both parallel paths has been very successfully applied in the Dräger Vapor vaporizer (Fig. 3.23) which incorporates two laminar flow annulae, one in the bypass with a variable aperture to permit automatic temperature compensation, and one in the outlet from the plenum chamber to provide manual control of the vaporizer output. Performance curves, both in relation to temperature and flow, are shown in Fig. 3.24 for two different temperatures.

The presence of laminar flow in a pipe, annulus, or other shape of duct can be made predictable by satisfying two conditions. Firstly, the flow needs to be uniform over a length of ducting which is much greater than its width. By 'uniform' we mean that a cross-sectional slice of the duct will appear the same at all points along its length. It tends to be only for uniform flows that less stringent restrictions on the second condition will permit laminar flow to appear. The second condition is that the Reynolds number of the flow must be below some critical value.

Reynolds number Re is the following dimensionless group of flow variables: $\rho \bar{u} d / \mu$, where ρ is the fluid density, $\bar{u}$ its mean velocity, d a measure of the width of the ducting and μ the fluid viscosity. The critical Reynolds number always depends to some extent upon the roughness of the walls adjacent to the flow. For a circular pipe with d equal to the diameter, the

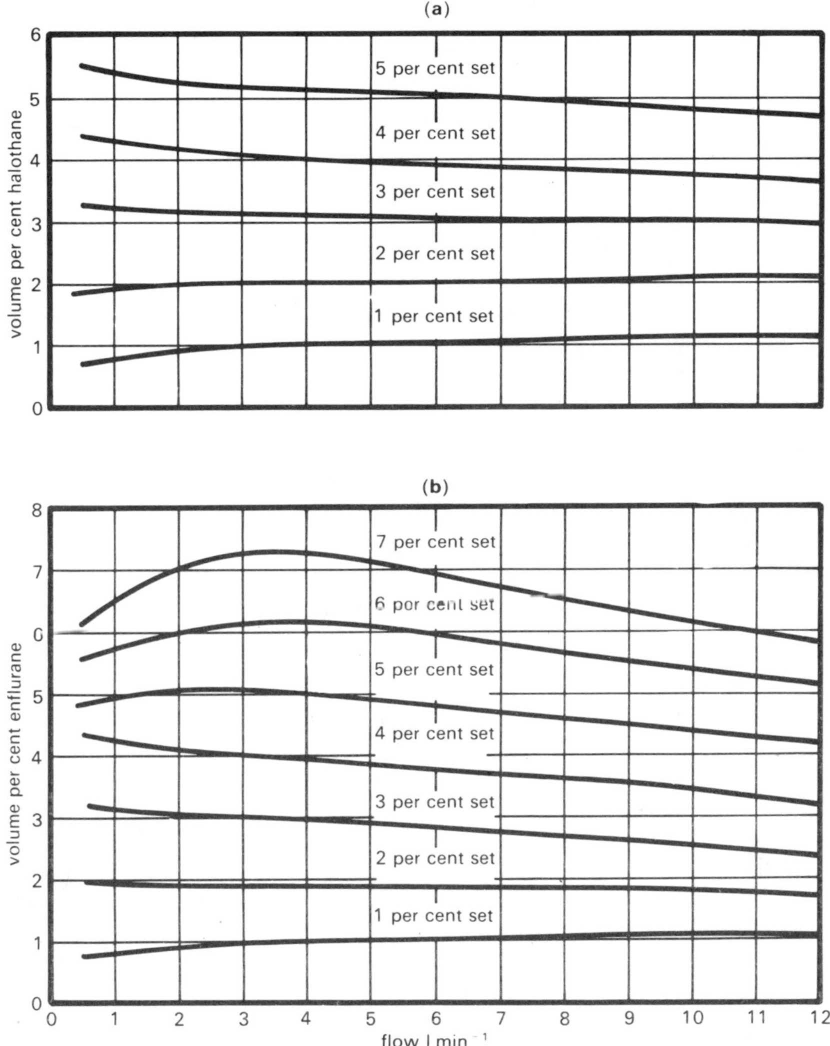

Fig. 3.22. Variation of PPV output with flow at 22 °C: (a) halothane model, (b) enflurane model. Data as provided by manufacturer. Gas not specified.

critical Reynolds number is found experimentally to be around 3000. Thus, to calculate the diameter of a pipe for which an air flow of 4 l min⁻¹ at 20 °C and atmospheric pressure is transitional between laminar and turbulent flow we set

$$\frac{\rho \bar{u} d}{\mu} = 3000. \tag{3.86}$$

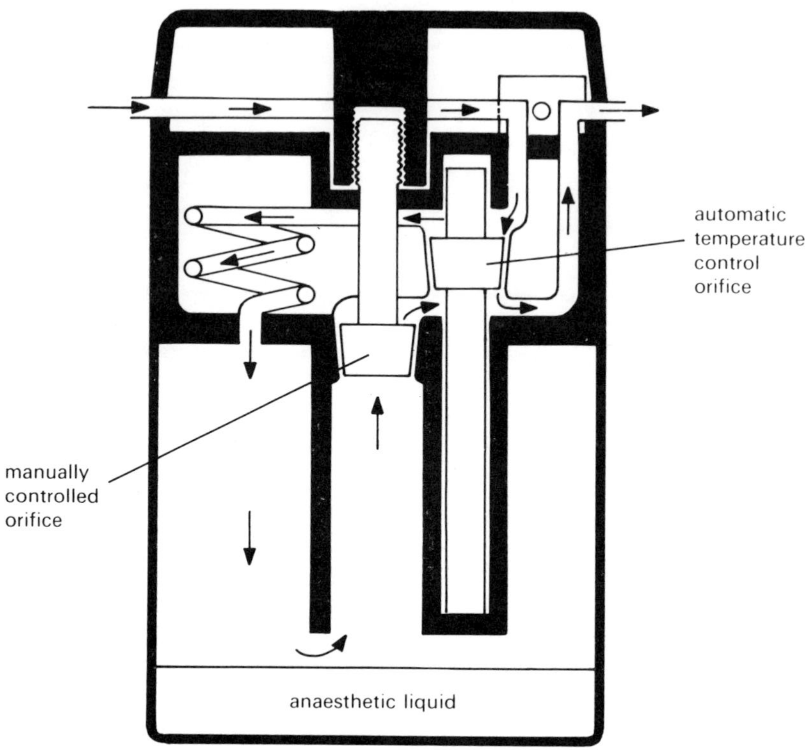

Fig. 3.23. Cross sectional view of the Dräger Vapor vaporizer. Arrows indicate the direction of gas flows. Variable resistances for both manual and automatic temperature control are designed to achieve laminar flow. Schematics as provided by manufacturer.

We note that $\rho = 1/v$, where v is the specific volume of the gas and is related by eqn (3.40) to p and T; also that $\Pi d^2 \bar{u}/4 = \dot{V}$. Equation (3.86) becomes

$$\frac{4p\dot{V}}{R_{kg}T\mu\Pi d} = 3000. \tag{3.87}$$

For air, $R_{kg} = 0.287\,\mathrm{kJ\,kg^{-1}\,K^{-1}}$ and $\mu = 18.1 \times 10^{-6}\,\mathrm{N\,s\,m^{-2}}$ at $20\,^{\circ}\mathrm{C}$ (293 K) and 101 kPa. For air flowing at $4\,\mathrm{l\,min^{-1}}$ eqn (3.87) thus gives

$$d = \frac{4 \times 101\,(\mathrm{kPa}) \times 4 \times 10^{-3}/60\,(\mathrm{m^3\,s^{-1}})}{0.287\,(\mathrm{kJ\,kg^{-1}\,K^{-1}}) \times 293\,(\mathrm{K}) \times 18.1 \times 10^{-6}\,(\mathrm{N\,s\,m^{-2})}} \times \frac{1}{3000}$$

$$= 6\,\mathrm{mm}. \tag{3.88}$$

The viscosities of all the major carrier gases at $20\,^{\circ}\mathrm{C}$ are given in Table 3.8. It can be seen that they vary sufficiently little not to change this result, for gases other than air, by more than one or two mm.

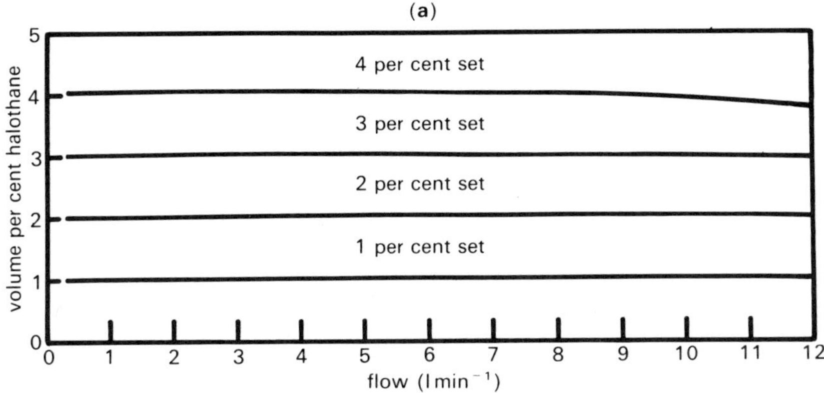

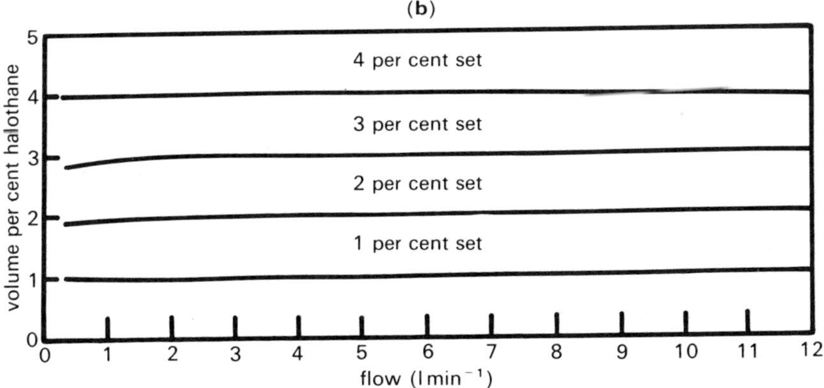

Fig. 3.24. Variation of output of the Vapor 19.1 with flow at (a) 22 °C and (b) 34 °C. Data as provided by manufacturer. Operation with air at pressure 101.3 kPa.

The particular result of eqn (3.88) appears relevant to the interpretation of the output–flow curves of the halothane 4 vaporizer (Fig. 3.21(b)). 6 mm is approximately the diameter of the long outlet tube from the plenum chamber in this model (position C in Fig. 3.7(b)). For flows below about 4 l min^{-1} this tube probably carries a predominantly laminar flow, giving rise to the fall in output with flow as discussed above. Above about 4 l min^{-1} the tube probably carries a mainly turbulent flow, similar to that across the bypass butterfly valve in this vaporizer. Because both bypass and plenum chamber flows are then in the same regime, at the higher flows the output remains independent of flow (Fig. 3.21(b)).

Table 3.8. *Dynamic viscosity μ for the major carrier gases at 20 °C*

Gas	$\mu\,(\mathrm{N\,s\,m^{-2}})$
Oxygen	20.2
Nitrogen	17.5
Air	18.3
Nitrous oxide	14.5

Data from Weast, R. C. (ed.) (1975). *Handbook of Chemistry and Physics* (56th edn). pp. F56–8. CRC Press, Cleveland, Ohio. Interpolation has been used to estimate data for 20 °C. Note that the kinetic theory of gases can readily be shown to predict that, for a given gas, $\mu \propto T^{\frac{1}{2}}$, where T is Kelvin temperature. μ is predicted to be independent of pressure and density. Experimental data conform well with these predictions, over a wide range of temperature.

In the Dräger Vapor vaporizer, laminar flow is maintained in both the bypass annulus and the annulus at exit from the plenum chamber right up to a flow of $15\,\mathrm{l\,min^{-1}}$, to maintain output largely independent of flow (Fig. 3.24). In applying the Reynolds number to these annular flows we note that its critical value remains approximately 3000 if d equals the annulus gap. Let D equal the mean large diameter of the annulus. Ignoring the slight taper and assuming $d \ll D$ we deduce

$$\bar{u} = \dot{V}/(\Pi D d). \tag{3.89}$$

Hence

$$\mathrm{Re} = \frac{\rho \bar{u} d}{\mu}$$

$$= \frac{\rho \dot{V}}{\mu \Pi D}, \tag{3.90}$$

which is a function of D but not d. Noting again that $\rho = p/(R_{\mathrm{kg}} T)$ and substituting values as for eqns (3.87) and (3.88), we calculate D for the critical condition at a flow $15\,\mathrm{l\,min^{-1}}$ to be

$$D = \frac{p \dot{V}}{3000\, R_{\mathrm{kg}}\, T \mu \Pi}$$

$$= \frac{101\,(\mathrm{kPa}) \times 15 \times 10^{-3}/60\,(\mathrm{m^3\,s^{-1}})}{0.287\,(\mathrm{kJ\,kg^{-1}\,K^{-1}}) \times 293\,(\mathrm{K}) \times 18.1 \times 10^{-6}\,(\mathrm{N\,s\,m^{-2}})} \times \frac{1}{3000}$$

$$= 5.5\ \mathrm{mm}. \tag{3.91}$$

Table 3.9. *Resistance to gas flow of 4 vaporizers. Measurements were made with oxygen flowing at 5 l min^{-1}, with 1 per cent set in each case.*

Vaporizer	Resistance (cm H$_2$O per l min^{-1})
Fluotec Mark 2	1.6
Fluotec Mark 3	3.2
*Vapor (Mark 1)	49
*Fluomatic	72

* vaporizers designed to achieve a high degree of laminar flow in both bypass and plenum chamber.

Data from Diaz, P. M. (1976). *British Journal of Anaesthesia* **48,** 387–91; Palayiwa, E., Sanderson, M. H., and Hahn, C. E. W. (1983). *British Journal of Anaesthesia* **55,** 1025–37.

For values of D greater than this eqn (3.90) predicts that Re will be less than 3000 and the annular flow well within the laminar region. The value of D adopted by the manufacturer of the Vapor is approximately 18 mm. The probable reason for this choice is that a calculation like that of eqn (3.91), but for a carrier gas containing a high proportion of nitrous oxide, yields a value of D around twice the value we have found for air.

We conclude that independence of vaporizer output with regard to gas flow seems to be achieved most successfully by the use of laminar flow resistances in both the bypass and chamber flows. The price paid for this is a considerably higher resistance to flow of the whole vaporizer. Data on this aspect of design is sparse but Table 3.9 provides an indication of the problem. We shall not examine this aspect further here, but note that a simple application of the equations for Couette flow would enable the reader to explore the effect on resistance of changes in d and D in eqns (3.89) and (3.90) for the Vapor design.

3.9   Other influences on the output from plenum vaporizers

Our analysis of the output of plenum vaporizers has so far concentrated on the effects of varying temperature and flow. In this section we mention briefly the multiple other factors known to participate in complicating the performance of what might at first (Fig. 3.7) have seemed to be a simple device.

Equation (3.85) suggests that changes in carrier gas density alone may vary the splitting ratio in a device in which different flow regimes exist in bypass and chamber flows. Attempts have been made to study this by varying the composition of mixtures of carrier gas feeding vaporizers. These attempts do not eliminate the effects of differences of viscosity between such mixtures and thus fail to vary ρ in isolation. ρ can be varied with virtually no change in μ by supplying carrier gas at different pressures.

Pressure changes are known to affect output, however, in a more profound way than is likely by changing splitting ratio alone. Equation (3.49) shows that F_{anaes} is highly dependent on $p_{\text{sat}}/p_{\text{c}}$ even in the presence of a fixed splitting ratio (Fig. 3.8). This arises because p_{sat} is the partial pressure of anaesthetic vapour in a chamber at pressure p_{c}. If p_{c} is reduced p_{sat} becomes a greater proportion; if p_{c} is increased the vapour fraction is reduced.

The presence of the chamber pressure p_{c} in eqn (3.49) is of importance for two reasons at least. Firstly, p_{c} may often be considerably greater than ambient atmospheric pressure, due either to a high resistance at the output from the chamber (point C in Fig. 3.7(b)) or due to the vaporizer being connected at the inlet of a breathing system or ventilator which has a high resistance to flow. With one widely used ventilator, for example, p_{c} is elevated above atmospheric pressure by around 16 per cent due to the ventilator alone*. Secondly p_{c} may vary considerably with altitude. At 3000 m where $p_{\text{atm}} \simeq 70\ \text{kPa}$, $p_{\text{sat}}/p_{\text{c}}$ will be increased by approximately 43 per cent above its value at sea level. The upwardly concave lines of Fig. 3.8 demonstrate that an even greater percentage rise in F_{anaes} will occur for a given rise in $p_{\text{sat}}/p_{\text{c}}$. F_{anaes} may easily rise by 50 per cent at this altitude. Since the anaesthetic effect of an agent probably depends upon its true partial pressure rather than its pressure relative to ambient atmosphere, this kind of inaccuracy may be of little clinical importance when vaporizers are used at high altitudes.

Progressive emptying of the plenum chamber as liquid evaporates causes a reduction with time in the output of most vaporizers. η_{vap} in eqn (3.49) falls progressively away from unity as more carrier gas finds a path through the chamber remote from anaesthetic liquid. Figure 3.25(a) shows the declining output of the Tec Mk 3 vaporizer measured by Synnott and Wren. Over 40 min the decrease was by 7 per cent of the initial setting.

The composition of the carrier gas has some influence in determining output. Figure 3.25(b) shows the output found by Synnott and Wren following a change in carrier gas composition from mainly nitrous oxide to 100 per cent oxygen. By subtracting data for the decline in output due to emptying alone (Fig. 3.25(a)) the effects of the change in carrier gas were isolated and are given in Fig. 3.25(c). The response displays the two features observed during many other experiments of this kind. Firstly, we note a transient change in output, in this case a rise over 1 min. Secondly, we see a steady state change in output, in this case a fall of 5 per cent. The transient and steady state changes in output are not always seen to occur in different

---

* Blease–Manley. The problem referred to here has recently been clarified in relation to clinical trials with isoflurane (Heneghan, C. P. H. (1986). *British Journal of Anaesthesia* **58**, 932).

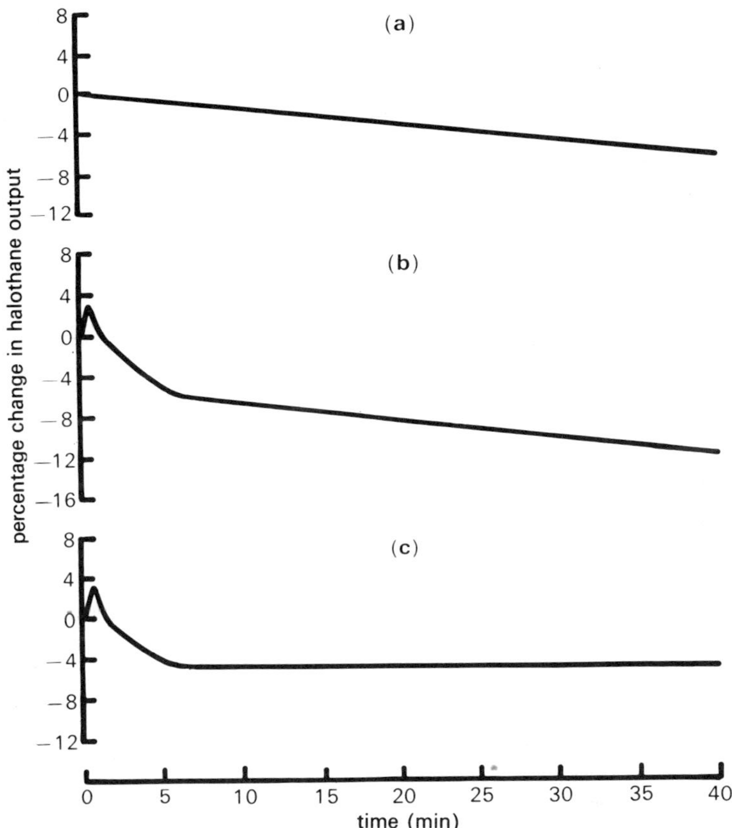

Fig. 3.25. Changes with time in output of halothane from a Tec 3 vaporizer (100 per cent oxygen was delivered at $9\,l\,min^{-1}$. Means taken of 3 vaporizers at both 1 per cent and 2 per cent settings.) (a) Effect of progressive emptying over 40 min, (b) output during the 40 min after a change in carrier gas composition from 66 per cent nitrous oxide/34 per cent oxygen to 100 per cent oxygen, (c) effect of change in carrier gas alone. This was calculated by subtracting the values in (a) from those in (b). From Synott, A. and Wren, W. S. (1986). *British Journal of Anaesthesia* **58,** 1055–8.

directions. Figure 3.26 gives the results of an experiment by Palayiwa, Sanderson and Hahn, also on a Tec Mk 3 vaporizer in which the transient and steady state changes both occur in the same direction, that of a reduction in output.

The explanation for the transient change has only recently been clarified. It appears that nitrous oxide has a high solubility in liquid halothane and enflurane (4 and 5 ml N_2O ml^{-1} respectively) and probably other agents as well. Consequently, the uptake or release of nitrous oxide by anaesthetic liquid can briefly reduce or increase the output flow from the plenum

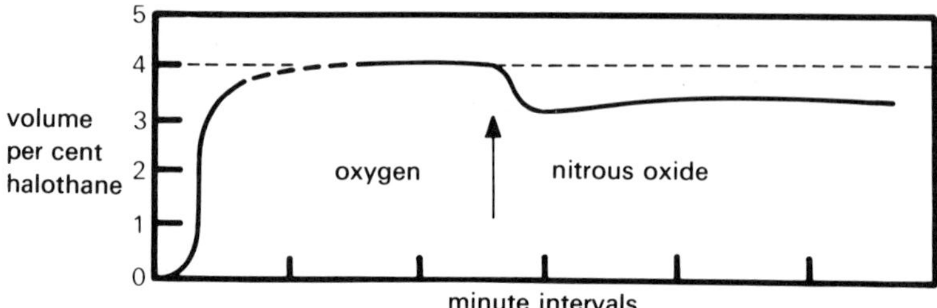

Fig. 3.26. Change in halothane output of a Tec Mk 3 vaporizer on changing the carrier gas from oxygen to nitrous oxide. Gas flow 5 1 min⁻¹. Dial set to 4 per cent. From (1984). *British Journal of Anaesthesia* **55**, 1025–38.

chamber and in some cases markedly modify the vaporizer output. The effect is most pronounced at low flows. Figure 3.27 depicts the results of an experiment by Scheller and Drummond, using an Ohio vaporizer with carrier gas flows of $3\,l\,min^{-1}$ in which the transient response has a maximum rise in output of enflurane from 1 per cent to over 2.5 per cent, and lasts for over 15 min. Such changes are of clinical importance.

The steady state response to changes in carrier gas composition is more controversial. Three factors, at least, are of immediate importance: density ρ, *dynamic* viscosity μ, and the ratio μ/ρ which is known as *kinematic* viscosity. When one carrier gas is exchanged for another of different composition the changes which may occur in these three parameters are of importance for the

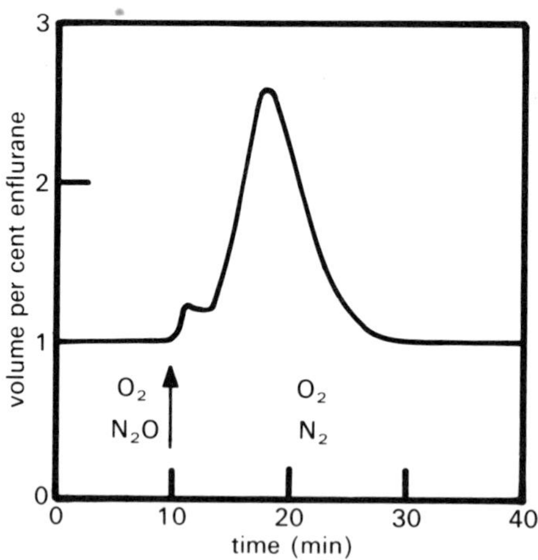

Fig. 3.27. Change in enflurane output of an Ohio vaporizer on changing the carrier gas from oxygen 30 per cent/nitrous oxide 70 per cent to oxygen 30 per cent/nitrogen 70 per cent. Gas flow $3\,l\,min^{-1}$. Dial set to 1 per cent. Temperature 21 °C. From Scheller, M. S. and Drummond, J. C. (1986). *Anesthesia and Analgesia* **65**, 88–90. (Reprinted with permission from the International Anesthesia Research Society.)

following reasons. Firstly, the resistance in regions of turbulent flow is a function of ρ (eqns (3.75) and (76)). Secondly, the resistance in regions of laminar flow is proportional to μ. Thirdly, the determinant of whether flow is more nearly turbulent or laminar is the Reynolds number which is proportional to μ/ρ (eqn (3.86)). In examining the change in splitting ratio accompanying the steady state response of a vaporizer to a change in carrier gas composition we therefore require the following approach. A change in μ/ρ must be calculated to estimate whether a transition may occur in the flow regime in either bypass or plenum chamber flow. Individual changes in the bypass and chamber resistances will then need to be estimated from the known changes in ρ and μ.

The clinical relevance of a knowledge of the steady state changes which occur with a change in gas composition, from 66 per cent nitrous oxide/34 per cent oxygen to 100 per cent oxygen, in three vaporizers can be gauged from Table 3.10.

Table 3.10. *Steady state changes in output of halothane from three vaporizers occurring during a change in carrier gas composition from 66 per cent nitrous oxide/34 per cent oxygen to 100 per cent oxygen. (Other parameters as for Fig. 3.25.)*

Vaporizer	Percentage change in output
Tec Mk 3	− 5
Vapor 19	− 1
Abingdon	− 15

From Synnott, A. and Wren, W. S. (1986). *British Journal of Anaesthesia* **58**, 1055–8. Note that there is considerable disagreement between authors in results of this kind, even using the same model of vaporizer.

Finally, it is appropriate to mention two further determinants of output. Intermittent back pressure may reverse plenum chamber flow and load the bypass with anaesthetic vapour, and tilting or inversion may load the bypass with liquid. A variety of cunning design features have been introduced to reduce these hazards.

3.10   Other forms of vaporizer

In 1978 a new anaesthetic delivery system was described which has been termed the Boston Anesthesia System. Mixtures of oxygen and nitrous oxide are produced by pulsed flow through sonic valves which give a fixed steady flow for the measured fraction of a second for which they remain open. Liquid anaesthetic is injected into the gas stream in metered volumes in much the same way as fuel injection is achieved in engines. The reliability and safety of such injection systems demands a high standard of microprocessor control.

In 1986 a somewhat simpler system, more reminiscent of a conventional carburettor, was shown to deliver predictable and accurate vapour concentrations in the clinical range. Figure 3.28 shows the prototype of a vaporizer now incorporated into a commercially available anaesthetic machine. In this device, a constant small volume (10 ml) of halothane is maintained in the

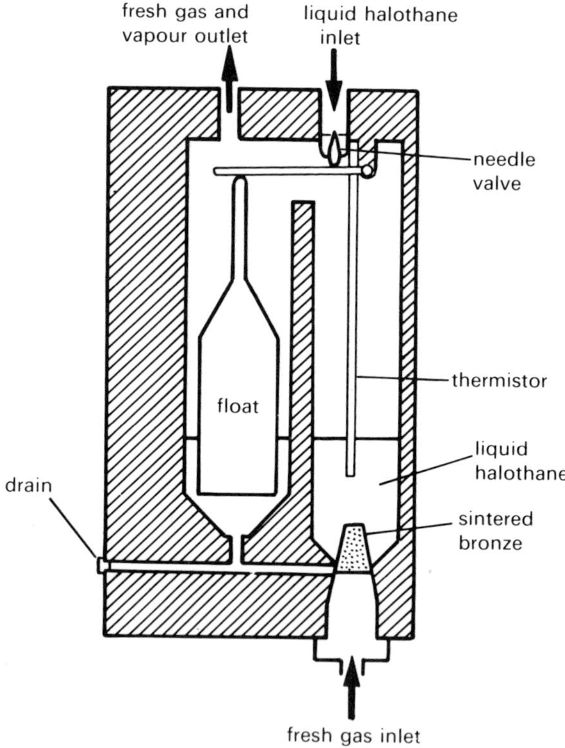

Fig. 3.28. The vaporization chamber of the halothane anaesthetic vaporizer described by Hahn, Palayiwa, Sugg and Lindsay-Scott (1986). *British Journal of Anaesthesia* **58**, 1161–6. The splitting ratio of the device is controlled using pulsed sonic valves by a microprocessor which is programmed to use the Antoine equation.

vaporizer by a float which activates a needle valve, through which the halothane is replenished. This small volume of liquid ensures that transient changes in output due to the solubility of nitrous oxide in halothane are kept to a minimum. Carrier gas is bubbled through the liquid to achieve a high degree of saturation. Temperature changes are dampened by manufacturing the device out of a thick cylindrical copper rod. Temperature is measured by a thermistor immersed in the liquid and this measurement is used to control the splitting ratio of the whole vaporization system. The microprocessor which controls the splitting ratio is programmed to use the saturated vapour pressure–temperature relationship of eqn (3.46) (the Antoine equation). It remains to be seen whether newer forms of vaporizer will make headway in replacing the traditional plenum vaporizer.

3.11 Vapour reception by the patient

Anaesthetics work by getting to the brain. Much of the rest of the body, however, particularly muscles and fat, acts as a huge sink capable of monopolizing most of the anaesthetic which gets taken up by the patient.

The rate at which an anaesthetic vapour or gas begins to be taken up from the alveoli into the blood perfusing the pulmonary capillaries is proportional to its alveolar partial pressure P_{AG} and the solubility it has in blood α. α is usually measured in ml of vapour (at STP) per ml of blood per bar of partial pressure. The greater the solubility of an anaesthetic, the more rapidly it will be soaked up from the alveoli by the blood and the lower will be its alveolar

Table 3.11. *Blood solubility α of nine inhalational anaesthetics. Also included is the product of α and the minimal alveolar concentration MAC (expressed as a percentage of atmospheric pressure).*

Agent	α (ml (STP) ml^{-1} bar^{-1})	$\alpha \times$ MAC
Nitrous oxide	0.41	42
Cyclopropane	0.48	4.5
Ether	10.6	20
Enflurane	1.7	2.8
Isoflurane	1.2	1.5
Halothane	2.1	1.6
Chloroform	7.0	3.5
Trichloroethylene	7.9	1.6
Methoxyflurane	9.7	1.6

Data from Stewart, A., Allott, P. R., Cowles, A. L. and Mapleson, W. W. (1973). *British Journal of Anaesthesia* **45**, 282–93; values derived from data pertaining to 37 °C.

partial pressure P_{AG} in comparison with its inspired partial pressure P_{IG}. The wide range of blood solubilities of the nine agents discussed earlier is shown in Table 3.11.

We can illustrate this influence of blood solubility by recalling Fig. 1.4, which depicts the entry with inspiration of a bolus of gas (volume V) into the alveolus and the exit with expiration of a corresponding bolus (volume V') of alveolar gas. Our model allowed for the uptake by the blood of a fraction ϕ of the volume V. For alveolar gas we thus have

$$\frac{P_{AG}}{P_{atm}} = \left(\frac{P_{IG}}{P_{atm}} - \phi\right)\frac{V}{V'}. \tag{3.92}$$

Assuming for a first approximation that $R = 1$ in eqn (1.15) we find $V' = V(1 - \phi)$ and write

$$\frac{P_{AG}}{P_{atm}} = \frac{(P_{IG}/P_{atm} - \phi)}{(1 - \phi)},$$

or

$$\frac{P_{IG} - P_{AG}}{P_{atm} - P_{AG}} = \phi. \tag{3.93}$$

ϕ is proportional to α and also a function of P_{AG}. During the early stages of an anaesthetic (induction) blood returning to the lungs will contain little anaesthetic and we may expect ϕ to be proportional to P_{AG}. Set $\phi = k\alpha P_{AG}$ and obtain

$$\frac{(P_{IG}/P_{AG} - 1)}{(P_{atm} - P_{AG})} = k\alpha. \tag{3.94}$$

For both the induction and subsequent hypothetical course of anaesthesia over hours, days and weeks, Mapleson used an extension of this reasoning to model the relationship between P_{AG} and a constant P_{IG} for a range of anaesthetics. Figure 3.29 shows the results of his analysis, which demonstrates that equilibrium can be approached in around one hour with insoluble agents such as nitrous oxide, but may not be reached even within a week with less soluble agents such as methoxyflurane! For all vapours $P_{IG}/P_{AG} \gg 1$ at induction. Since P_{atm} usually greatly exceeds P_{AG} it follows that eqn (3.94) may be approximated by

$$P_{IG}/P_{AG} \simeq kP_{atm}\alpha. \tag{3.95}$$

Now the brain is known rapidly to equilibrate with alveolar gas, so P_{AG} will need to approximate MAC (expressed in units of partial pressure) for anaesthesia to be attained. Equation (3.95) suggests that to achieve this P_{IG} will need to exceed MAC according to

$$P_{IG}/\text{MAC} \simeq kP_{atm}\alpha. \tag{3.96}$$

There is reason to believe that k will be similar for all agents. The anaesthetic

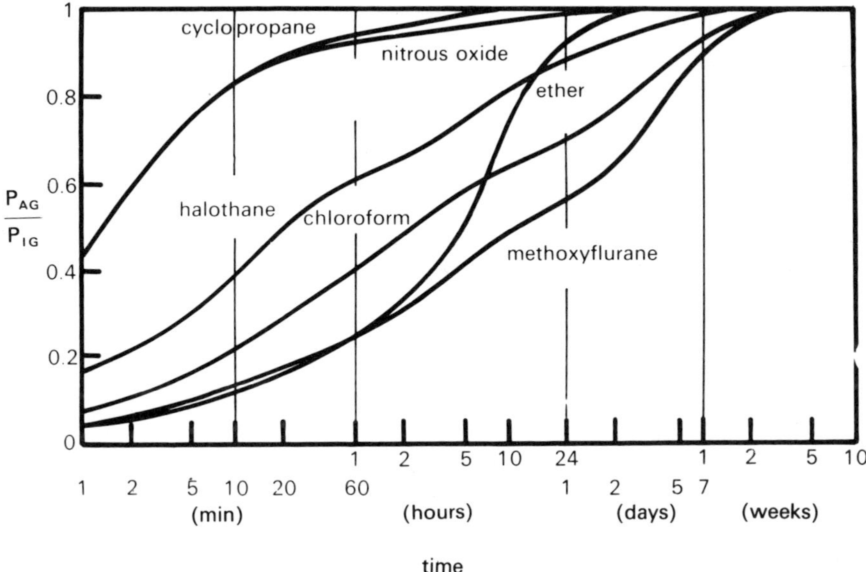

Fig. 3.29. The approach of alveolar partial pressure of anaesthetic P_{AG} towards a constant inspired partial pressure P_{IG} for six inhalated anaesthetics. These curves were derived by Mapleson from a model accounting for uptake of anaesthetic into several distinct body compartments: fat, muscle, and so on. The model does not allow for metabolic elimination of the anaesthetics, and thus tends to overpredict values of P_{AG}. From Chenoweth, M. B. (ed.) (1972). *Modern Inhalational Anesthetics*, p. 334. Springer-Verlag, Berlin.

requirement for induction thus simplifies to

$$P_{IG} \propto \alpha \text{MAC}. \tag{3.97}$$

Simply stated, to attain a brain partial pressure sufficient for anaesthesia (MAC) within a few minutes of commencing administration of a vapour, it is necessary to administer a vapour partial pressure (P_{IG}) much greater than MAC. To a first approximation this P_{IG} is proportional to α. For the highly soluble methoxyflurane, Mapleson used his model to compute the way in which it would necessary to vary P_{IG} during a very long anaesthetic to achieve a brain partial pressure of MAC within 10 min and then to maintain it constant thereafter. Figure 3.30 shows the result. P_{IG}/MAC equals 10 for the first 10 min, thereafter is lowered to about 4.5, but closely approaches 1 only after a week.

3.12 Thermodynamic difficulty of generating anaesthetic vapours for induction and maintenance of anaesthesia

Equation (3.5) provided us with a measure of the volume ΔV of an anaesthetic vapour at pressure p_{sat} which is required to provide a volume V of gas

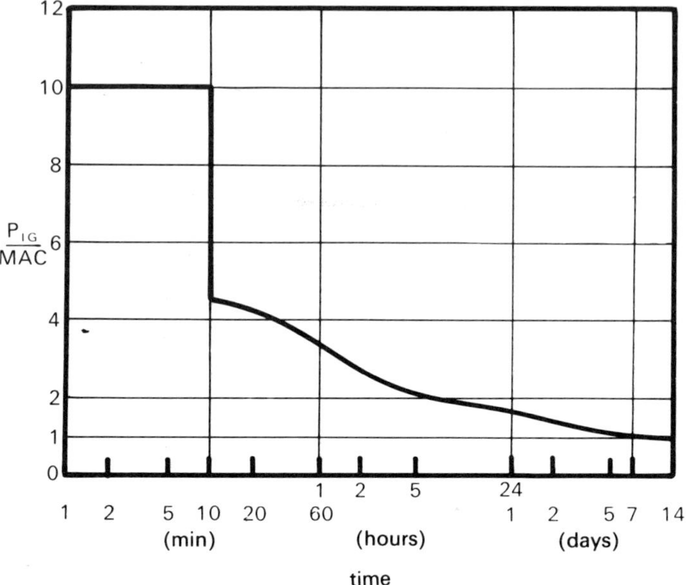

Fig. 3.30. The way in which the inspired partial pressure of methoxyflurane P_{IG} needs to be varied with time in order to achieve a brain tension of MAC (in pressure units) in 10 min and then to maintain it constant. The curve was derived by Mapleson using the same model as for Fig. 3.29. From Chenoweth, M. B. (ed.) (1972). *Modern Inhalational Anesthetics*, p. 336. Springer-Verlag, Berlin.

containing a minimal alveolar concentration of the vapour:

$$\left(\frac{\Delta V}{V}\right)_{\text{MAC}} = \left(\frac{\text{MAC}}{p_{\text{sat}}}\right)\left(\frac{P_{\text{atm}}}{100}\right). \tag{3.5}$$

We used this equation to compare agents in Fig. 3.4 with regard to the difficulty which might be experienced in generating the necessary $(\Delta V/V)_{\text{MAC}}$ for maintaining anaesthesia.

In an assessment of the practical difficulty of vaporizing anaesthetic agents the need to supply heat to the plenum chamber is likely to be of greater importance than the volume of agent required in unit time. Let ΔV be the volume of anaesthetic vapour generated at pressure p_{sat} in unit time for production of a mixture at MAC. The corresponding mass of vapour equals $m_2 - m_1$ in eqn (3.62). Replace $K(T_0 - T)$ in that equation by Q_{MAC}, set $m_1 c_{\text{p}}(T - T_0) = 0$ and $\Delta T = 0$ to get

$$Q_{\text{MAC}} = (m_2 - m_1)h_{\text{fg}}. \tag{3.98}$$

The ideal gas equation (eqn 3.40) relates ΔV to $(m_2 - m_1)$:

$$(m_2 - m_1) = \frac{p_{sat}\,\Delta V}{R_{kg}\,T_0}.$$

(3.99)

Since $R_{kg} = R_{mol}/M_{vap}$ eqn (3.98) can now be written

$$Q_{MAC} = \left(\frac{p_{sat}\,h_{fg}\,M_{vap}}{R_{mol}\,T_0}\right)\Delta V.$$

(3.100)

With eqn (3.5) this becomes

$$Q_{MAC} = \left(\frac{p_{sat}\,h_{fg}\,M_{vap}}{R_{mol}\,T_0}\right)\left(\frac{MAC}{p_{sat}}\right)\left(\frac{P_{atm}}{100}\right)V$$

$$= h_{fg}\,M_{vap}\,MAC\left(\frac{P_{atm}\,V}{R_{mol}\,T_0\,100}\right).$$

(3.101)

V is here the volume of gas–vapour mixture generated in unit time.

The bracketed term in eqn (3.101) may be regarded as constant. Different agents can now be compared with regard to the heat required per unit time to generate a mixture of potency 1 MAC, by listing the product $h_{fg}\,M_{vap}\,MAC$

Table 3.12. *League tables for difficulty in vaporizing anaesthetic agents during induction and maintenance of anaesthesia from a thermodynamic point of view is given by the magnitudes of the products* $\alpha h_{fg}\,M_{vap}\,MAC$ *and* $h_{fg}\,M_{vap}\,MAC$ *respectively. Constituent data from Tables 3.1, 3.4, 3.6 and 3.11.*

Agent	$\alpha h_{fg}\,M_{vap}\,MAC$ (order re-induction)	$h_{fg}\,M_{vap}\,MAC$ (order re-maintenance)
Ether	575 000 (1)	54 200 (2)
Enflurane	93 800 (3)	55 200 (1)
Isoflurane	40 600 (7)	33 900 (3)
Halothane	46 900 (6)	22 300 (4)
Chloroform	103 000 (2)	14 700 (5)
Trichloroethylene	49 600 (5)	6280 (6)
Methoxyflurane	52 500 (4)	5410 (7)

as in Table 3.12. Enflurane and ether come out worst; trichloroethylene and methoxyflurane are best.

In the previous section we saw that the demands of induction of anaesthesia differ from those of maintenance of anaesthesia. The partial pressure of anaesthetic vapour needed early on during induction is approximately proportional to αMAC (eqn (3.97)) rather than MAC. The relevant heat flow requirement becomes proportional to $\alpha h_{fg} M_{vap}$ MAC, which is also tabulated in Table 3.12. With regard to induction, ether comes out to be far more difficult to vaporize than any other agent. Isoflurane, halothane, trichloroethylene and methoxyflurane all have similar relatively favourable heat flow requirements.

Problems

3.1   A plenum vaporizer is supplied with $10\,l\,min^{-1}$ of a carrier gas mixture of 50 per cent oxygen–50 per cent nitrogen at 17°C. The plenum chamber contains isoflurane. When delivering 2 per cent isoflurane the steady state temperature of the liquid isoflurane is found to be 13.5°C.

Use the Antoine equation for isoflurane to estimate the saturation pressure in the plenum chamber. Calculate the splitting ratio at this setting. What is the specific heat capacity of the carrier gas?

A new setting is made on the vaporizer dial and the steady state liquid temperature becomes 10°C. By assuming that the heat transfer coefficient K for the delivery of heat to the liquid remains constant, and that ambient conditions are unchanged, estimate the new percentage output from the device.

3.2   A plenum vaporizer contains $200\,ml$ of liquid enflurane at 20°C which has become contaminated by nitrous oxide during delivery of 1 per cent enflurane in a mixture of 30 per cent oxygen–70 per cent nitrous oxide flowing at $5\,l\,min^{-1}$.

The carrier gas composition is changed abruptly to 100 per cent oxygen. The dissolved nitrous oxide is discharged over the subsequent 10 min. Estimate the percentage change in output concentration of enflurane from the vaporizer assuming that the contaminating nitrous oxide is discharged at a constant rate, that the solubility of 100 per cent nitrous oxide in enflurane is $5\,ml\,(STP)\,ml^{-1}$, and that the splitting ratio remains constant.

3.3   The enthalpy of vaporization for ether can be approximated over the range -20 to $+30$°C by the equation

$$h_{fg} = a - b(T - T_0).$$

Show that the Clausius–Clapeyron equation in this case predicts a relationship of the form (Dupré's equation):

$$p_{sat} = p_0\, T^{(-b/R_{kg})} \exp\left(-\frac{(a + bT_0)}{R_{kg}\,T}\right).$$

Assuming that this equation and the Antoine equation (parameters in Table 3.2) agree at $T_0 = 293.15\,\text{K}$ (20 °C), calculate p_0 by taking $a = 385\,\text{kJ}\,\text{kg}^{-1}$ and $b = 0.398\,\text{kJ}\,\text{kg}^{-1}\,\text{K}^{-1}$.

Examine the deviation of the above equation from the Antoine equation at 313.15 K (40 °C) and 253.15 K (-20 °C), and suggest why it coincides less accurately with measured values of p_{sat} (Fig. 3.6) despite modelling measured values of h_{fg} more precisely (Fig. 3.5).

Further reading

Antoine, C. (1888). Tensions des vapeurs: nouvelle relation entre les tensions et les températures. *Compte Rendus des Seance de l'Academie des Sciences* **107**, 681–4.

Cooper, J. B., Newbower, R. S., Moore, J. W. and Trautman, E. D. (1978). A new anesthesia delivery system. *Anesthesiology* **49**, 310–18. (Boston Anesthesia System.)

Dorrington, K. L. (1985). Splitting ratio. *Anaesthesia* **40**, 704–5.

Dorsch, J. A. and Dorsch, S. E. (1984). *Understanding Anesthesia Equipment* (2nd edn). Williams and Wilkins, Baltimore, Maryland.

Gould, D. B., Lampert, B. A. and MacKrell, T. N. (1982). Effect of nitrous oxide solubility on vaporizer aberrance. *Anaesthesia and Analgesia* **61**, 938–40.

Leigh, J. M. (1985). Variations on a theme: splitting ratio. *Anaesthesia* **40**, 70–2.

Lin, C-Y. (1980). Assessment of vaporizer performance in low-flow and closed-circuit anaesthesia. *Anaesthesia and Analgesia* **59**, 359–66.

Nawaf, K. and Stoelting, R. K. (1979). Nitrous oxide increases enflurane concentrations delivered by Ethrane vaporizers. *Anesthesia and Analgesia* **58**, 30–2.

Petty, C. (1987). *The Anesthesia Machine*. Churchill Livingstone, New York.

Prins, L., Strupat, J., Clement, J. and Hill, R. L. (1980). An evaluation of gas density dependence of anaesthetic vaporizers. *Canadian Anaesthetists' Society Journal* **27**, 106–110.

Schlichting, H. (1960). *Boundary Layer Theory* (4th edn). McGraw-Hill, New York (Turbulent and laminar flow.)

Schreiber, P. (1972). *Anaesthesia Equipment*. Springer-Verlag, Berlin.

Ward, C. S. (1985). *Anaesthetic Equipment* (2nd edn). Baillière Tindall, London.

4 Mechanical ventilation of the lungs

4.1 Introduction

Anaesthesia permitted massive advances in surgery from the 1840s. With the introduction of asepsis (elimination of contaminating micro-organisms) in the 1880s, surgery within the abdomen became relatively free from the hazard of infection for the first time. Extension to surgery within the chest encountered a problem which was only to be solved around the turn of the century by the introduction of mechanical ventilation of the lungs.

Normal breathing requires an intact chest wall (Fig. 4.1). Air is drawn into the lungs during inspiration by the downward movement of the muscular diaphragm, which separates the chest from the abdomen, and by the expansion of the chest volume which results from hingeing movements of the ribs. This is achieved even though the lungs are not adherent to the inside of the chest wall. Between the outer lining of the lung and the closely applied inner lining of the chest wall lies a potential space known as the pleural cavity. At rest (at the end of a normal expiration, Fig. 4.1(a)) the average pressure within this cavity is approximately 5 cm H_2O below atmospheric. The pressure is subatmospheric on account of the elastic tendency of the lung to recoil away from the chest wall. During an inspiration (Fig. 4.1(b)) the movements of the diaphragm and rib cage generate an even lower pressure in the pleural cavity, around 10 cm H_2O below atmospheric. In the presence of any disruption in the integrity of the chest wall this mechanism of breathing is compromised (Fig. 4.1(c)). The lung on the affected side collapses under the recoil of its elastic components and ceases to function. The maintenance of breathing is further embarrassed by the shift of midline structures in the chest (the heart, oesophagus, and so on) towards the intact side of the chest, thereby reducing the effectiveness of the lung which has not collapsed. Early operations within the chest, even in anaesthetized patients, were a race against asphyxia from this phenomenon of 'pneumothorax'.

In 1896 the French surgeons Tuffier and Hallion published a description of operations inside the chest of dogs, achieved by rhythmic insufflation of the lungs through a tube passed through the mouth into the trachea. This kind of artificial ventilation (Fig. 4.2(a)) had apparently been widely known among surgeons since the seventeenth century as a means of keeping animals alive, but only slowly became adopted around the turn of this century for use with patients because of the difficulty surgeons experienced in intubating the trachea.

The difficulty of tracheal intubation meant that other attempts to overcome the pneumothorax problem attained a vogue in the early years of this

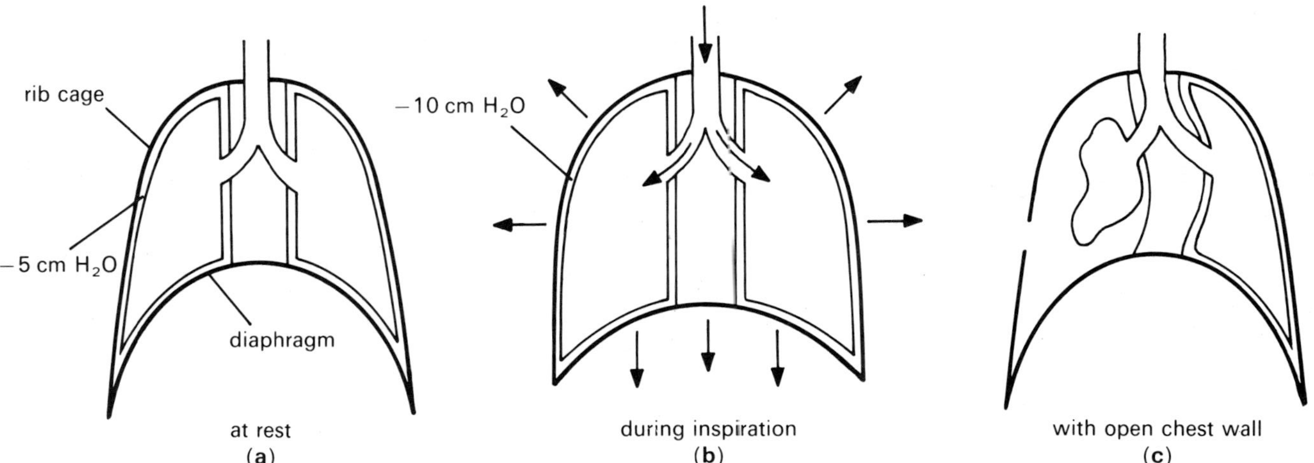

Fig. 4.1. Normal mechanical function of the lungs and the phenomenon of pneumothorax: (a) at rest, a subatmospheric pressure in the pleural cavity holds the lungs expanded against the chest wall; (b) during inspiration the chest volume increases and the pressure in the pleural cavity becomes more subatmospheric; (c) breathing is compromised by a leak in the chest wall.

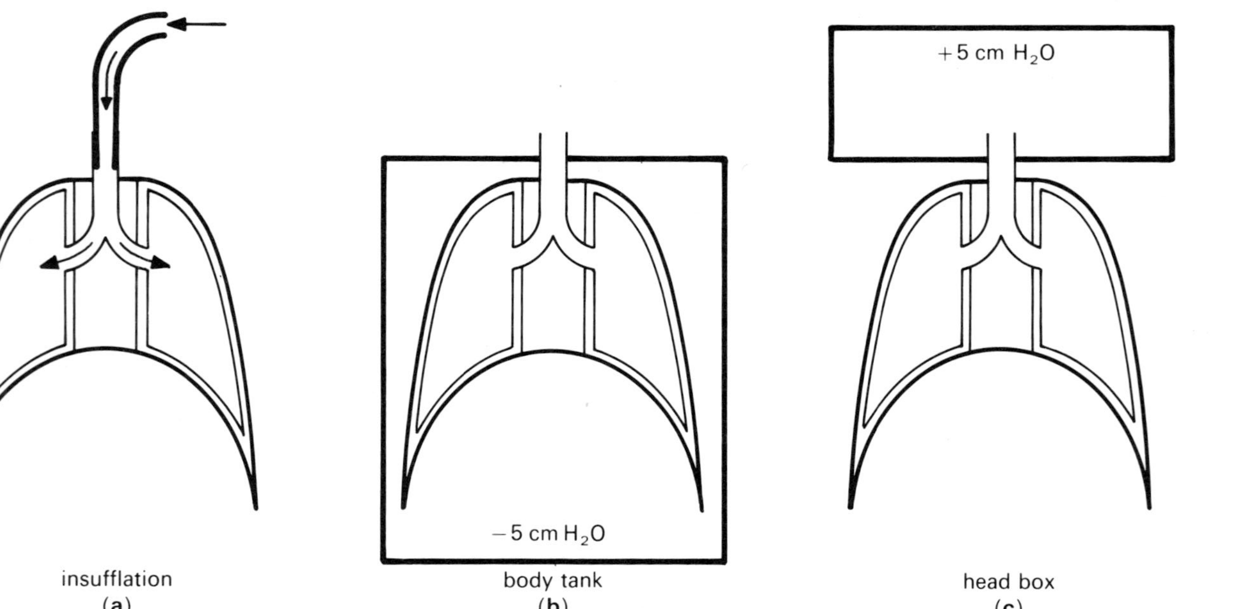

Fig. 4.2. Solutions to the pneumothorax problem: (a) insufflation of gas into the lungs via an endotracheal tube; (b) subatmospheric ('negative') pressure chamber surrounding the patient's trunk; (c) 'positive' pressure chamber surrounding the patient's head.

century. In 1904 Sauerbruch introduced the use of a large 'negative' (sub-atmospheric) pressure chamber in which the whole of the patient's body was contained (along with the surgeon performing the operation), except the head which lay outside exposed to normal atmospheric pressure. This arrangement is depicted diagrammatically in Fig. 4.2(b). With the large chamber held at a constant negative pressure the tendency for collapse of an exposed lung could certainly be reduced, but survival depended upon normal respiratory movements of the lung in the intact side of the chest.

It was in the very different context of respiratory insufficiency due to poliomyelitis (which affects the nerves which activate the muscles of breathing) that a negative pressure chamber proved to be a highly effective means of artificial ventilation. The 'iron lung' or tank ventilator was much smaller than the room-sized chamber devised by Sauerbruch, sufficient only to contain the patient's body from the neck down. Unlike the latter it was evacuated rhythmically at a normal respiratory rate yielding pressures of up to 60 cm H_2O below atmospheric. In 1938 Lord Nuffield, the great engineer philanthropist, turned over part of his motor-car factory in Cowley, Oxford, to the production of tank ventilators and donated one on request to any hospital in the British Commonwealth. These ventilators still find occasional use today in patients requiring intermittent assistance with their breathing because of neuromuscular weakness.

Another early means of overcoming the pneumothorax problem during surgery within the chest was the application of a 'positive' pressure to a small chamber which contained only the patient's head, and utilized an airtight seal around the neck. Such an arrangement is depicted in Fig. 4.2(c). An apparatus of this kind using a hand-operated compressor was introduced by Brauer in 1905. As with the Sauerbruch negative pressure chamber, this device merely applied constant pressure rather than the rhythmic assistance which is required to take over from normal breathing. It would, however, have similarly assisted respiratory movements of the lung in the intact side of the chest whilst a thoracotomy was performed on the opposite side. As an alternative to a whole-head chamber a well-fitting mask also came to be used to apply positive pressure to the lungs, either constantly or rhythmically, without the need for tracheal intubation. Most of these various techniques continue to have applications in respiratory intensive care and anaesthesia for surgery, but currently by far the most prominent form of mechanical ventilation of the lungs is via a tube passed into the trachea by direct vision, using a laryngoscope.

Two developments had a profound influence on the widespread acceptance of mechanical ventilators in the middle years of this century: the introduction of curare into anaesthetic practice in 1942, and the catastrophic epidemic of poliomyelitis in Copenhagen in 1952.

Curare had been known since the sixteenth century as an arrow poison used by South American Indians. By 1850 its mode of action had become understood as a reversible inhibitor of the transmission of nerve impulses arriving at muscle cells. Over the next hundred years it found occasional use in experimental pharmacology, the treatment of tetanus and convulsions, and even during abdominal surgery, but its modern widespread application to anaesthesia dates from its use in Montreal in 1942. It rapidly became apparent that paralysis facilitated the use of much lighter levels of anaesthesia than would otherwise have been possible, and achieved the additional benefit of eliminating the muscle tone which hampers surgery, particularly in the abdomen. The prerequisite of the use of paralysis is of course the provision of adequate artificial ventilation of the lungs, be it driven by hand or automatically by machine.

If curare orchestrated the frequent use of mechanical ventilation of the lungs during anaethesia, poliomyelitis demonstrated the need for automation. So large was the number of victims of this disease in Copenhagen in 1952 that the manpower required to ventilate patients by hand occupied 1400 university students, almost the entire student body. The prospect of similar epidemics elsewhere in Europe stimulated engineering design and production of the family of ventilators which now seems an indispensible part of modern hospital medicine.

4.2   Manually controlled ventilation using anaesthetic breathing systems with a single pressure-release valve

The early use of mechanical ventilation during anaesthesia was often a form of 'assisted' ventilation during which the anaesthetist squeezed the reservoir bag of the breathing system in time with the patient's own breathing, to promote more rapid uptake of anaesthetic vapour and speed the process of induction. The situation frequently arises in current anaesthetic practice (for example, after temporary paralysis to aid intubation of the trachea) in which one of the rebreathing systems in Fig. 2.26 is used for artificial ventilation by hand. In this chapter we examine the rebreathing characteristics of the Mapleson A, B, C, D, and F systems. These are the rebreathing systems incorporating a one-way valve.

In contrast to our assessment in chapter 2 of the performance of these systems during spontaneous ventilation, here we shall assume that gas leaves the breathing system only during inspiration rather than during expiration. The reason for this is as follows: during manually controlled ventilation the operator generates an inspiratory flow by manually squeezing the reservoir bag. To prevent loss of most of the gas from the system via the expiratory valve it is necessary to increase resistance to flow through the valve by tightening the valve mechanism. Some inspiratory flow is then directed into the patient whilst some passes through the valve. During expiration it is

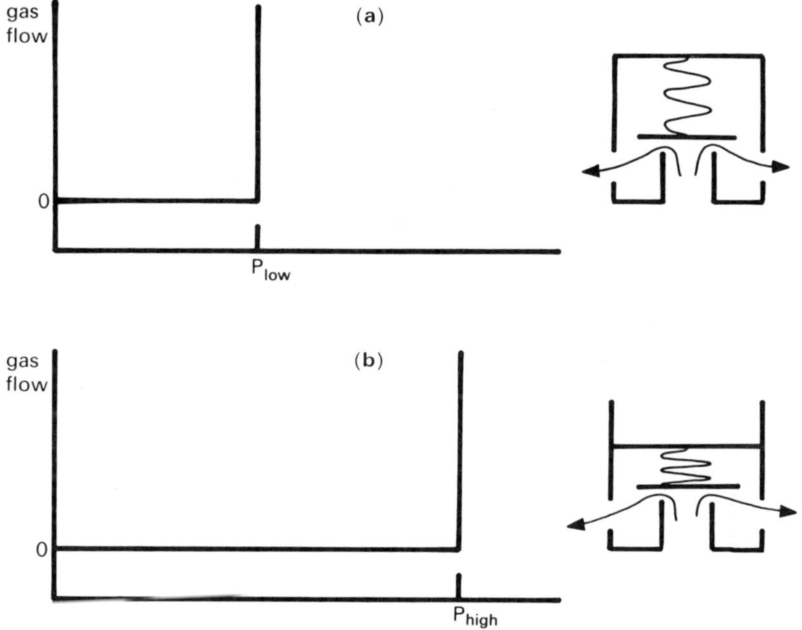

Fig. 4.3. The ideal of a constant pressure generating valve. At all pressures below some threshold no flow occurs; at the threshold any flow is available. The pressure threshold is low when the spring is slack (a) and high when the spring is compressed (b). Practical valves approximate to this behaviour over a limited range of gas flow.

desirable for there to be minimal resistance to expiratory flow and it is desirable for a sufficient capacity within the reservoir bag to permit all expiratory gas to enter the system, not to be forced to pass through the expiratory valve.

Expiratory valves commonly approximate to constant pressure generators (Fig. 4.3) through which zero flow occurs until a pressure threshold is reached, at which any flow can proceed through the valve. This pressure threshold is varied by screwing down, to a variable degree, the spring which is applied to the valve disc. The technique of assisted ventilation requires the operator to adjust the valve to a constant setting such that the volume of gas leaking through the valve during inspiration is just equal to the volume of gas entering the system during one ventilatory cycle. We now apply these considerations to the individual systems.

4.3   Controlled ventilation with Mapleson A (Magill, Lack) systems

The Mapleson A systems are depicted in Figs. 2.22, 2.26 and 4.4. Before the beginning of an inspiration the patient-end of the breathing system, including

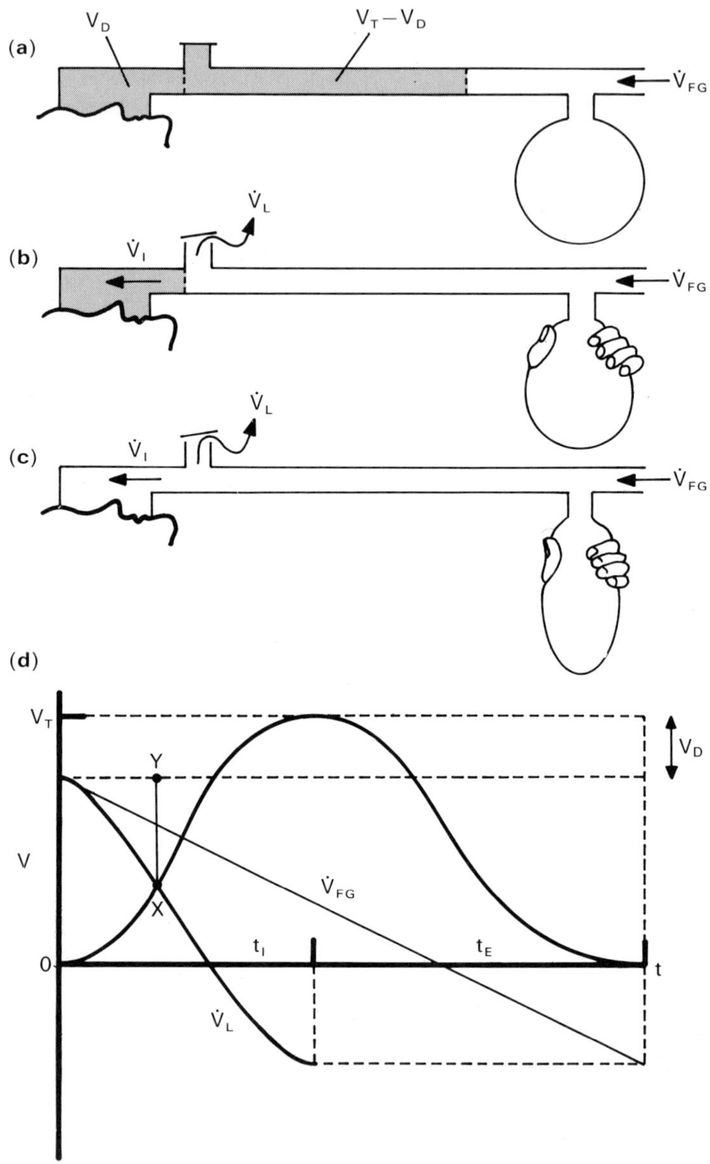

Fig. 4.4. Rebreathing properties of the Mapleson A system during controlled ventilation. (a) Immediately prior to inspiration (inflation); (b) reservoir tube just cleared of CO_2-containing gas (point X during inspiration in Fig. 4(d)); (c) late inspiration; (d) the respiratory waveform with a construction depicting the constant fresh gas flow $\dot{V}_{FG}$ and the leak flow $\dot{V}_L$ through the valve. XY is the volume of fresh gas reaching the alveoli.

the dead space, contains a volume V_T of gas derived from the alveoli during the previous expiration. This volume contains some CO_2.

Inspiration is assisted by manual squeezing of the reservoir bag, which generates a leak flow $\dot{V}_L$ through the expiratory valve (Fig. 4.4(b)). $\dot{V}_L$ may vary as inspiration proceeds. In Fig. 4.4(d) the leakage of gas through the expiratory valve is depicted by a curve labelled $\dot{V}_L$ on a V–t plot of the respiratory waveform. The magnitude of the gradient of this line at any time equals the flow $\dot{V}_L$. Note the following features of the line. Firstly, it is present only for the duration t_1 of inspiration. Secondly, its vertical height equals the vertical height of the straight line labelled $\dot{V}_{FG}$, the gradient of which gives the flow of fresh gas which enters the system through the whole respiratory cycle. The reason for this is that the volume of gas which leaks from the valve during inspiration must equal the volume of fresh gas which enters the system during both inspiration and expiration (assuming that the patient breathes out the same volume of gas he breathes in).

No gas devoid of CO_2 enters the equipment dead space until a volume $V_T - V_D$ of CO_2-containing gas leaves the reservoir tube, either via the valve or into the equipment dead space (Fig. 4.4(a)). The moment at which this occurs is represented on the V–t plot by the point X where the leak volume line crosses the inspiratory limb of the respiratory waveform. At X the inspired volume and the leaked volume sum to $V_T - V_D$. As inspiration proceeds after X only fresh gas enters the equipment dead space *en route* to the alveoli (Fig. 4.4(c)). It follows that the line XY in Fig. 4.4(d) gives the volume of fresh gas entering the alveoli during assisted ventilation with the Mapleson A system.

To recap: inspiration necessarily involves rebreathing a volume V_D of CO_2-containing gas into the alveoli plus a proportion of the volume $V_T - V_D$ which entered the reservoir tube during the preceding expiration. Line XY in Fig. 4.4(d) represents the volume of this bolus which is forced out of the expiratory valve and consequently the volume of fresh gas reaching the alveoli during inspiration.

Figure 4.5 represents the case of the idealized respiratory waveform which consists of constant inspiratory and expiratory flows together with an assumed constant leak flow. Again assuming that the total volume leaked by the valve during inspiration equals the total volume of fresh gas delivered throughout the cycle, we have

$$\dot{V}_L t_1 = \dot{V}_{FG}(t_1 + t_E)$$

or

$$\dot{V}_1 = \dot{V}_{FG}(1 + t_E/t_1). \tag{4.1}$$

If X lies at a time τ into inspiration, then τ is the time required for flows $\dot{V}_L$ and $\dot{V}_I$ to empty a volume $V_T - V_D$ of CO_2-containing gas from the reservoir

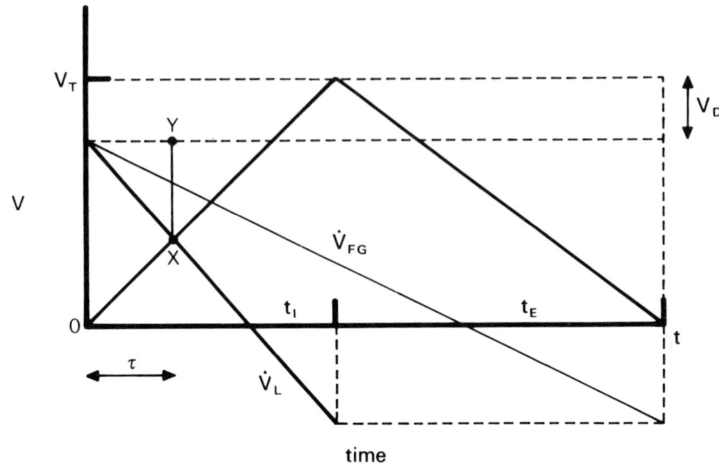

Fig. 4.5. The equivalent construction to Fig. 4.4(d) for the idealized respiratory waveform that consists of constant inspiratory and expiratory flows.

tube:

$$\tau = (V_T - V_D)/(\dot{V}_L + \dot{V}_I). \tag{4.2}$$

The volume of gas depicted by line XY in Fig. 4.5 equals the volume leaving the valve in time τ:

$$V_{XY} = \dot{V}_L \tau. \tag{4.3}$$

Substituting from eqns (4.1) and (4.2) into (4.3) we obtain the volume of fresh gas reaching the alveoli:

$$V_{XY} = (V_T - V_D)/\{1 + \dot{V}_I/[\dot{V}_{FG}(1 + t_E/t_I)]\}. \tag{4.4}$$

The result is more succinctly stated in terms of the ventilation $\dot{V}$ $(= \dot{V}_I/(1 + t_E/t_I);$ eqn 2.9) as

$$V_{XY} = (V_T - V_D)/(1 + \dot{V}/\dot{V}_{FG}). \tag{4.5}$$

The fraction of fresh gas in the breath is thus

$$F_{IFG} = V_{XY}/V_T$$
$$= (1 - V_D/V_T)/(1 + \dot{V}/\dot{V}_{FG}). \tag{4.6}$$

The concepts of rebreathing index ($\dot{V}/\dot{V}_0$) and CO_2 retention index (F'_{ECO_2}/F_{ECO_2}), introduced in chapter 2 in relation to spontaneous ventilation, remain pertinent to the behaviour of breathing systems during controlled ventilation. Recall that the rebreathing index is the ratio of the ventilation $\dot{V}$ required at a given fresh gas flow to the ventilation $\dot{V}_0$ at a very high fresh gas flow, such that in both cases the F_{ECO_2} is identical. Inspired and expired fractions of CO_2 have been related by eqns (2.16) and (2.62). They combine with eqn (4.6) to yield the result

$$\frac{\dot{V}}{\dot{V}_0} = \frac{1}{[1 - (\dot{V}_0/\dot{V}_{\text{FG}})(1 - V_{\text{D}}/V_{\text{T0}})]},\qquad (4.7)$$

where V_{T0} is the tidal volume at ventilation $\dot{V}_0$. As for derivations of rebreathing index in chapter 2, we have here assumed that the respiratory rate is constant throughout ($\dot{V}/\dot{V}_0 = V_{\text{T}}/V_{\text{T0}}$). Equation 4.7 is plotted in Fig. 4.6. This provides a striking comparison with the performance of the system during spontaneous ventilation shown in Fig. 2.24. The efficiency of the system during spontaneous ventilation contrasts with its inefficiency

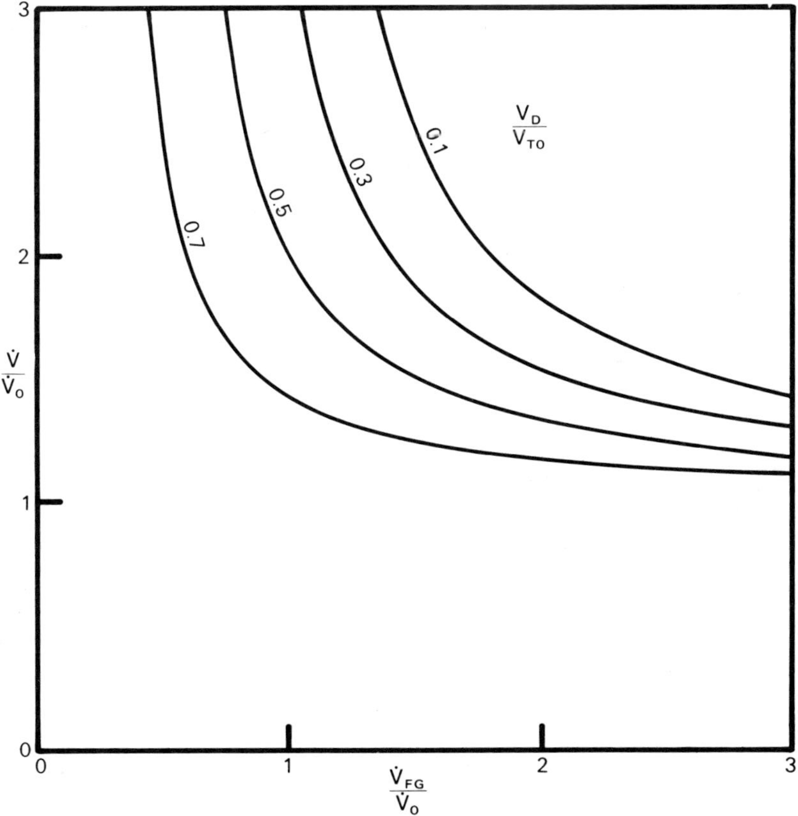

Fig. 4.6. The rebreathing index for the Mapleson A (Magill, Lack) system during controlled ventilation, plotted for different values of the relative dead space $V_{\text{D}}/V_{\text{T0}}$. Constant $\dot{V}_{\text{I}}$ and $\dot{V}_{\text{E}}$ assumed; $t_{\text{E}}/t_{\text{I}}$ may take any value; respiratory rate assumed constant.

during controlled ventilation, when fresh gas flows around $3\dot{V}_0$ are needed to bring the rebreathing index to around 1.3 for moderate dead space volumes ($V_D/V_{T0} \simeq 0.3$).

Recall that the CO_2 retention index is the ratio of the fraction of CO_2 in the expired breath F'_{ECO_2} at a given fresh gas flow to the fraction of CO_2 in the expired breath F_{ECO_2} at a very high fresh gas flow, such that in both cases the ventilation $\dot{V}_0$ is identical. We again make use of the relationship between inspired and expired fractions of CO_2 given in eqns (2.16) and (2.62). Combining these with eqn (4.6) we find the result

$$\frac{F'_{ECO_2}}{F_{ECO_2}} = \frac{1}{(1 + \dot{V}_0/\dot{V}_{FG})}. \tag{4.8}$$

Equation 4.8 is plotted in Fig. 4.7, which presents a different aspect of the

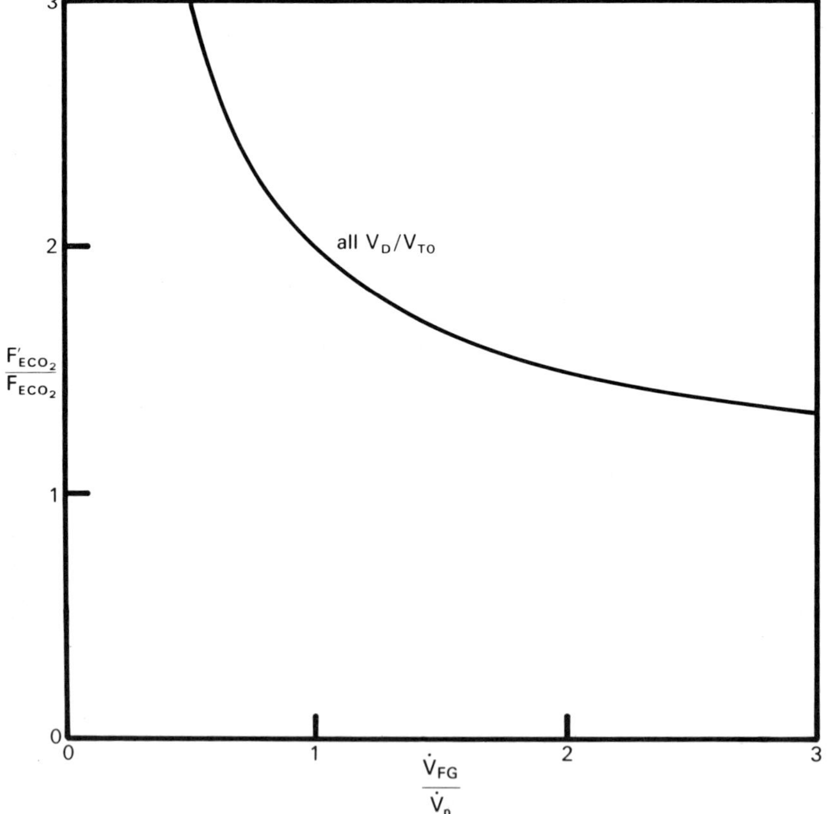

Fig. 4.7. The CO_2 retention index for the Mapleson A (Magill, Lack) system during controlled ventilation. V_D/V_{T0} and t_E/t_I may take any value. Constant $\dot{V}_I$ and $\dot{V}_E$ assumed.

inefficiency during assisted ventilation which we have already noticed in Fig. 4.6. Even at a fresh gas flow three times the ventilation ($\dot{V}_{FG}/\dot{V}_0 = 3$) the expired CO_2 fraction remains 33 per cent raised above the asymptotic value to which it tends as $\dot{V}_{FG} \rightarrow \infty$. Figure 4.7 differs markedly from the CO_2 retention index observed during spontaneous ventilation (Fig. 2.25). In particular note that the plot is independent of V_D/V_{T0} during assisted ventilation, but dependent on V_D/V_{T0} during spontaneous ventilation.

We conclude that the Mapleson A system is not well suited to controlled ventilation on account of the marked rebreathing, even at high fresh gas flows. A modification to the system which overcomes this limitation (the Miller system) is described later in this chapter.

4.4 Controlled ventilation with the Mapleson B and C systems

The Mapleson B and C systems are depicted in Fig. 2.26. The C system is repeated in Fig. 4.8 with one important modification to make it suitable for controlled ventilation: the fresh gas entry port still lies immediately adjacent to the valve, but it is closer to the patient than the valve. This arrangement avoids the excessive spillage of fresh gas which would occur if the valve were closer to the patient than the fresh gas entry port. For spontaneous breathing the relative positions of these components is unimportant.

Consider first the behaviour of the C system during controlled ventilation (Fig. 4.8). Immediately before the beginning of inspiration the system dead space contains gas breathed out of the alveoli during the previous expiration (Fig. 4.8(a)). Fresh gas flows into the reservoir bag and mixes with gas already present in the bag, some of which is presumed to be CO_2.

Inspiration is achieved by manual squeezing of the reservoir bag which generates a leak flow through the valve. The first gas to reach the patient's alveoli will be the volume V_D of dead space gas. As this begins to flow into the alveoli the initial flow into the dead space region will be fresh gas only. The inspiratory flow is initially less than the fresh gas flow (Fig. 4.8(b)) and some fresh gas flow spills from the valve together with gas from the bag. When the gradient of the V–t respiratory waveform reaches $\dot{V}_{FG}$, as at point A in Fig. 4.8(i), all fresh gas is directed towards the patient (Fig. 4.8(c)). After this moment inspiratory flow exceeds fresh gas flow and some gas from the reservoir bag is directed towards the patient (Fig. 4.8(d)). Inspiration proceeds and reaches the point at which a total volume $V_T - V_D$ has been inspired. This is represented by Z in Fig. 4.8(i). The remaining part of inspiration involves the flow of a volume V_D of gas into the dead space. This gas does not reach the alveoli and so its composition is not directly of relevance at this stage.

It follows then that the volume of fresh gas passing directly into the alveoli during inspiration is given by the line XY in Fig. 4.8(i), where Y lies on a

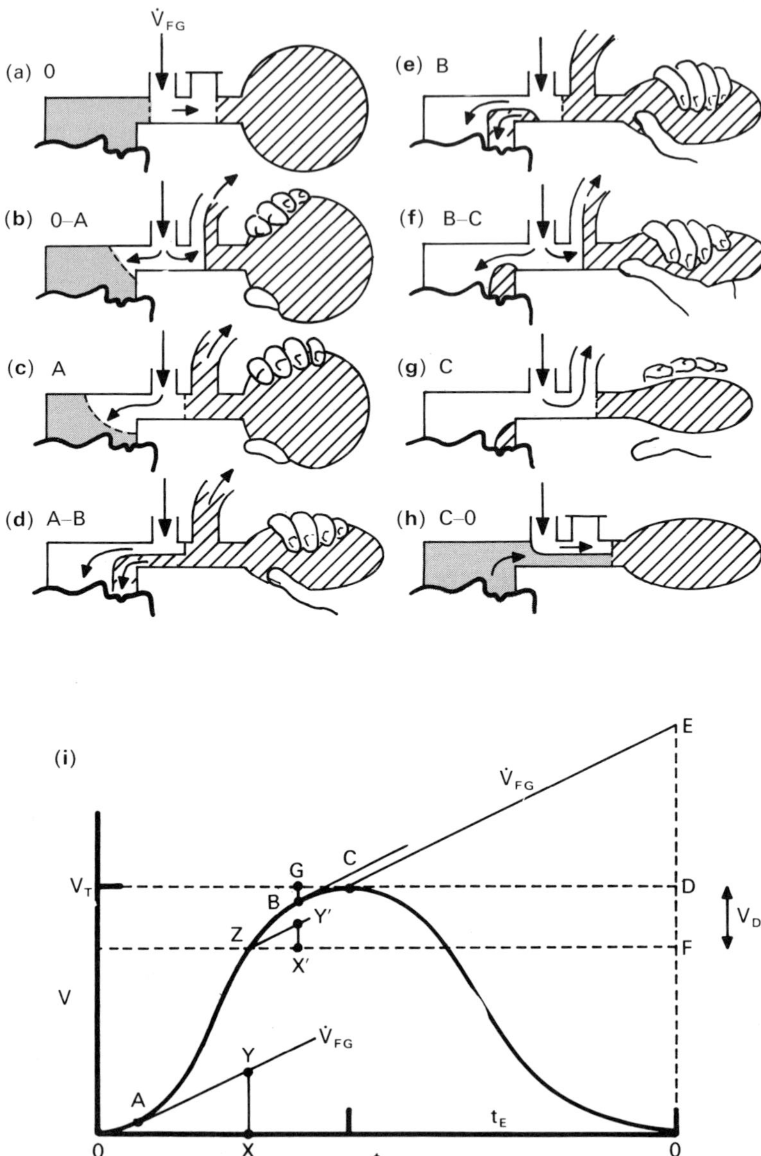

Fig. 4.8. Rebreathing properties of the Mapleson C system during controlled ventilation. (a) immediately prior to inspiration (inflation); (b) $\dot{V}_I < \dot{V}_{FG}$; (c) $\dot{V}_I = \dot{V}_{FG}$; (d) $\dot{V}_I > \dot{V}_{FG}$; (e) $\dot{V}_I = \dot{V}_{FG}$ again; (f) $\dot{V}_I < \dot{V}_{FG}$ again; (g) end of inspiration; (h) expiration; (i) the respiratory waveform with constructions depicting system performance. XY represents the volume of fresh gas reaching the alveoli directly. YZ represents the volume of gas reaching the alveoli from the reservoir bag. Shaded gas is expired alveolar gas. Cross-hatched gas is that in, or from, the reservoir bag.

tangent to the inspiratory limb of gradient $\dot{V}_{FG}$ and lies vertically below Z. Furthermore, line YZ gives the volume of gas inspired into the alveoli from the reservoir bag. The remaining volume V_D of inspired gas is that rebreathed directly from the dead space. We conclude that rebreathing in excess of the volume V_D can only be eliminated if the fresh gas flow line has a gradient equal to the steepest part of the inspiratory limb between 0 and Z. This will usually mean that $\dot{V}_{FG}$ must equal the peak inspiratory flow.

Calculation of the exact fraction of CO_2 in the inspired gas when $\dot{V}_{FG}$ is less than peak inspiratory flow is complicated by the problem of finding the CO_2 content of the volume YZ of gas breathed into the alveoli from the reservoir bag. This can be deduced from the remaining constructions on Fig. 4.8(i), as follows.

We assume perfect mixing in the bag of the C system. The composition of gas leaving the bag is that of the mixture entering the bag. The bag fills only during expiration when the valve is shut (Fig. 4.8(h)). It takes in the following gases: the volume $\dot{V}_{FG}t_E$ of fresh gas entering the system during expiration ($=$ DE in Fig. 4.8(i)); the volume V_D of gas from the dead space ($=$ DF); a volume $V_T - V_D$ of gas expired from the alveoli ($=$ F0). Only the dead space volume DF is not uniform in composition. The key to finding its composition is to note the significance of the point B.

Inspiratory flow is less than $\dot{V}_{FG}$ after B, so between B and C only fresh gas enters the dead space (volume BG). Prior to moment B the gas entering the dead space is a volume X′Y′ of fresh gas together with a volume Y′B of reservoir gas. If we express the CO_2 fraction of reservoir gas as F_{RCO_2} and retain the term F_{ECO_2} for the fraction of CO_2 in expired alveolar gas, we can now deduce that

$$F_{RCO_2} = \frac{F_{RCO_2}Y'B + F_{ECO_2}F0}{DE + DF + F0}$$

$$= \frac{Y'BF_{RCO_2} + (V_T - V_D)F_{ECO_2}}{\dot{V}_{FG}t_E + V_T}. \tag{4.9}$$

Solving for F_{RCO_2} we obtain

$$F_{RCO_2} = F_{ECO_2}\left[\frac{(V_T - V_D)}{\dot{V}_{FG}t_E + V_T - Y'B}\right]. \tag{4.10}$$

Note that unlike the Mapleson A system, the pattern of leakage flow from the valve does not directly influence the rebreathing characteristics of the C system.

Figure 4.9 represents the case of the idealized respiratory waveform consisting of constant inspiratory and expiratory flows. The fraction of CO_2 in the inspired gas is given by

$$F_{ICO_2}V_T = F_{ECO_2}V_D + F_{RCO_2}YZ, \tag{4.11}$$

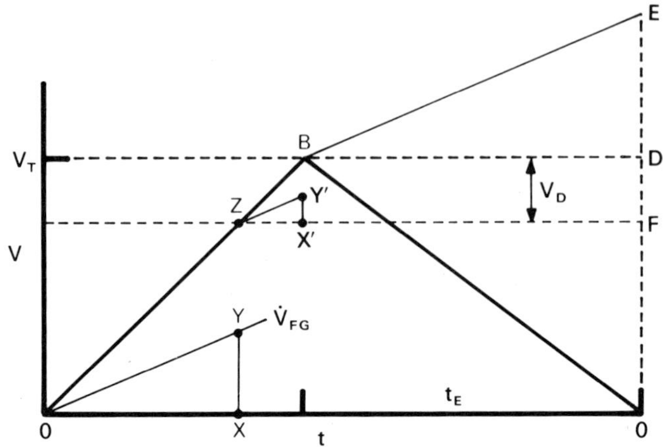

Fig. 4.9. The equivalent construction to figure 4.8(i) for the idealized respiratory waveform that consists of constant inspiratory and expiratory flows.

where $YZ = (\dot{V}_I - \dot{V}_{FG})(V_T - V_D)/\dot{V}_I$ (Fig. 4.9). We note that $Y'B = (\dot{V}_I - \dot{V}_{FG})V_D/\dot{V}_I$ and substitute for YZ and $Y'B$ in eqns. (4.10) and (4.11):

$$F_{ICO_2} = F_{ECO_2} \left\langle \frac{V_D}{V_T} + \left(1 - \frac{V_D}{V_T}\right) \left\{ \frac{V_T - V_D[1 - (\dot{V}_{FG}/\dot{V}_I)] - \dot{V}_{FG}t_I}{V_T - V_D[1 - (\dot{V}_{FG}/\dot{V}_I)] + \dot{V}_{FG}t_E} \right\} \right\rangle. \quad (4.12)$$

The rebreathing index is calculated using eqn (2.16) to relate the ventilation $\dot{V}$ at any fresh gas flow (less than $\dot{V}_I$) to the ventilation $\dot{V}_0$ where rebreathing is eliminated ($\dot{V}_{FG} = \dot{V}_I$) for the same F_{ECO_2}. The resulting relation between $\dot{V}/\dot{V}_0$, V_D/V_{T0} and $\dot{V}_{FG}/\dot{V}_0$ is as follows:

$$\frac{\dot{V}}{\dot{V}_0} - \frac{V_D}{V_{T0}} = \left(1 - \frac{V_D}{V_{T0}}\right)\left(\frac{\dot{V}_0}{\dot{V}_{FG}}\right)$$

$$\times \left\{ \frac{\dot{V}}{\dot{V}_0} - \left(\frac{V_D}{V_{T0}}\right)\left[1 - \frac{\dot{V}_{FG}}{\dot{V}_0} \times \frac{\dot{V}_0}{\dot{V}} \times \frac{1}{(1 + t_E/t_I)}\right] \right.$$

$$\left. + \left[\frac{\dot{V}_{FG}}{\dot{V}_0} \times \frac{1}{(1 + t_I/t_E)}\right] \right\}. \quad (4.13)$$

Equation 4.13 is plotted in Fig. 4.10 for the case $t_I = t_E$ for four values of V_D/V_{T0}. In contrast to the behaviour of the Mapleson A system during assisted ventilation (Fig. 4.6) we see that rebreathing can be eliminated from the C system by setting $\dot{V}_{FG} = 2\dot{V}_0$. Even at low fresh gas flows the rebreathing may be minimal in the presence of a sizeable ratio V_D/V_{T0}.

The CO_2 retention index for the system is derived by combining eqns (2.16) and (4.12) to find the ratio between expired CO_2 fraction for all $\dot{V}_{FG}(F'_{ECO_2})$

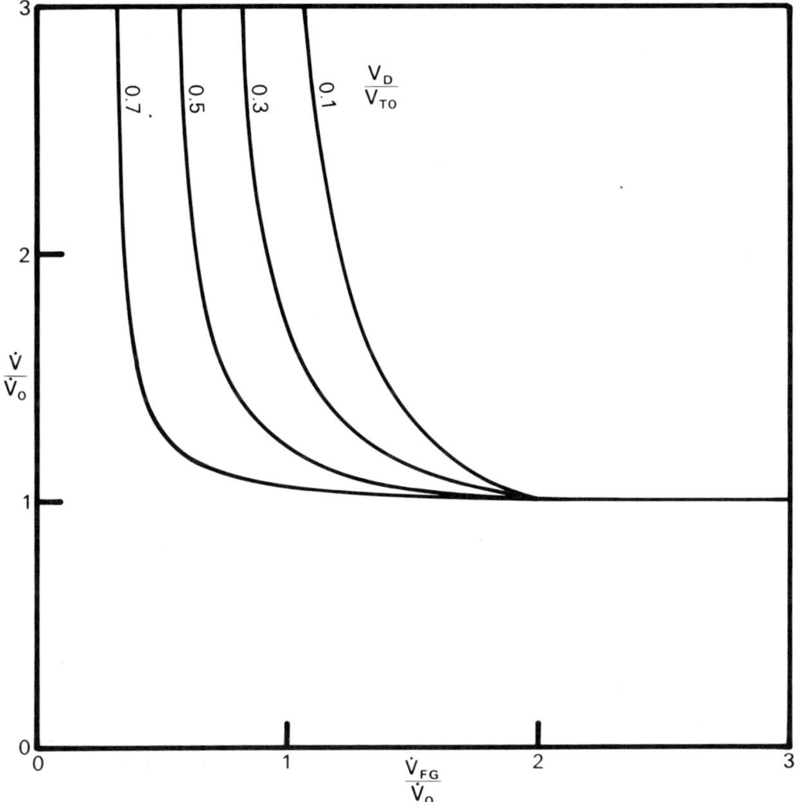

Fig. 4.10. The rebreathing index for the Mapleson C system during controlled ventilation, plotted for different values of the relative dead space V_D/V_{TO}. Constant $\dot{V}_I$ and $\dot{V}_E$ assumed, with $t_I = t_E$ (and $\dot{V}_I = \dot{V}_E$).

and that for absent rebreathing (F_{ECO_2} when $\dot{V}_{FG} \geq 2\dot{V}_0$) both for the same ventilation $\dot{V}_0$:

$$\frac{F'_{ECO_2}}{F_{ECO_2}} = \left(\frac{\dot{V}_0}{\dot{V}_{FG}}\right)\left(1 - \frac{V_D}{V_{TO}}\right) + \left(\frac{1}{1 + t_E/t_I}\right)\left(1 + \frac{V_D}{V_{TO}}\right). \qquad (4.14)$$

Equation (4.14) is plotted in Fig. 4.11 for the case $t_I = t_E$. We note that the index remains quite low even when the fresh gas flow is only equal to the ventilation ($\dot{V}_{FG}/\dot{V}_0 = 1$). This contrasts with the inefficiency during assisted ventilation of the Mapleson A system (Fig. 4.7). A further difference is that, unlike the A system, the C system has a CO_2 retention index which depends upon V_D/V_{TO}. We conclude that the Mapleson C system is well suited to controlled ventilation if fresh gas flows are utilized in the approximate range $1.5 < (\dot{V}_{FG}/\dot{V}_0) < 2.5$.

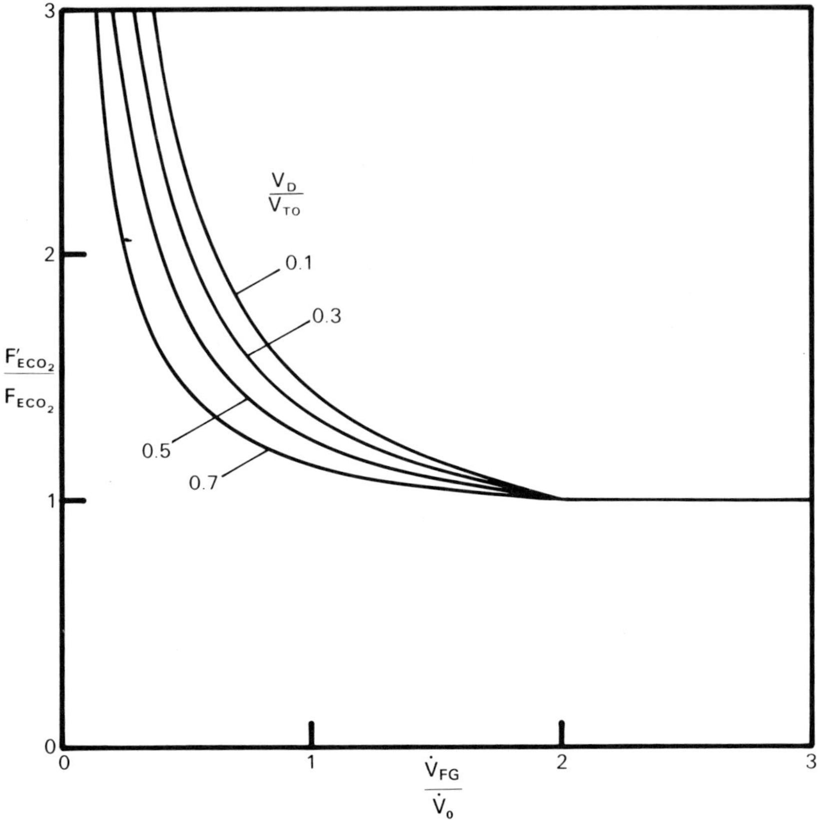

Fig. 4.11. The CO_2 retention index for the Mapleson C system during controlled ventilation, plotted for different values of the relative dead space V_D/V_{TO}. Constant $\dot{V}_I$ and $\dot{V}_E$ assumed, with $t_I = t_E$ (and $\dot{V}_I = \dot{V}_E$).

In what respect does the performance of the Mapleson B system differ from what we have deduced for the C system? In the B system (Fig. 2.26) gas is expired not into a reservoir bag but into a reservoir tube in which axial mixing can be assumed not to occur. The composition of the gas which reaches the alveoli during the following inspiration (ZY in Fig. 4.8(i)) cannot then be deduced by assuming perfect mixing between expired gas and fresh gas arriving during expiration (eqn (4.9)). The stratification of gases along the tube will modify the composition of reservoir gas entering the alveoli in comparison with the perfectly mixed reservoir gas of the C system. Where $\dot{V}_I$ and $\dot{V}_E$ are constants, the C system will use a given fresh gas flow slightly more efficiently than the B system on account of its mixing in the reservoir bag of a volume V_D of dead space gas which is relatively rich in fresh gas (X'B in Fig. 4.9). In the B system a smaller proportion of this ultimately reaches the alveoli. In only one circumstance can we expect identical theoretical performances between the two systems: when $\dot{V}_E$ is a constant and $V_D = 0$ gas at any section of the reservoir tube of the B system will be identical to the mixed gases in the bag of the C system in the proportions $\dot{V}_{FG}:\dot{V}_E$, fresh gas:expired gas. Under all other circumstances we may expect only a very small difference between the performance of these systems.

4.5 Controlled ventilation with the Mapleson D and F systems

The Mapleson D and F systems are depicted in Fig. 2.26. They are the forms of T-piece systems which include a reservoir bag, which makes it possible to assist ventilation by manually squeezing the bag. Recall from chapter 2 that the Bain system is a coaxial form of the Mapleson D type, and the F system is otherwise known as the Jackson Rees modification to Ayres T-piece (Fig. 2.9). The two systems are functionally identical during controlled ventilation. We consider the performance of the D system as depicted in Fig. 4.12.

Immediately before inspiration begins the dead space contains gas breathed out during the previous expiration and the reservoir tube contains a mixture of expired gas and fresh gas, stratified along the tube according to the relative flows with which these two components arrive at the T-piece throughout expiration (Fig. 4.12(a)). Early in inspiration fresh gas accumulates at the patient end of the reservoir tube (Fig. 4.12(b)). At moment A, depicted in Figs. 4.12(c) and (e), the volume of fresh gas which has arrived since the beginning of inspiration exactly equals the volume of gas which has entered the patient. At this moment, therefore, some CO_2-containing gas from the reservoir tube enters the dead space region. All gas which enters the dead space before point Z in Fig. 4.12(e) will be inspired into the alveoli. Gas entering the dead space after point Z will not reach the alveoli and is consequently of no functional significance.

It follows then that a volume of fresh gas which is not mixed in the reservoir tube and reaches the alveoli is given by the line XY in Fig. 4.12(e). Here Y lies directly below Z on a line of gradient $\dot{V}_{FG}$ which passes through the origin. Line YZ gives the CO_2-containing volume of gas which reaches the alveoli from the reservoir tube. The remaining inspired volume, V_D, is that rebreathed directly from the dead space.

The exact composition of the volume YZ is easily derived. Construction Y'Z' on the right-hand side of Fig. 4.12(e) gives the composition of the final volume YZ of gas deposited at the patient end of the reservoir tube at the end of expiration. The portion of the vertical line Y'Z' lying above the horizontal axis gives the volume which is expired gas; the portion lying below the axis gives the volume of fresh gas in this mixture.

Figure 4.13 represents the case of the idealized respiratory waveform consisting of constant inspiratory and expiratory flows. From this con-

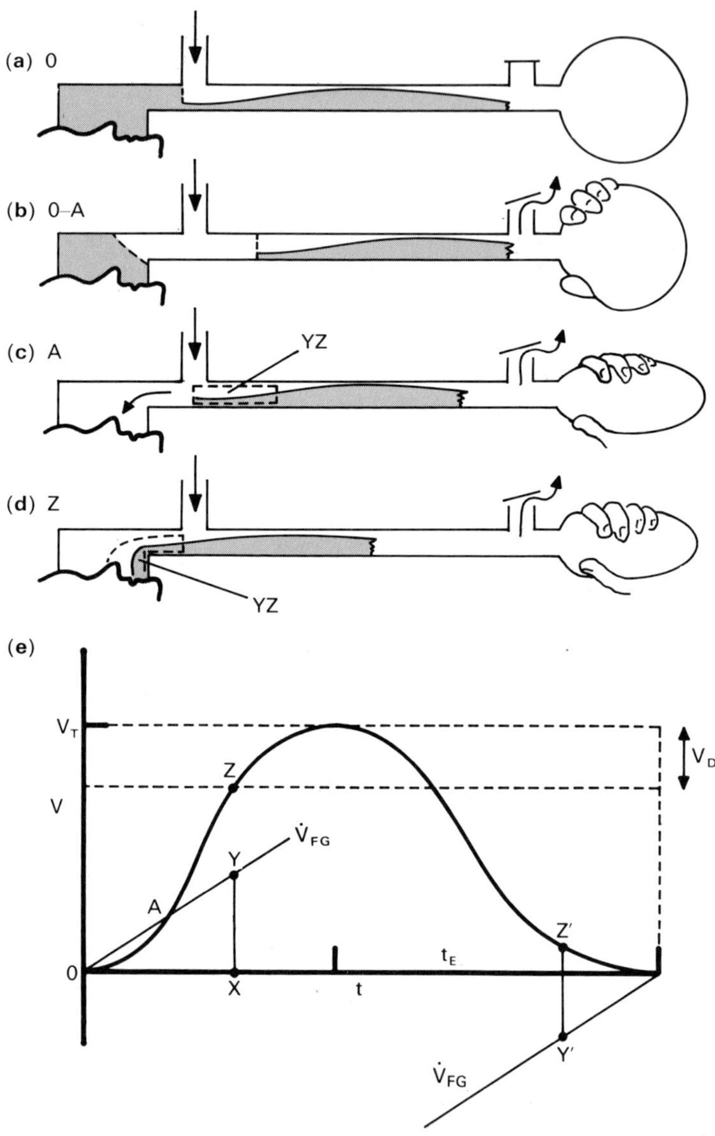

Fig. 4.12. Rebreathing properties of the Mapleson D and F systems during controlled ventilation. (a) immediately prior to inspiration (inflation); (b) fresh gas delivery exceeds inspired volume; (c) fresh gas delivery equals inspired volume; (d) volume $V_T - V_D$ inspired; (e) the respiratory waveform with constructions depicting system performance. XY is the volume of fresh gas reaching the alveoli without mixing in the reservoir tube with expired gas. YZ is the volume of CO_2-containing gas which is inspired into the alveoli from the reservoir tube. Y'Z' = YZ. (For a similar approach see Dorrington, K. L. and Lehane, J. R. (1989) *Anaesthesia*, in press.)

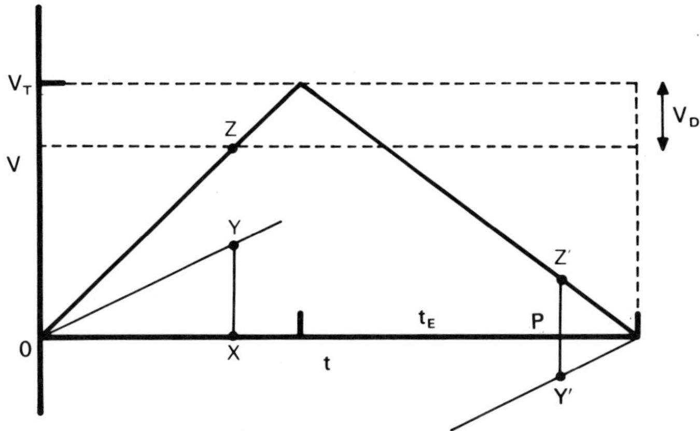

Fig. 4.13. The equivalent construction to Fig. 4.12(e) for the idealized respiratory waveform which consists of constant inspiratory and expiratory flows.

struction we deduce that the fraction of the inspired gas which is fresh (not rebreathed) is given by

$$F_{\text{IFG}} = \frac{\text{XY} + \text{Y}'\text{P}}{V_{\text{T}}}$$

$$= \frac{1}{V_{\text{T}}}\left[\dot{V}_{\text{FG}}\left(\frac{V_{\text{T}} - V_{\text{D}}}{\dot{V}_{\text{I}}}\right) + \dot{V}_{\text{FG}}\left(\frac{\dot{V}_{\text{I}} - \dot{V}_{\text{FG}}}{\dot{V}_{\text{FG}} + \dot{V}_{\text{E}}}\right)\left(\frac{V_{\text{T}} - V_{\text{D}}}{\dot{V}_{\text{I}}}\right)\right]$$

$$= \left(\frac{V_{\text{T}} - V_{\text{D}}}{V_{\text{T}}}\right)\left(\frac{\dot{V}_{\text{FG}}}{\dot{V}_{\text{I}}}\right)\left(1 + \frac{\dot{V}_{\text{I}} - \dot{V}_{\text{FG}}}{\dot{V}_{\text{FG}} + \dot{V}_{\text{E}}}\right). \tag{4.15}$$

The rebreathing index is derived by combining eqns (2.16), (2.62) and (4.15). The result is identical to that found in chapter 2 for spontaneous breathing with the T-piece system:

$$\frac{\dot{V}}{\dot{V}_0} = \frac{1}{(1 + t_{\text{I}}/t_{\text{E}})} \times \frac{(\dot{V}_{\text{FG}}/\dot{V}_0)[1 + (V_{\text{D}}/V_{\text{T0}})(t_{\text{I}}/t_{\text{E}})]}{[(\dot{V}_{\text{FG}}/\dot{V}_0) - 1 + (V_{\text{D}}/V_{\text{T0}})]}. \tag{2.30}$$

Equation (2.30) is plotted in Fig. 2.12 for the case $t_{\text{I}} = t_{\text{E}}$.

Why do we find the same rebreathing index for the T-piece systems during both controlled and spontaneous ventilation but markedly different rebreathing indices for the Mapleson A system in these two situations? The relevant crucial difference between the systems is as follows: only in the Mapleson A system does the action of controlling ventilation by squeezing the reservoir bag eject gas from the valve which would otherwise (during spontaneous ventilation) reach the alveoli. We must emphasize that we are momentarily comparing controlled and spontaneous ventilation on the assumption that the shape of the respiratory waveform generated by the two mechanisms is identical, and trying to account for differences in performance which are unrelated to differences in the waveform alone.

For the idealized respiratory waveform, comparison of Figs. 2.12 and 4.10 leads to an interesting conclusion regarding the relative merits of the D/E/F systems, and the C system. The rebreathing index during controlled ventilation of the C system is always lower than for the D/E/F systems. They become identical only for the limiting case $V_D/V_{TO} = 0$ for which both eqns (2.30) and (4.13) reduce to

$$\frac{\dot{V}}{\dot{V}_0} = \frac{1}{(1 - \dot{V}_0/\dot{V}_{FG})(1 + t_I/t_E)}. \tag{4.16}$$

Whether this advantage of the C system over the D/E/F systems is retained for other respiratory waveforms can be determined by the appropriate analyses depicted in Figs. 4.8 and 4.12.

The CO_2 retention index for the D and F systems is derived by combining eqns (2.16), (2.62) and (4.15). Recall that the result applies only to our idealized respiratory waveform.

$$\frac{F'_{ECO_2}}{F_{ECO_2}} = \frac{1}{(1 + t_I/t_E)} + \left(\frac{\dot{V}_0}{\dot{V}_{FG}}\right). \tag{4.17}$$

The result (Fig. 4.14 for $t_I = t_E$) is independent of V_D/V_{TO}, unlike that for the C system (Fig. 4.11) to which it becomes identical for the case $V_D/V_{TO} = 0$ (compare eqns (4.14) and (4.17)). For all non-zero values of V_D/V_{TO} the C system has a lower CO_2 retention index and thus a greater economy of fresh gas.

We may draw the following conclusions from the foregoing analyses. The performance of the Mapleson A system during controlled ventilation is very different from its performance during spontaneous ventilation. It is worst and best of the Mapleson systems in these two situations respectively. The B and C systems are more efficient during spontaneous ventilation than controlled ventilation. Though our analysis of these systems has been incomplete, we can conclude from Figs. 2.29 and 4.8 that elimination of rebreathing requires a larger fresh gas flow when ventilation is controlled. The D and F systems behave identically during controlled and spontaneous ventilation. (The E system cannot be used for controlled ventilation because it has no reservoir bag; during spontaneous ventilation its behaviour is the same as the D and F systems if its reservoir tube is sufficiently long to avoid entrainment of air into the alveoli.)

For our idealized respiratory waveform ($\dot{V}_I$ and $\dot{V}_E$ constant), in the limiting unphysiological case of zero dead space the performance of the B, C, D, E and F systems during controlled ventilation is the same. For more

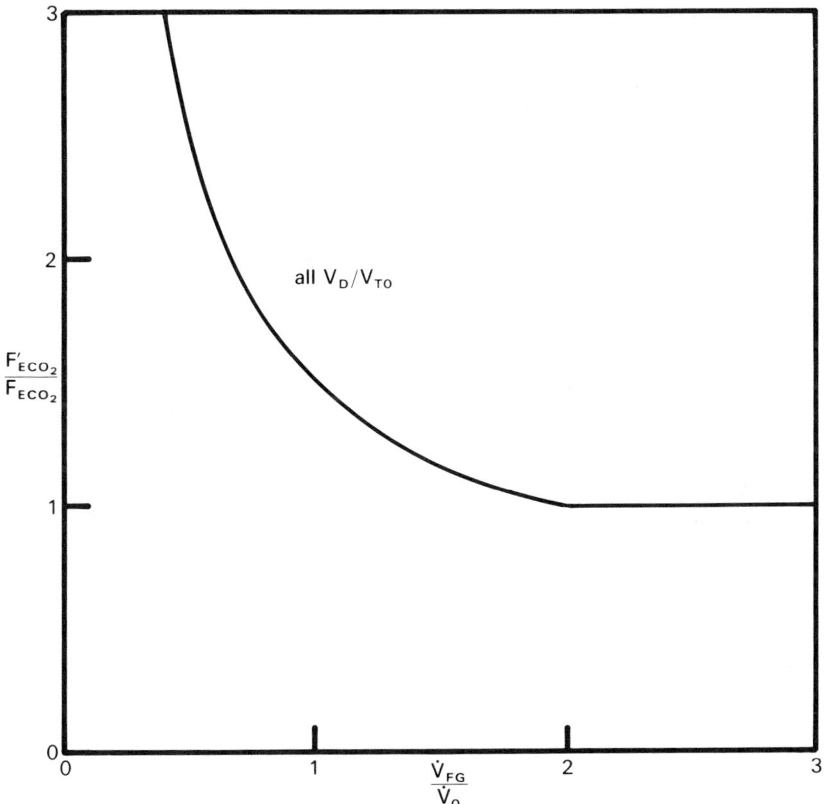

Fig. 4.14. The CO_2 retention index for the Mapleson D and F systems during controlled ventilation. Constant $\dot{V}_I$ and $\dot{V}_E$ assumed with $t_I = t_E$ (and $\dot{V}_I = \dot{V}_E$).

realistic waveforms and physiological values of dead space the C system will often be more efficient than the D/E/F systems. These T-piece systems will tend to have a higher efficiency than the C systems in the presence of long end-expiratory pauses.

The unfavourable performance of the Mapleson A system during controlled ventilation can be overcome by the use of a cunning modification described by Millar and Millar (Millar, D. M. and Millar, J. C. (1988). *British Journal of Anaesthesia* **60**, 469–75). The arrangement is depicted in Fig. 4.15. The reservoir bag on the inlet limb of the system is enclosed by a reservoir which is connected to the expiratory valve at the patient end. This secondary reservoir itself connects to another expiratory valve and another reservoir bag. During spontaneous ventilation the Millar system behaves as a normal Mapleson A system. During controlled ventilation the action of squeezing the secondary reservoir bag not only compresses the inner, primary, reservoir

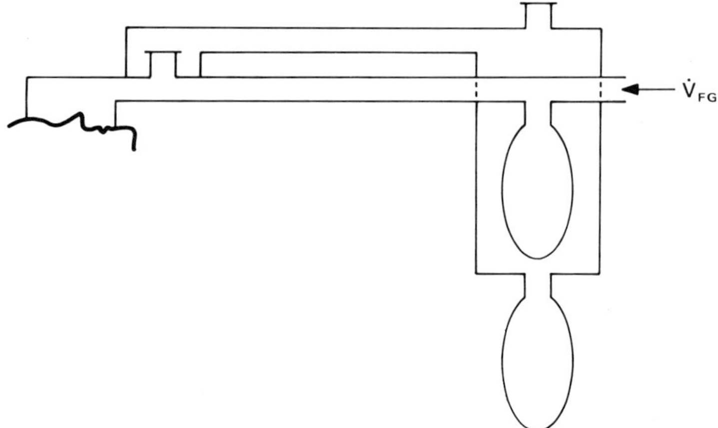

Fig. 4.15. The Millar modification to the Mapleson A system. The efficiency with which this system handles the fresh gas flow is the same during both spontaneous and controlled ventilation.

bag, but also closes the primary expiratory valve. Because this valve remains closed during inspiration the system performance becomes identical to that during spontaneous ventilation. This performance is depicted for the case of an idealized respiratory waveform in Figs. 2.24 and 2.25.

4.6   Automatic ventilation of the lungs

This is achieved by the use of a machine to deliver gas at regular intervals into a breathing system. In patients who are unable to breathe unaided this obviates the need for manual control of their ventilation. It also introduces a need for additional safety features such as alarms and pressure-release valves to prevent harm to the patient in the event of equipment failure.

Two types of ventilator can be distinguished according to the way the fresh gas supply is handled. In type I ventilators the fresh gas supply enters the breathing system as a constant flow which can reach the patient without passing through any valves (Fig. 4.16). The ventilator generates a respiratory waveform at the patient end of the system by varying the degree of occlusion of the expiratory valve alone (Fig. 4.16(a)) or by combining control of the valve with intermittent displacement of gas elsewhere in the system (Fig. 4.16(b)). Arrangements of this kind can be envisaged which are similar to all breathing systems used with manual control (for example, Figs. 4.8 and 4.12) except that a reservoir bag is replaced by a machine which displaces gas and also provides control over the expiratory valve. In practice only the T-piece system (Mapleson D/E/F) is in common use in this type of automatic ventilation. The new Millar system may become popular.

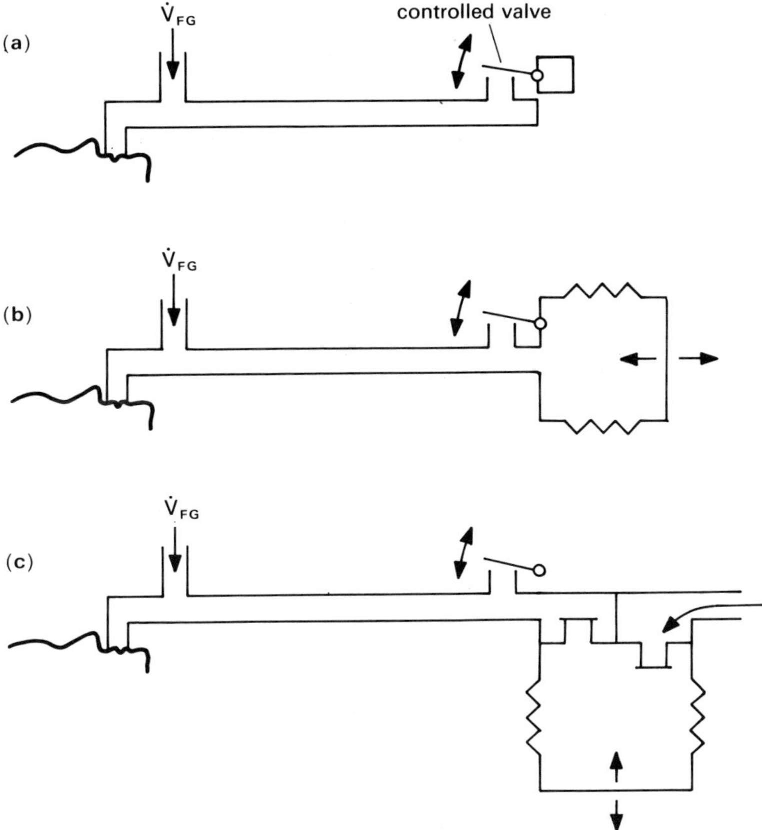

Fig. 4.16. Ventilators classified here as type I, on account of the fresh gas delivery being directly available to the patient, include T-piece systems with (a) expiratory valve control alone; (b) valve and bellows control; (c) valve control plus intermittent gas delivery from a secondary supply. (Note that patients who are connected to automatic ventilators are depicted in this and subsequent figures with oral endotracheal tube connections, rather than face masks.)

In type II ventilators the supply of fresh gas does not pass uninterrupted to the patient. It is intermittently chopped into boluses of gas before delivery to the patient through a system of valves (Fig. 4.17). A ventilator of this kind may deliver fresh gas intermittently from a supply at very high pressure (Fig. 4.17(a)) or make use of a steady flow of fresh gas conserved at a lower pressure in a reservoir bag (Fig. 4.17(b)). The former system is rarely used because it is usually desirable to supply the patient with a combination of gases which do not come ready-mixed in a high pressure supply, but are delivered at low pressure by an anaesthetic machine or mixing valve. Ventilators which use a bellows to draw gas from a low pressure supply require a

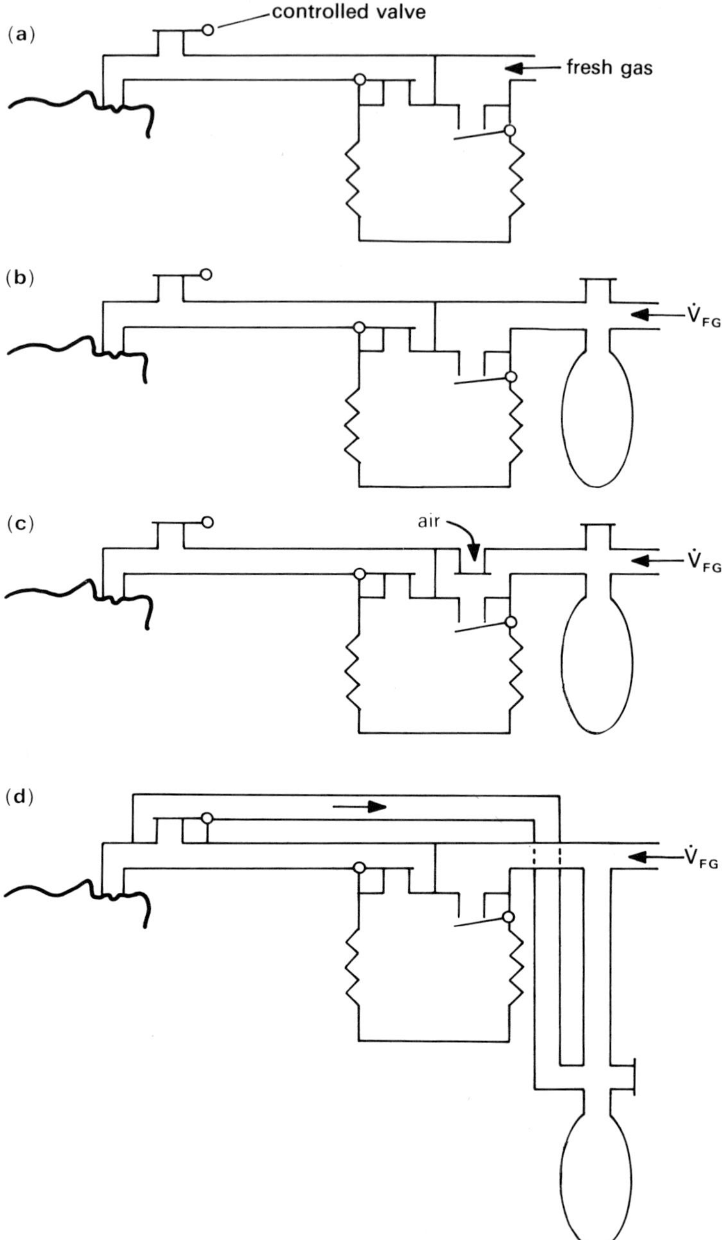

Fig. 4.17. Ventilators classified here as type II, on account of the intermittent parcelling of the fresh gas supply before its arrival at the patient, include devices which (a) draw fresh gas intermittently from a high pressure source; (b) use a generous constant flow of fresh gas; (c) supplement a constant flow of fresh gas with air; (d) permit rebreathing of expired alveolar gas.

one-way valve at inlet to prevent retrograde pumping of gas into the supply. Maintenance of the one-way flow also requires a one-way valve at outlet from the bellows (Fig. 4.17(b)).

The ventilator depicted in Fig. 4.17(b) will only function so long as the fresh gas flow $\dot{V}_{FG}$ equals or exceeds the ventilation $\dot{V}$ delivered by the bellows to the patient. Excess fresh gas ($\dot{V}_{FG} - \dot{V}$) is spilled from a valve close to the reservoir bag. To prevent failure in the event of inadequate fresh gas flow most devices allow for entrainment of air by the bellows to supplement the fresh gas supply (Fig. 4.17(c)). An alternative arrangement is to supplement the fresh gas supply with expired gas, thus allowing rebreathing to occur via the ventilator (Fig. 4.17(d)).

The power required to drive ventilators can be provided by a supply of high pressure gas (sometimes the fresh gas flow itself) or some other source which is usually electrical. Where a gas supply alone is used, it is common to incorporate valves with sonic orifices to control the 'fluid logic' of the ventilator. These provide a flow of gas which is independent of downstream pressures and make it possible for the gas supply alone to cycle the ventilator in a predictable preset manner.

Ventilators may be further classified according to the manner in which they cycle, firstly from inspiration to expiration, and secondly from expiration to inspiration. The cycling may simply be determined by time intervals set by the operator. Alternatively, cycling may occur upon delivery of a set volume of gas. Sometimes changes in pressure are used to this end, particularly in ventilators which attempt to synchronize themselves with a patient's own efforts to breathe.

Finally, differences between ventilators can be defined according to whether they are mainly generators of flow or pressure during each of the phases of inspiration and expiration. Thus, for example, a machine incorporating a powerful motor which drives a bellows to displace gas at a constant rate will tend to generate a constant flow into the patient regardless of the resistance and compliance offered by the patient's lungs. This system offers the advantage of providing measured tidal volumes but carries the risk of generating dangerously high pressures. Conversely, a machine containing a bellows which is compressed during inspiration by a weight will tend to generate a constant pressure. The volume of gas delivered will then be dependent on the resistance and compliance of the patient's lungs as well as the time for which the pressure is permitted to act. This arrangement offers the safety of limiting pressure to physiological levels but leaves the tidal volume somewhat unpredictable. Controls of flow and pressure can similarly be achieved during expiration. In the following sections we consider the characteristics of some of these ventilators.

4.7   Type I ventilators with T-piece configuration

The principle of controlling ventilation with the use of a single valve (Fig. 4.16(a)) is used in the Inter Med Bear Cub infant ventilator (Figs. 4.18 and 4.19). This device is electrically powered but also requires a fresh gas supply at a pressure of 200 kPa. It uses a very high fresh gas flow with the aim of avoiding rebreathing, apart from the irreducible dead space of the patient and endotracheal tube connectors. The ventilator is time cycled. During inspiration it develops a waveform which depends on a maximum pressure set by the operator. The fraction of the inspiratory time taken to reach this pressure in turn depends upon the fresh gas flow and the resistance and compliance of the patient's lungs. To clarify its behaviour we need to consider these terms in more detail.

We define the *resistance* of a patient's lungs to be the ratio of the pressure required to generate a flow of gas to the flow itself:

$$\eta = \frac{p}{\dot{V}_{\mathrm{I}}}, \tag{4.18}$$

here writing the flow as that pertaining to inspiration. Typical values in normal patients range from around $30\ \mathrm{cm\,H_2O\,l^{-1}\,s^{-1}}$ in the newborn to about $1\ \mathrm{cm\,H_2O\,l^{-1}\,s^{-1}}$ in adults.

Lung *compliance* is defined as the ratio of the volume to which the lungs are inflated to the pressure required to achieve the inflation in the absence of flow:

$$C = \frac{V}{p}. \tag{4.19}$$

Typical values in normal patients are $5\ \mathrm{ml\,cm\,H_2O^{-1}}$ in the newborn and $200\ \mathrm{ml\,cm\,H_2O}$ in adults.

It follows from these definitions that the inflation pressure applied to the lungs will generally be the sum of the two contributions

$$p = \eta\dot{V}_{\mathrm{I}} + \frac{V}{C}. \tag{4.20}$$

η and C are not necessarily constants; they may themselves vary with both $\dot{V}_{\mathrm{I}}$ and V. The influence of lung tissue viscoelasticity introduces a further difficulty in making C to some extent time-dependent. Despite these complications, however, η and C can often be regarded as constant for approximate qualitative work.

We consider an infant with a lung compliance of $5\ \mathrm{ml\,cm\,H_2O^{-1}}$ and resistance $30\ \mathrm{cm\,H_2O\,l^{-1}\,s^{-1}}$ connected to a ventilator of the kind shown in Fig. 4.16(a) with a fresh gas flow $10\ \mathrm{l\,min^{-1}}$. Assume that the ventilator operates as follows: inspiration is initiated by occluding the ex-

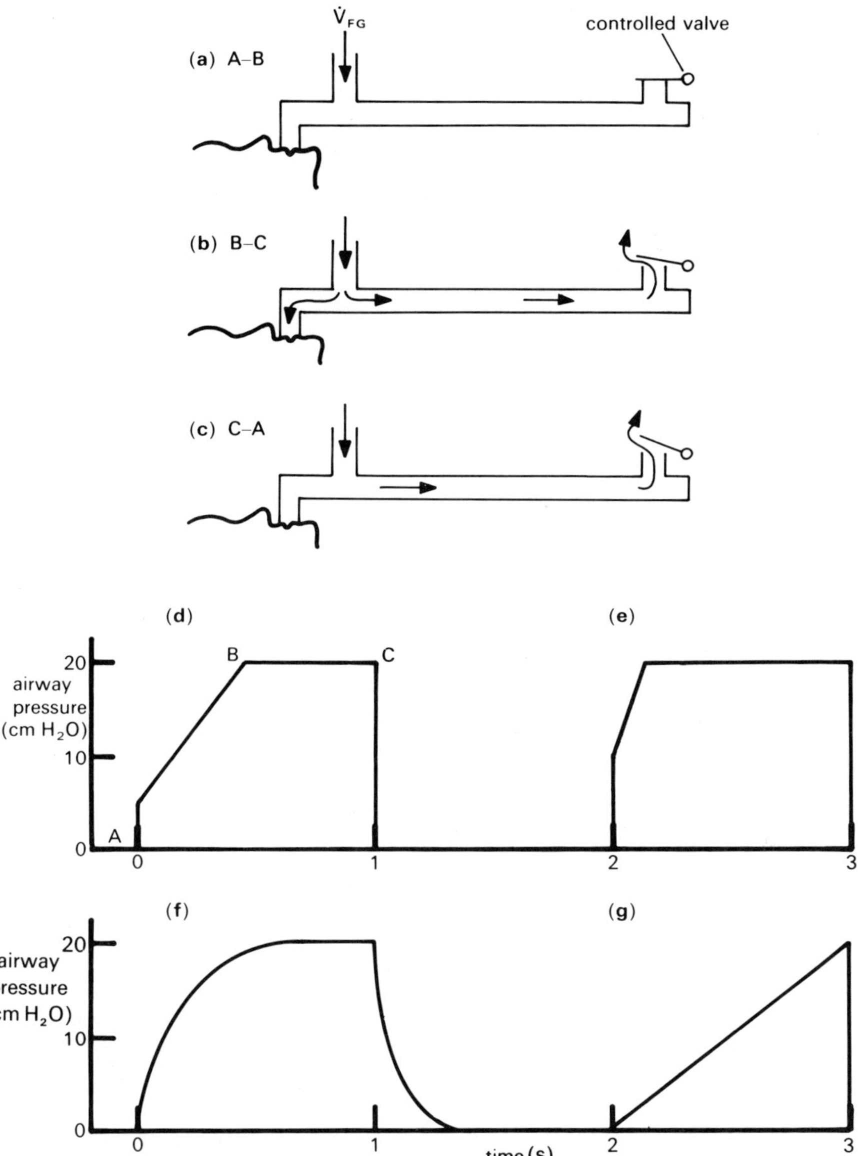

Fig. 4.18. Type I ventilator of the T-piece kind using control of an expiratory valve alone to generate inspiratory and expiratory flows and limit the airway pressure to 20 cm H_2O. (a) Early inspiration ($p < 20$ cm H_2O); (b) late inspiration ($p = 20$ cm H_2O); (c) expiration; (d) pressure waveform for $\dot{V}_{FG} = 10\,\mathrm{l\,min^{-1}}$, $\eta = 30$ cm $H_2O\,l^{-1}\,s^{-1}$, $C = 5$ ml cm H_2O^{-1}; (e) as (d) except $\dot{V}_{FG} = 20\,\mathrm{l\,min^{-1}}$; (f) typical measured waveform ($\dot{V}_{FG} = 10\,\mathrm{l\,min^{-1}}$); (g) $\dot{V}_{FG} = 6\,\mathrm{l\,min^{-1}}$, $\eta = 0$, $C = 5$ ml cm H_2O^{-1}.

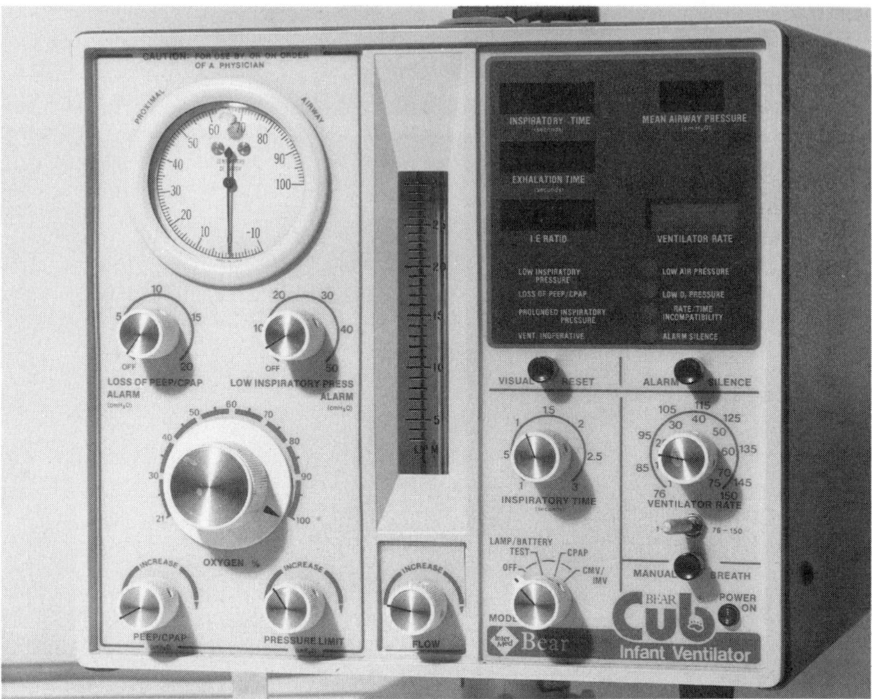

Fig. 4.19. The Inter Med Bear Cub infant ventilator.

piratory valve in such a way that it permits no flow from the system until the pressure within the system reaches 20 cm H_2O. Thereafter it permits any flow whilst maintaining this constant ceiling of pressure (see Fig. 4.3).

The initial flow of gas into the patient generates a pressure within the system of $p = \eta \dot{V_I} = \eta \dot{V}_{FG} = 30$ cm $H_2O\,l^{-1}s^{-1} \times (10/60)\,l\,s^{-1} = 5$ cm H_2O (Fig. 4.18(a)). As lung volume increases there is a contribution from the second term of eqn (4.20) which elevates p by $\dot{V}_{FG}/C$ for every second that inspiration proceeds (Fig. 4.18(b)). $\dot{V}_{FG}/C = (10 \times 1000/60)$ ml s^{-1}/ 5 ml cm $H_2O^{-1} = 33.3$ cm H_2O. Clearly the airway pressure rises from 5 to 20 cm H_2O in under 1 s, in fact in only $(20 - 5)/33.3 = 0.45$ s (Fig. 4.18(d)).

On reaching the ceiling airway pressure of 20 cm H_2O our model predicts that the inspiratory flow will fall exponentially as the pressure due to flow resistance falls towards zero and the pressure resulting from the lung compliance alone rises towards 20 cm H_2O. The tidal volume will approach 100 ml (20 cm $H_2O \times 5$ ml cm H_2O^{-1}). In the example depicted in Fig. 4.18(d), $t_I = t_E = 1$ s and the duration of the inspiratory plateau of pressure is $1 - 0.45 = 0.55$ s. A more nearly square pressure waveform is advocated for some patients in order to maximize the tidal volume in the presence of high resistance. This can be achieved by the use of even higher fresh gas flows. Fig. 4.18(e) shows the theoretical response when $\dot{V}_{FG} = 20\,l\,min^{-1}$.

In practice the measured pressure waveform does not show the sudden changes of gradient envisaged by our simple analysis. The waveform during both inspiration and expiration takes a more rounded form as depicted in Fig. 4.18(f) for a fresh gas flow of $10\,l\,min^{-1}$. The reasons for this include the following. Firstly, our assumption that η and C are constant is imprecise. Secondly, the tubing of the breathing system has a resistance and compliance of its own. Thirdly, no valve can operate precisely with the proposed characteristic of maintaining a fixed pressure difference for a wide range of flows. Fourthly, inertial effects contribute to measured pressures. The rapid oscillations of flow are inseparable from forces of acceleration and deceleration which appear as pressure gradients within the breathing system.

Because some of these factors may lead to considerable differences in pressure between the patient end and valve end of the breathing system, the designers of the Bear Cub infant ventilator have ensured that the valve is controlled on the basis of pressures sensed by the machine at the patient end.

In the example given above, the fresh gas flow of $10\,l\,min^{-1}$ is 3.3 times greater than the ventilation of $3\,l\,min^{-1}$ which would be achieved if inspiratory flow were to cease by the end of the inspiratory plateau in pressure ($V_T = 20\,cm\,H_2O \times 5\,ml\,cm\,H_2O^{-1}$; $r = 30\,min^{-1}$). Is there a minimum desirable fresh gas flow? Because the lungs fill exponentially in the presence of an airway resistance and constant inflating pressure, a reduction in $\dot{V}_{FG}$ will produce a fall in V_T. In the limiting case of zero resistance the minimum fresh gas flow which could fill the lungs in this case is $6\,l\,min^{-1}$ (100 ml every second). This case is illustrated in Fig. 4.18(g). In general, for variable t_I this critical minimum fresh gas flow is given by

$$\dot{V}_{FG} = \frac{V_T}{t_I} = \frac{p_{max}C}{t_I}, \tag{4.21}$$

where p_{max} is the pressure ceiling generated by the ventilator. Since ventilation $V = V_T r = V_T/(t_I + t_E)$ we may write eqn (4.21) as follows:

$$\dot{V}_{FG} = \dot{V}(1 + t_E/t_I). \tag{4.22}$$

If the fresh gas flow falls below this value ventilation can only be maintained by adding to the system a means of displacing gas from the reservoir tube into the patient.

This can be achieved as in Fig. 4.16(b) by the intermittent displacement of a closed bellows which acts like the manually controlled reservoir bag of Fig. 4.12. Alternatively, a ventilator more commonly used as a type II device can be used to deliver a bolus of gas into the end of the reservoir tube which is distant from the patient (Fig. 4.16(c)). If in all cases the reservoir tube has a sufficiently large volume to prevent gas from passing retrogradely against the fresh gas flow along its whole length, both of these methods will be functionally identical. If the arrangement of Fig. 4.16(c) is adopted then the bellows can be supplied with any convenient gas, for example air, since this 'driving gas' of the system never reaches the patient. A commonly used arrangement of this kind is the combination of a Penlon Nuffield 200 Series ventilator (Fig. 4.20) with a coaxial Bain T-piece system (Fig. 2.9(d)). The ventilator can be driven by a high pressure supply (340 kPa) of oxygen alone and requires no electrical input. It delivers a measured bolus of oxygen using sonic valves, contains no bellows, and is consequently very compact.

The functional analysis of these T-piece systems is identical to that given in Figs. 4.12 and 4.13, which we found in fact to be identical to that given in Fig. 2.11. For the case of the idealized respiratory waveform, the rebreathing index is given in Fig. 2.12 and the CO_2 retention index in Fig. 4.14. Recall that the functional similarity between the T-piece systems during spontaneous, manually controlled, and now automatic ventilation refers to identical behaviour for a given respiratory waveform. In the three different situations the relationship between valve opening and volumes displaced by the bag or ventilator may be quite different, but for any given respiratory waveform the rebreathing characteristics of the systems will be the same. In practice marked differences in behaviour are experienced between T-piece systems during spontaneous, manually controlled and automatic ventilation because the three different uses tend to give rise to quite different respiratory waveforms. We now examine one aspect of this in the last part of this section.

Probably the most important practical difference between the respiratory waveform during spontaneous ventilation and automatic ventilation concerns not the shape of the waveform but its amplitude. The ventilation $\dot{V}$ on an automatic ventilator may well exceed the ventilation $\dot{V}_0$ achieved during normal spontaneous ventilation. If this occurs then the fraction of CO_2 in expired alveolar gas F_{ECO_2} will fall unless the ventilator induces rebreathing, that is the addition to the alveoli of CO_2-containing gas of a greater volume than V_D. The T-piece arrangement which incorporates a Bain coaxial system and a Nuffield Series 200 ventilator is used in some centres in such a mode. Hyperventilation is combined with deliberate rebreathing of expired alveolar gas. The F_{ECO_2} is adjusted by varying both the ventilation provided by the ventilator and the fresh gas flow delivered at the T-piece. One of the reasons given for using hyperventilation is the possibility that large tidal volumes may reduce the collapse of lung alveoli which is known to occur during anaesthesia.

In its most general form the relationship between F_{ECO_2}, $\dot{V}$ and $\dot{V}_{FG}$ can be deduced from the construction of Fig. 4.12(e). We examine it in detail for the idealized respiratory waveform (Fig. 4.13), the performance of which is summarized in eqn (4.15). A combination of eqns (2.16) and (2.62) yields the

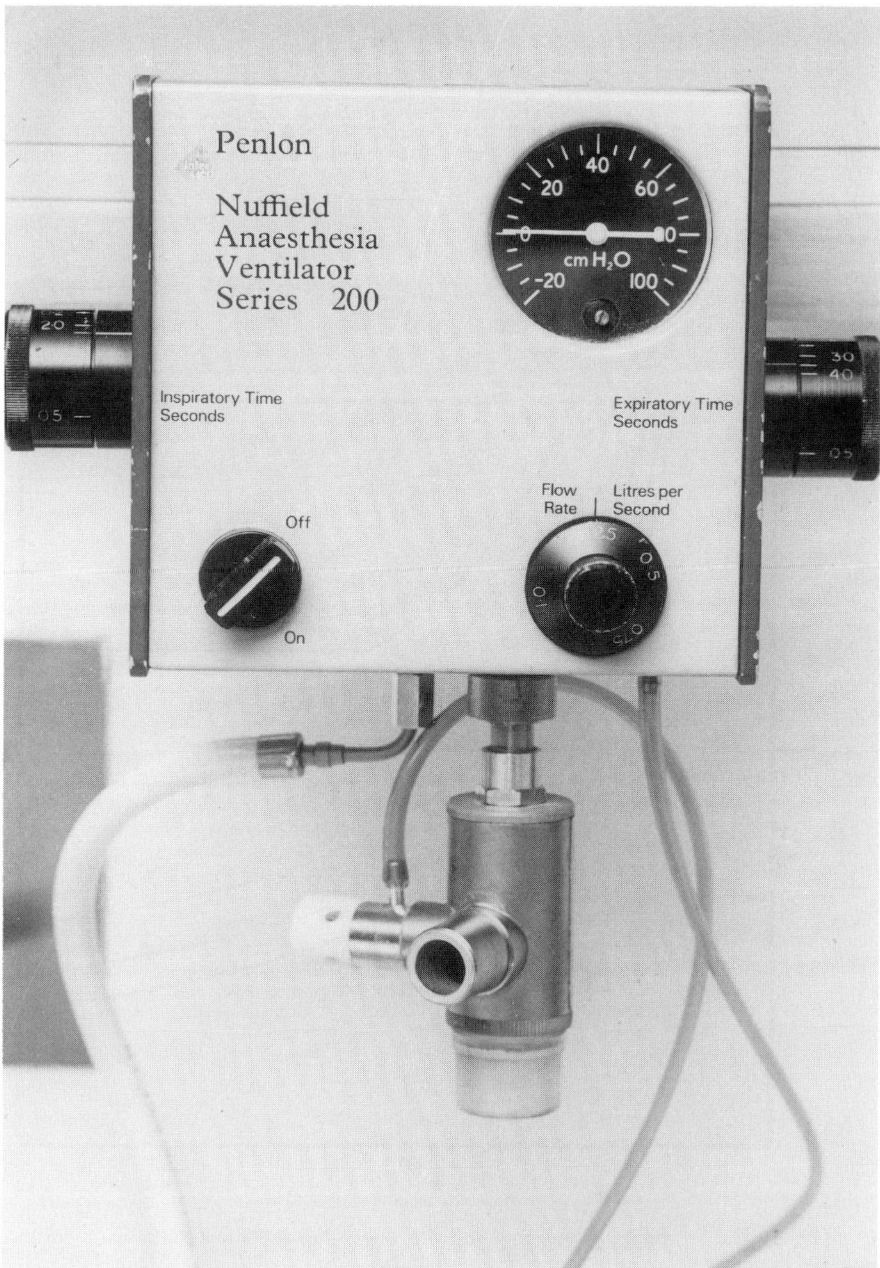

Fig. 4.20. The Penlon Nuffield 200 Series ventilator.

result

$$F_{ECO_2} F_{IFG} = \frac{\dot{V}_{CO_2}}{\dot{V}}. \qquad (4.23)$$

By substituting in this equation for F_{IFG} from eqn (4.15) we generate the equation

$$\frac{F_{ECO_2}}{(\dot{V}_{CO_2}/\dot{V}_0)} = \left[\frac{1/(1 + t_I/t_E) + (\dot{V}/\dot{V}_0)/(\dot{V}_{FG}/\dot{V}_0)}{(\dot{V}/\dot{V}_0 - V_D/V_{T0})} \right]. \qquad (4.24)$$

We again assume for the purposes of this analysis that the respiratory rate $(r = 1/(t_I + t_E))$ remains constant. $V_{T0} = \dot{V}_0/r$.

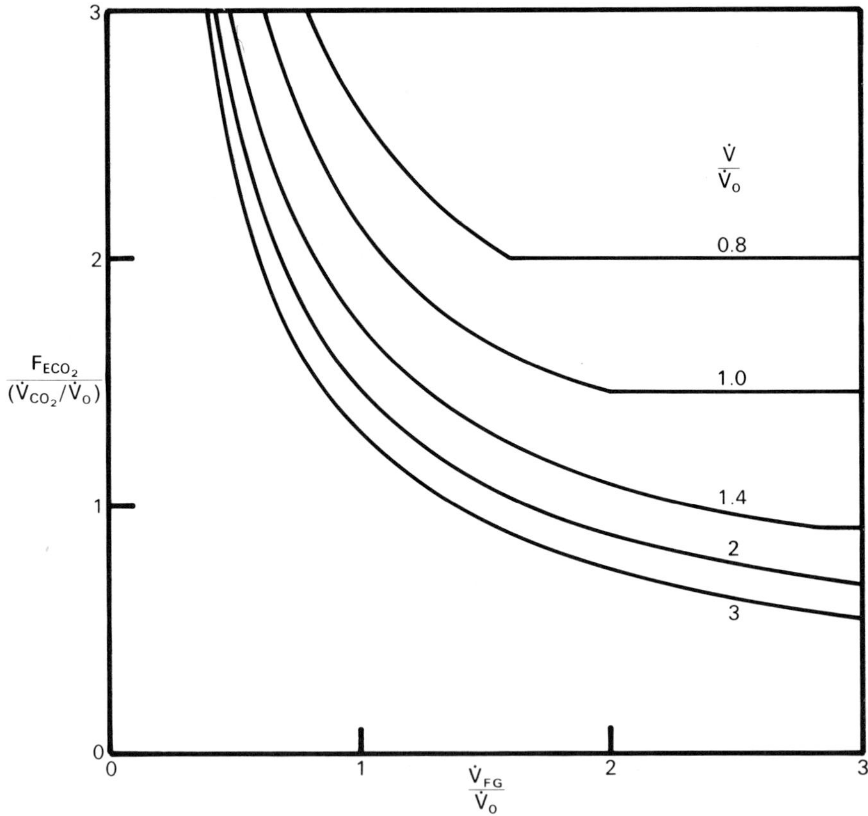

Fig. 4.21. T-piece breathing system combined with automatic ventilation. Performance for the idealized respiratory waveform with $\dot{V}_I = \dot{V}_E =$ constant, $t_I = t_E$, $V_D/V_{T0} = 0.3$ (eqn (4.24)). The dimensionless CO_2 concentration in expired alveolar gas is plotted vertically as a function of fresh gas flow for different ventilations. The break points on the upper three graphs coincide with the limit of validity of the solution given by eqn (4.24) for which $\dot{V}_{FG} < \dot{V}_I = \dot{V}(1 + t_E/t_I)$.

Figure 4.21 presents the relationship between $F_{ECO_2}/(\dot{V}_{CO_2}/\dot{V}_0)$ and $\dot{V}_{FG}/\dot{V}_0$ for a range of values of $\dot{V}/\dot{V}_0$. The case depicted is for $t_E = t_I$ and $V_D/V_{TO} = 0.3$. Note that eqn (4.24) becomes invalid when $\dot{V}_{FG} = \dot{V}_I$ (F_{IFG} becomes $1 - V_D/V_T$ and rebreathing is at a minimum). Thus a 'break point' occurs on the solutions, beyond which the fresh gas flow has no further influence on F_{ECO_2}.

We need to give some physiological significance to the dimensionless variable $F_{ECO_2}/(\dot{V}_{CO_2}/\dot{V}_0)$. For a normal F_{ECO_2} of 0.05 ($P_{aCO_2} \simeq 5\,kPa$) at metabolic CO_2 production $\dot{V}_{CO_2}$ of 200 ml min^{-1} and a normal ventilation of 6000 ml min^{-1} the dimensionless variable equals $0.05/(200/6000) = 1.5$. In some circumstances it is desirable to lower F_{ECO_2} to around 0.03 ($P_{aCO_2} \simeq 3\,kPa$, for example, during brain surgery). $F_{ECO_2}/(\dot{V}_{CO_2}/\dot{V}_0)$ then equals 0.9. The range of clinical interest therefore lies near the centre of the vertical axis in Fig. 4.21.

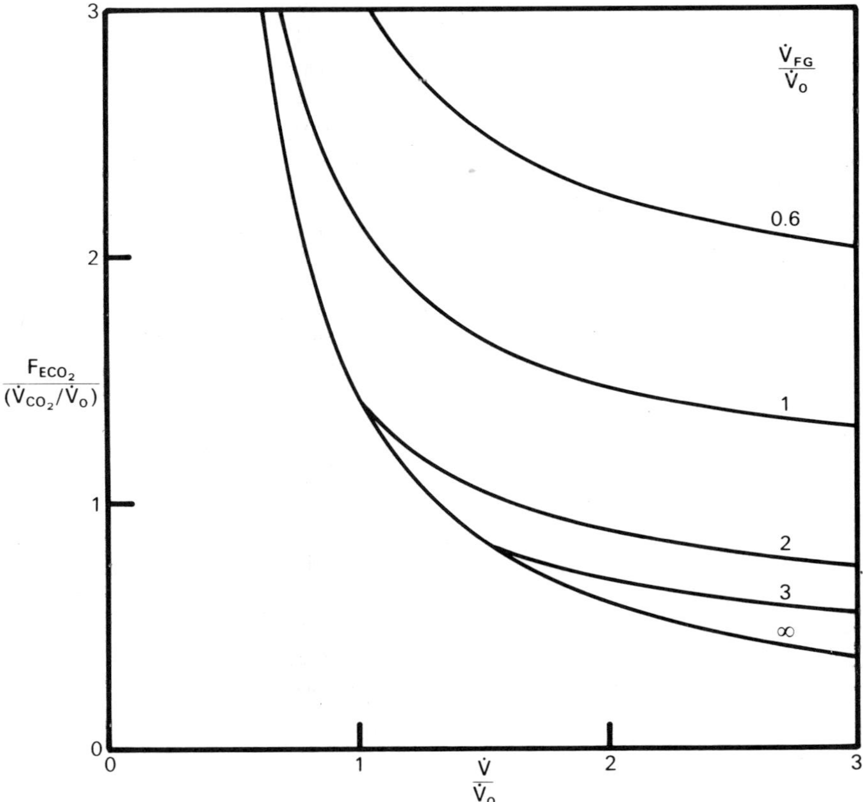

Fig. 4.22. Theoretical data of Fig. 4.21 plotted with ventilation as the independent variable for different values of fresh gas flow.

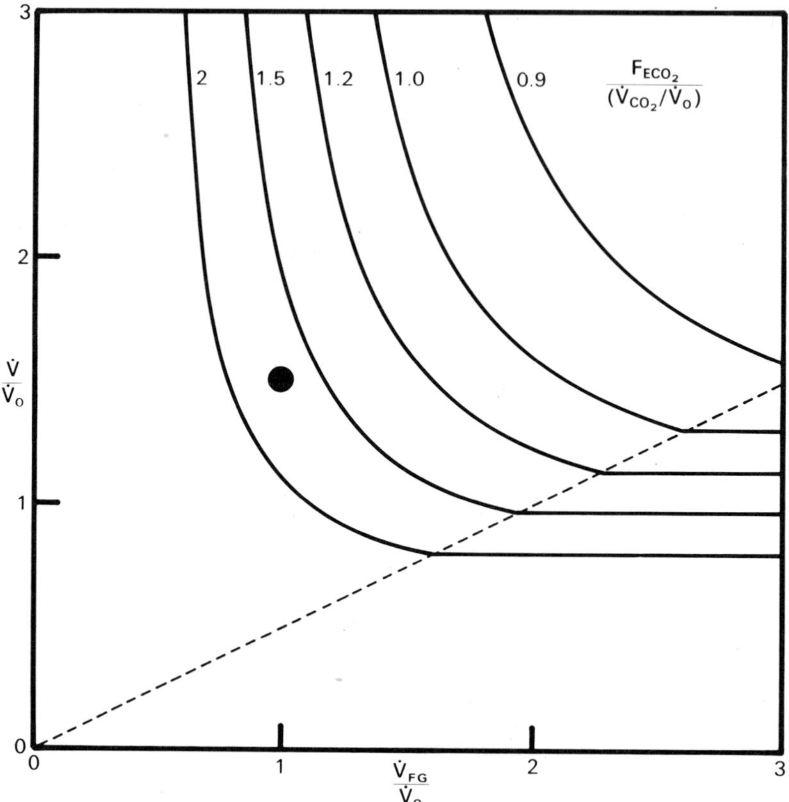

Fig. 4.23. Theoretical data of Figs. 4.21 and 4.22 plotted as isocapnia lines (lines of constant $F_{ECO_2}/(\dot{V}_{CO_2}/\dot{V}_0)$). The filled circle locates the approximate working values for $\dot{V}_{FG}$ and $\dot{V}$ which have been recommended for achieving normocapnia, on the basis of clinical studies.

Figure 4.22 contains similar information to Fig. 4.21 but with $\dot{V}/\dot{V}_0$ plotted horizontally and lines depicting constant $\dot{V}_{FG}/\dot{V}_0$. Both of these figures illustrate that F_{ECO_2} is heavily dependent upon both $\dot{V}_{FG}$ and $\dot{V}$ for most of the range of practical interest. This is most strikingly depicted in a plot of the form in Fig. 4.23 where lines of constant $F_{ECO_2}/(\dot{V}_{CO_2}/\dot{V}_0)$ are plotted on a graph of $\dot{V}/\dot{V}_0$ against $\dot{V}_{FG}/\dot{V}_0$. We refer to these as *isocapnia* lines.* We again note the presence of break points representing the condition $\dot{V}_{FG} = \dot{V}_I$.

The influence of varying t_I/t_E on the normal isocapnia line ($F_{ECO_2}/(\dot{V}_{CO_2}/\dot{V}_0) = 1.5$ approximately) is shown in Fig. 4.24. The effect of quite large changes in the range 0.5–2 is not great. Finally, the influence of varying V_D/V_{TO} on the normal isocapnia line is shown in Fig. 4.25. This has a relatively large effect on performance.

* The term 'isopleth' is sometimes used.

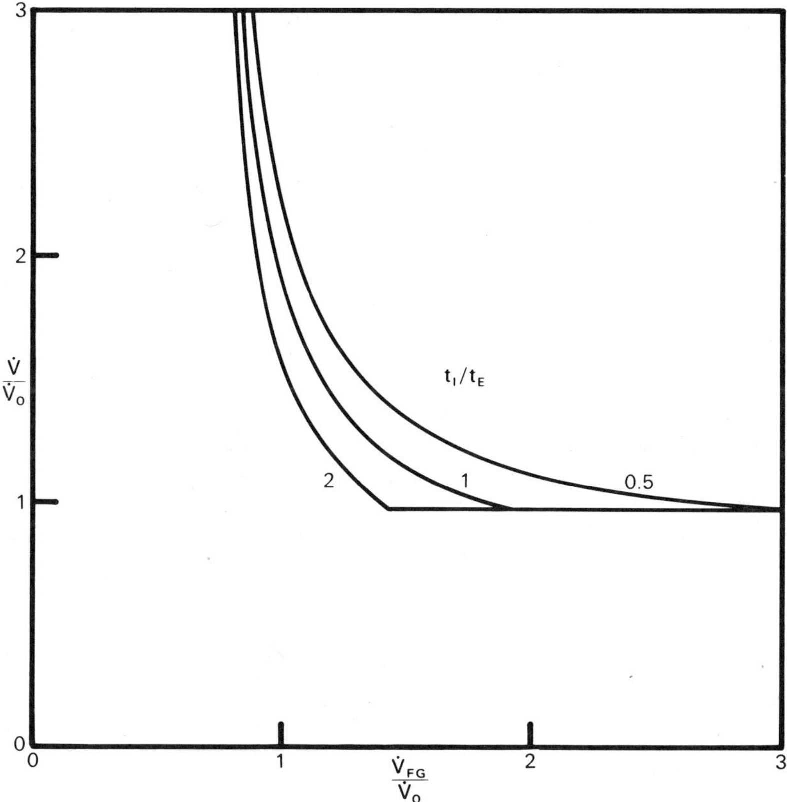

Fig. 4.24. The normal isocapnia line ($F_{ECO_2}/(\dot{V}_{CO_2}/\dot{V}_0) = 1.5$, approximately) plotted for different values of t_1/t_E.

Precision can clearly be improved by generating the equivalent of Figs. 4.21 to 25 for a shape of respiratory waveform which more accurately models that measured during automatic ventilation. During inspiration the Nuffield Series 200 ventilator closely approximates to a generator of constant $\dot{V}_I$. In this respect our idealized waveform is a good model. Expiration, however, tends with this system to be passive. The expiratory flow against resistance η is generated by the elastic recoil of the lungs which have compliance C. Expiration thus approximates to an exponential change in volume with a time constant given by ηC ($\simeq 0.2$ sec). Such an exponential expiratory waveform will lie below the expiratory line of Fig. 4.13. Gas rebreathed from the reservoir tube will thus be relatively richer in fresh gas and the system more efficient in its handling of fresh gas than the above analysis suggests. The theoretical data of Figs. 4.21 to 25 therefore give a lower limit, or conservative estimate, of the efficiency of the system.

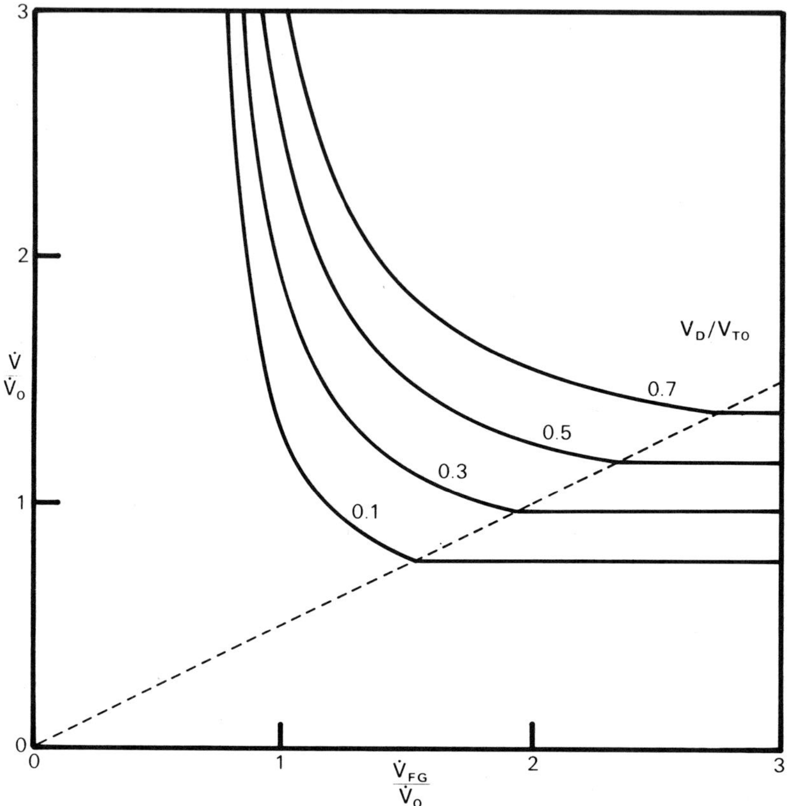

Fig. 4.25. The normal isocapnia line ($F_{ECO_2}/(\dot{V}_{CO_2}/\dot{V}_0) = 1.5$, approximately) plotted for different values of V_D/V_{TO}.

A number of clinical studies on T-piece systems used for automatic ventilation have measured the relationship between P_{aCO_2} and $\dot{V}_{FG}$. Figure 4.26 relates some of these measurements to eqn (4.24). Some authors have recommended working values for $\dot{V}_{FG}$ and $\dot{V}$ during anaesthesia. The usual recommendation for achieving normocapnia is a fresh gas flow close to $\dot{V}_{FG}/\dot{V}_0 = 1$ and a ventilation close to $\dot{V}/\dot{V}_0 = 1.5$. These values are plotted as a filled circle in Fig. 4.23. The agreement with theory is fair. Two factors probably account for the discrepancy in the direction of hypercapnia: firstly, as stated earlier, eqn (4.24) overestimates $\dot{V}/\dot{V}_0$ for a given $\dot{V}_{FG}/\dot{V}_0$ because it fails to model an approximately exponential expiratory waveform. Secondly, recommendations for anaesthetized subjects must allow for reduced $\dot{V}_{CO_2}$. Normocapnia during anaesthesia probably corresponds with a value of $F_{ECO_2}/(\dot{V}_{CO_2}/\dot{V}_0)$ nearer to 2.0 than to 1.5 (see legend to Fig. 4.26).

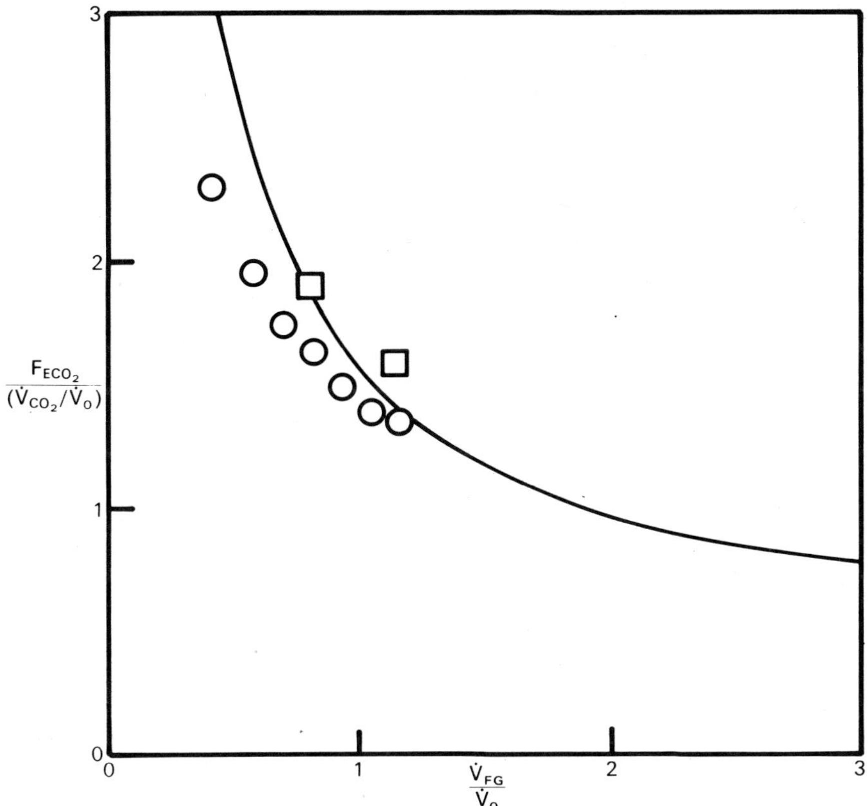

Fig. 4.26. T-piece breathing system combined with automatic ventilation. Comparison of eqn (4.24) with data from two studies: ○ Bain, J. A. and Spoerel, W. E. (1975). *Canadian Anaesthetists' Society Journal* **22**, 34–8; □ Henville, J. D. and Adams, A. P. (1976). *Anaesthesia* **31**, 247–56. Both studies were in adults of both sexes, with mean values of $\dot{V}$ around $10\,\mathrm{l\,min^{-1}}$. t_I/t_E is given in neither study. $F_{ECO_2}/(\dot{V}_{CO_2}/\dot{V}_0)$ is derived from the published data by assuming an atmospheric pressure of $101.3\,\mathrm{kPa}$ and a value of $170\,\mathrm{ml}$ (BTPS) $\mathrm{min^{-1}}$ (i.e., $150\,\mathrm{ml}$ (STP) $\mathrm{min^{-1}}$) for $\dot{V}_{CO_2}$ of anaesthetized adults (Nunn, J. F. (1987). *Applied Respiratory Physiology* (3rd edn) p. 366. Butterworths, London). $\dot{V}_0$ is set to $6\,\mathrm{l\,min^{-1}}$. The solid line represents eqn (4.24) for $t_I/t_E = 1$, $V_D/V_{TO} = 0.3$, $\dot{V}/\dot{V}_0 = 10/6 = 1.7$.

We emphasize, finally, a possible pitfall in the application of the theory represented by eqn (4.24). $\dot{V}_{FG}$, $\dot{V}$ and F_{ECO_2} all appear normalized to a baseline ventilation $\dot{V}_0$. We have taken this to equal a normal adult spontaneous ventilation of $6000\,\mathrm{ml\,min^{-1}}$. This is, however, an arbitrary choice which is not essential to the application of the theory. Equation (4.24) can in fact be rewritten without $\dot{V}_0$:

$$\frac{F_{ECO_2}}{\dot{V}_{CO_2}} = \frac{1/(1 + t_I/t_E) + (\dot{V}/\dot{V}_{FG})}{\dot{V} - V_D r}. \tag{4.25}$$

It follows that any value of $\dot{V}_0$ may be chosen in the application of eqn (4.24) (for example Fig. 4.23) so long as the same value is used throughout for computations of $\dot{V}_{FG}/\dot{V}_0$, $\dot{V}/\dot{V}_0$ and $F_{ECO_2}/(\dot{V}_{CO_2}/\dot{V}_0)$.

4.8   Type II ventilators with and without rebreathing

Figure 4.17 depicts some of the arrangements which can be adopted for the intermittent uptake of fresh gas by a ventilator and its subsequent delivery to the patient. In Fig. 4.17(b) we envisaged a steady flow of fresh gas $\dot{V}_{FG}$ being partly conserved by a reservoir bag whilst the ventilator inlet valve was closed (during the inspiratory phase). So long as $\dot{V}_{FG}$ equals or exceeds the delivered ventilation $\dot{V}$ no supplement to the fresh gas flow will be required. The volume of reservoir bag required is readily derived. It must be capable of storing all fresh gas delivered during inspiration for subsequent release into the ventilator. This bag volume V_B is thus:

$$V_B \geq \dot{V}_{FG}\, t_I. \tag{4.26}$$

This relationship assumes that the bellows fills with gas during the whole of the expiratory phase at a flow which exceeds $\dot{V}_{FG}$. If this condition is not satisfied then a larger V_B is required.

When $\dot{V}_{FG}$ falls below $\dot{V}$ supplemental gas is needed at inlet to the ventilator. An air inlet valve (Fig. 4.17(c)) is a safe way of achieving this in that it both provides oxygen and avoids excess rebreathing. During anaesthesia, however, it introduces a risk of diluting anaesthetic gases and thereby allowing a patient to wake up. Avoidance of 'awareness' in paralysed patients who may be suffering the pain of surgery is a major concern of anaesthesia, but balanced against this risk is the need for ventilators to be 'fail safe' by continuing to deliver an acceptable concentration of oxygen in the event of a failure in the fresh gas supply.

A way of minimizing the dilution of anaesthetic gases is to permit supplementation of the fresh gas flow with expired gas (Fig. 4.17(d)), but this is at the expense of allowing rebreathing of CO_2. As mentioned in the previous section, there are occasions when hyperventilation of the lungs combined with rebreathing may offer the advantage of minimizing alveolar collapse during anaesthesia. We shall now explore the characteristics of one such rebreathing system.

A system which permits rebreathing of expired gas will benefit fully from the fresh gas flow only if no fresh gas is spilled from the system before it enters the ventilator. A reservoir is needed, similar to that of Fig. 4.17(c), to collect fresh gas during the inspiratory phase of the ventilator cycle. Expired gas must also be available at the ventilator inlet. If a tube connects it directly from the expiratory valve to the fresh gas inlet, then expired gas may be entrained by the ventilator in preference to fresh gas from the reservoir bag.

This would result in excessive rebreathing. One way of overcoming this difficulty is to use the arrangement of Fig. 4.17(d) in which a tube is used as a reservoir for the fresh gas flow, and expired gas is directed into the reservoir tube well away from the fresh gas inlet. The performance of the system is analysed in Fig. 4.27.

At the end of the inspiratory phase (Fig. 4.27(a)) a volume $\dot{V}_{FG}\, t_I$ of fresh gas has collected in the reservoir tube. We assume that the ventilator fills at a constant flow V_T/t_E throughout expiration. During early expiration (Fig.

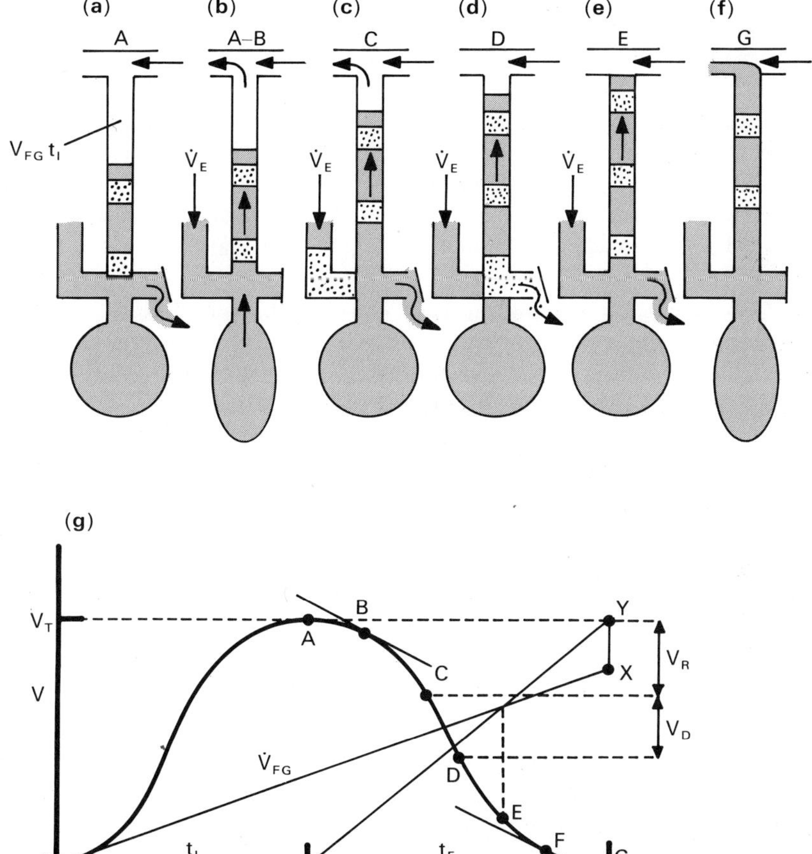

Fig. 4.27. Performance of the type II ventilator with rebreathing, connected in the mode of Fig. 4.17(d). The reservoir tube is depicted at six stages in the expiratory cycle: (a) beginning of expiration, (b) bag reduces in volume until expiratory flow equals flow out of the reservoir tube, (c) dead space gas (dotted) begins to enter reservoir tube, (e) ventilator begins to entrain expired gas from reservoir tube, (f) expiration ends. The respiratory waveform is shown in (g).

4.27(b)) and during late expiration (FG in Fig. 4.27(g)) the expiratory flow is likely to be lower than the flow into the ventilator. At these times the valve on the reservoir tube will remain shut and the reservoir bag will discharge some of its contents into the reservoir tube. As expiration proceeds the ventilator takes in only fresh gas until point E is reached (Fig. 4.27(e)), at which time the $\dot{V}_{FG}$ and V_T/t_E lines cross. From this moment on expired gas enters the ventilator. At the end of expiration a volume XY (Fig. 4.27(g)) of expired gas has left the reservoir tube to enter the ventilator.

The precise composition of the volume XY of rebreathed gas depends upon the disposition within the reservoir tube of gas from the dead space. Having not reached the alveoli this gas retains the characteristics of inspired gas and therefore has low CO_2 concentration. The progress of the expired dead space gas is followed in Fig. 4.27 in which it is represented with coarse dots. We denote the volume of the tube through which expired gas reaches the reservoir tube by V_R. At point C in Fig. 4.27(g) a volume V_R of gas has been expired and so dead space gas reaches the reservoir tube (Fig. 4.27(c)). If this occurs in mid-expiration when the valve is open none of this gas will enter the reservoir bag; some will leave the system via the valve and some will enter the reservoir tube proper. The volume entering the tube depends upon the time for further expiration of a volume V_D (CD in Fig. 4.27(g)). If $V_R \geq V_T$ a similar construction is appropriate using $V_R - V_T$ or $V_R - 2V_T$ and so on as required.

Precise considerations such as these regarding separate boluses of dead space gas are of little practical value for at least two reasons. Firstly, the assumption that there is no axial mixing in the system tubing becomes less tenable as the length of the tubing paths increase and the boluses of gas become smaller. Secondly, the relative magnitudes of V_T, V_R and V_D will be highly variable between patients and ventilator settings and it is impracticable to analyse every case in this manner. We therefore make the assumption that expired gas in the reservoir tube is perfectly mixed with a fraction $F_{\bar{E}CO_2}$ of CO_2 where

$$F_{\bar{E}CO_2} V_T = F_{ICO_2} V_D + F_{ECO_2}(V_T - V_D),$$

or

$$F_{\bar{E}CO_2} = F_{ICO_2}\left(\frac{V_D}{V_T}\right) + F_{ECO_2}\left(1 - \frac{V_D}{V_T}\right). \tag{4.27}$$

The tidal volume inspired to the alveoli is composed of a volume V_D of alveolar expired gas and a volume $V_T - V_D$ of the mixture which was entrained by the ventilator during the previous expiration. This mixture contained a volume $\dot{V}_{FG}(t_I + t_E)$ of fresh gas with a volume $V_T - \dot{V}_{FG}(t_I + t_E)$ of *mixed* expired gas. We deduce therefore

$$F_{ICO_2} V_T = F_{ECO_2} V_D + F_{\bar{E}CO_2}\left(\frac{V_T - V_D}{V_T}\right)[V_T - \dot{V}_{FG}(t_I + t_E)]$$

or

$$F_{\text{ICO}_2} = F_{\text{ECO}_2}\left(\frac{V_\text{D}}{V_\text{T}}\right) + F_{\bar{\text{E}}\text{CO}_2}\left(1 - \frac{V_\text{D}}{V_\text{T}}\right)\left(1 - \frac{\dot{V}_{\text{FG}}}{\dot{V}}\right). \tag{4.28}$$

Combine eqns (4.27), (4.28) and (2.16) to solve for F_{ECO_2}:

$$\frac{F_{\text{ECO}_2}}{\dot{V}_{\text{CO}_2}} = \frac{1}{\dot{V}_{\text{FG}}}\left[\frac{1}{(1 - V_\text{D}/V_\text{T})} - \left(\frac{V_\text{D}}{V_\text{T}}\right)\left(1 - \frac{\dot{V}_{\text{FG}}}{\dot{V}}\right)\right]. \tag{4.29}$$

Note that this solution is valid only if $\dot{V} \geq \dot{V}_{\text{FG}}$. For all cases in which $\dot{V} < \dot{V}_{\text{FG}}$ the relevant solution becomes

$$\frac{F_{\text{ECO}_2}}{\dot{V}_{\text{CO}_2}} = \frac{1}{\dot{V}(1 - V_\text{D}/V_\text{T})}. \tag{4.30}$$

For the limiting case of zero dead space eqn (4.29) predicts

$$\frac{F_{\text{ECO}_2}}{\dot{V}_{\text{CO}_2}} = \frac{1}{\dot{V}_{\text{FG}}}, \tag{4.31}$$

and F_{ECO_2} becomes independent of ventilation (if $\dot{V} \geq \dot{V}_{\text{FG}}$).

Using the same format as eqn (4.24), eqn (4.29) can be rewritten

$$\frac{F_{\text{ECO}_2}}{(\dot{V}_{\text{CO}_2}/\dot{V}_0)} = \frac{1}{(\dot{V}_{\text{FG}}/\dot{V}_0)}\left[\frac{1}{1 - (V_\text{D}/V_{\text{T0}})(\dot{V}_0/\dot{V})}\right.$$
$$\left. - \left(\frac{V_\text{D}}{V_{\text{T0}}}\right)\left(\frac{\dot{V}_0}{\dot{V}}\right)\left(1 - \frac{\dot{V}_{\text{FG}}/\dot{V}_0}{\dot{V}/\dot{V}_0}\right)\right]. \tag{4.32}$$

Equation (4.32) is plotted in Fig. 4.28 in the form of isocapnia lines for various values of V_D/V_{T0}.

Comparison between Figs. (4.25) and (4.28) shows firstly that the type II system with rebreathing is considerably more efficient in its use of fresh gas at all values of V_D/V_{T0} than the type I system with rebreathing via a T-piece. The comparison is strictly applicable within the restriction of an idealized respiratory waveform since Fig. 4.25 relates only to this case, but the conclusion is likely to have wider validity. A second possible advantage of the type II system is that F_{ECO_2} is less dependent on ventilation than with the type I system. So long as $\dot{V}$ exceeds $\dot{V}_{\text{FG}}$, the fresh gas flow almost exclusively determines F_{ECO_2}, particularly for small dead space volumes. This is not the case for the type I system for which the isocapnia lines are less steep, showing that both $\dot{V}$ and $\dot{V}_{\text{FG}}$ are important determinants of F_{ECO_2} over much of the useful performance range.

The arrangement shown in Fig. 4.17(d) can be connected with many ventilators. The Penlon Oxford Ventilator is one example (Fig. 4.29). This ventilator has no electrical connections; it is driven by a high pressure (320 kPa) source of gas, typically oxygen. It is predominantly time-cycled and

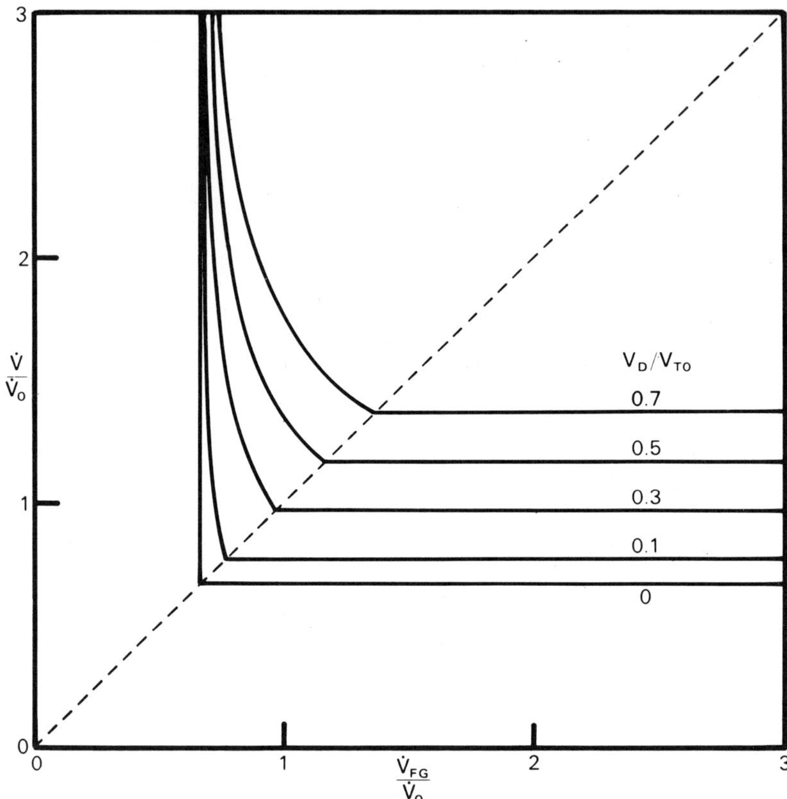

Fig. 4.28. Type II ventilator with rebreathing constituted as in Fig. 4.17(d). The normal isocapnia line ($F_{ECO_2}/(\dot{V}_{CO_2}/\dot{V}_0) = 1.5$, approximately) plotted for different values of V_D/V_{TO}. Performance for any respiratory waveform (eqn (4.32)).

generates an approximately constant flow from a bellows during inspiration. Two different sizes of bellows are available: for children and adults.

The rebreathing arrangements described above tend to be used only for automatic ventilation of patients with healthy lungs undergoing anaesthesia for surgery. Ventilators used for patients in intensive care wards rarely incorporate rebreathing, and those recently designed for the management of patients with severe lung disease now incorporate sophisticated electro-mechanical control of the respiratory volume and pressure waveforms, with multiple alarms to draw attention to malfunction.

One such device is the Siemens Servo 900C (Fig. 4.30) in which inspiratory and expiratory flow and pressure transducers and valves are used to maintain the various flow and/or pressure waveform options which can be selected by the operator. Devices of this kind invariably require an electrical power

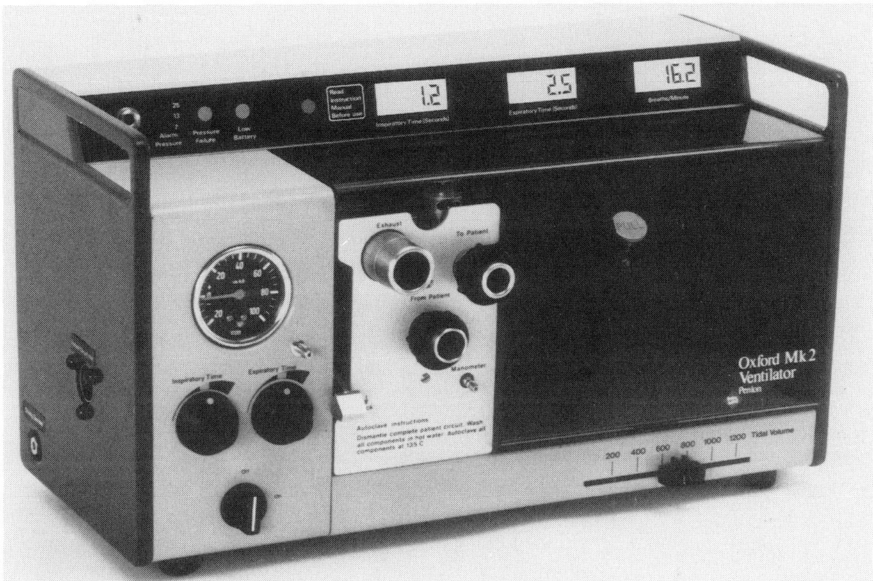

Fig. 4.29. The Penlon Oxford ventilator.

supply (sometimes a battery can be used in the short term) and usually need a high pressure supply of fresh gas. Further description of their transducers, information handling, effector mechanisms, and clinical application are beyond the scope of this section.

4.9   High frequency ventilation

Throughout chapters 2 and 4, breathing systems have been analysed on the basis of the assumption that no axial mixing occurs as gases flow along tubes. Boluses of gas which are stratified along the tubing of breathing systems have been regarded as separated abruptly by boundaries which lie at right angles to the flow (Fig. 4.31(a)), whether it be steady or oscillatory. One consequence of this assumption, illustrated by eqn (2.1), is that CO_2 exchange can only be maintained when the tidal volume is greater than the dead space volume ($V_T > V_D$).

The assumption of absent axial mixing flies in the face of our knowledge of boundary layers. We know that in both laminar and turbulent flows the velocity of gas at the wall of a tube is zero; that at the centre of a tube the velocity of flowing gas is greater than the mean velocity in the tube. This velocity profile (Fig. 4.31(b)) gives rise to a boundary between two species of gas, which extends along the tube and has a far greater surface area than any

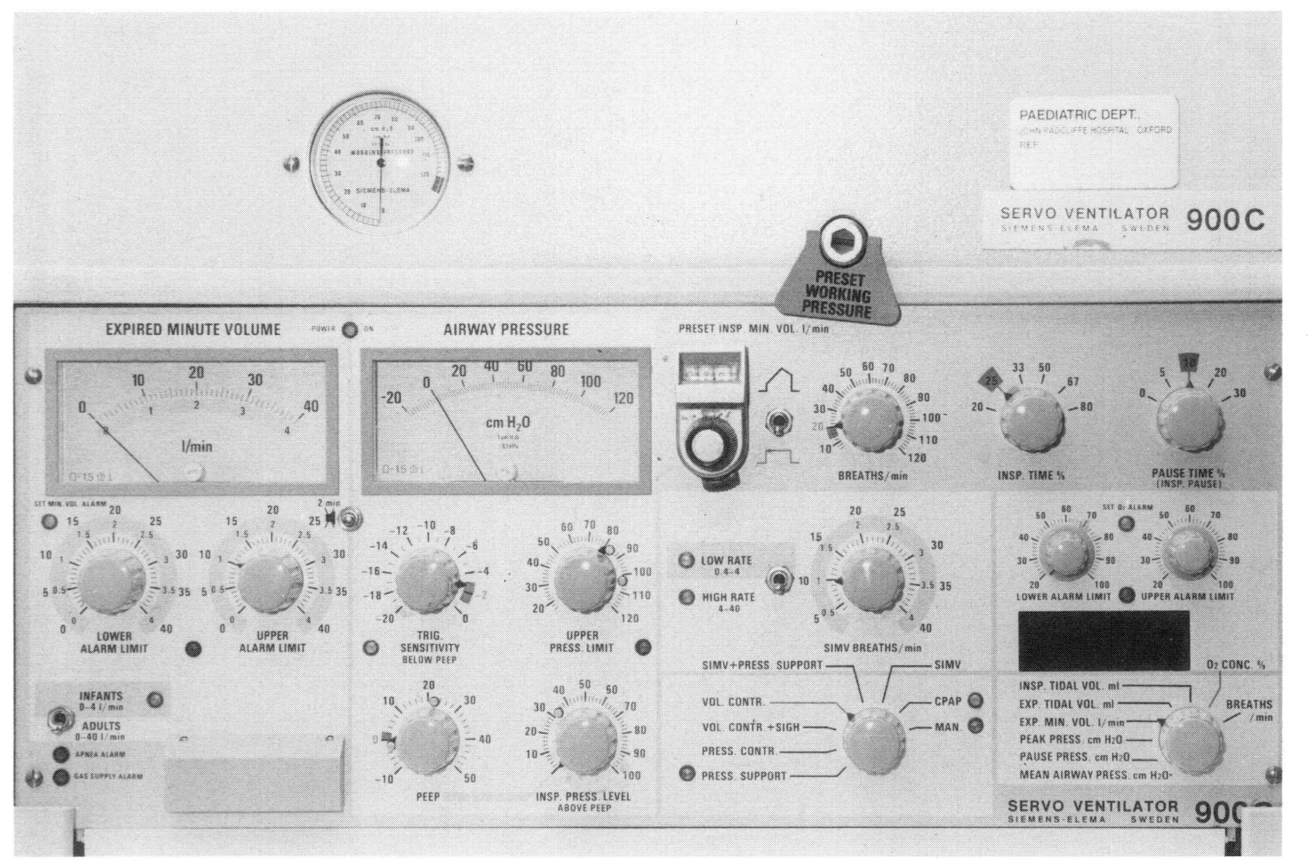

Fig. 4.30. The Siemens Servo 900C ventilator.

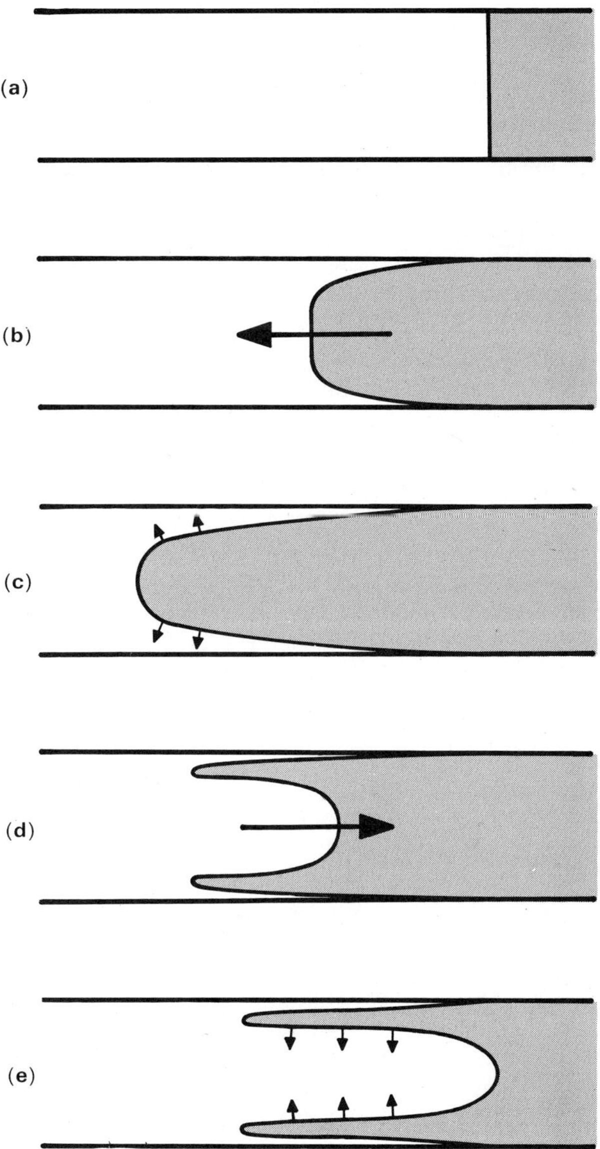

Fig. 4.31. Axial mixing of two species of gas in a tube due to diffusion combined with non-uniformity of the velocity profile. See text for description.

initial boundary across the section of the tube. Diffusion normal to this boundary then permits mixing of the two species of gas to a greater extent than would occur across a single tube section (Fig. 4.28(c)). If flow is oscillatory (Fig. 4.31(d)) the velocity profile deposits annular streaks of gas in the axial direction, increasing the area for diffusive mixing even more (Fig. 4.31(e)). The question we face is to what extent the foregoing analyses are limited in precision due to this phenomenon. In answering this question we shall find that the mixing process can actually be exploited to enhance gas exchange such that tidal volumes can be used which are smaller than the dead space volume ($V_T < V_D$), so long as ventilation is carried out at higher frequencies than those which occur physiologically.

We illustrate the axial dispersion of CO_2 in oscillatory flow along a tube using a simple model developed by Versprille (in Scheck, P. A., Sjöstrand, U. H., and Smith, R. B. (1983). *Perspectives in High Frequency Ventilation*, pp. 1–11. Martinus Nijhoff, Boston, Massachusetts). The velocity profile is simplified to a displacement of a cylinder of gas in the centre of the tube representing the forward motion of gas containing a fraction F_i of CO_2 into a region $i + 1$ of lower fraction F_{i+1} (Fig. 4.32(a) and (b)). The cylinder is taken to have cross-sectional area a. The pipe area is denoted by A. Perfect lateral mixing by diffusion is then assumed, which forms a compartment with mean CO_2 fraction $F_i a/A + F_{i+1}(1 - a/A)$ (Fig. 4.32(c)). When flow is reversed a cylinder of gas of this new concentration is carried back into compartment i (Fig. 4.32(d)). Perfect lateral mixing then leaves compartment i with a mean CO_2 fraction F_i' where

$$F_i' = \left[F_i \frac{a}{A} + F_{i+1}\left(1 - \frac{a}{A}\right) \right] \frac{a}{A}$$

$$+ \left[F_{i-1} \frac{a}{A} + F_i\left(1 - \frac{a}{A}\right) \right]\left(1 - \frac{a}{A}\right). \qquad (4.33)$$

In the steady state $F_i' = F_i$ and the resulting form of eqn (4.33) is

$$F_i = \left(\frac{F_{i+1} + F_{i-1}}{2} \right). \qquad (4.34)$$

The transfer of CO_2 from compartment i to the left in the forward phase of the flow is $F_i a x$, where x is the compartment width. The backward flow into compartment i from the left is $[F_i a/A + F_{i+1}(1 - a/A)]ax$. Noting that the tidal volume is $V_T = ax$, and allowing for r oscillations per unit time, we therefore predict a CO_2 flux of

$$\dot{V}_{CO_2} = F_i a x r - [F_i a/A + F_{i+1}(1 - a/A)]axr$$

$$= (F_i - F_{i+1})(1 - a/A)V_T r. \qquad (4.35)$$

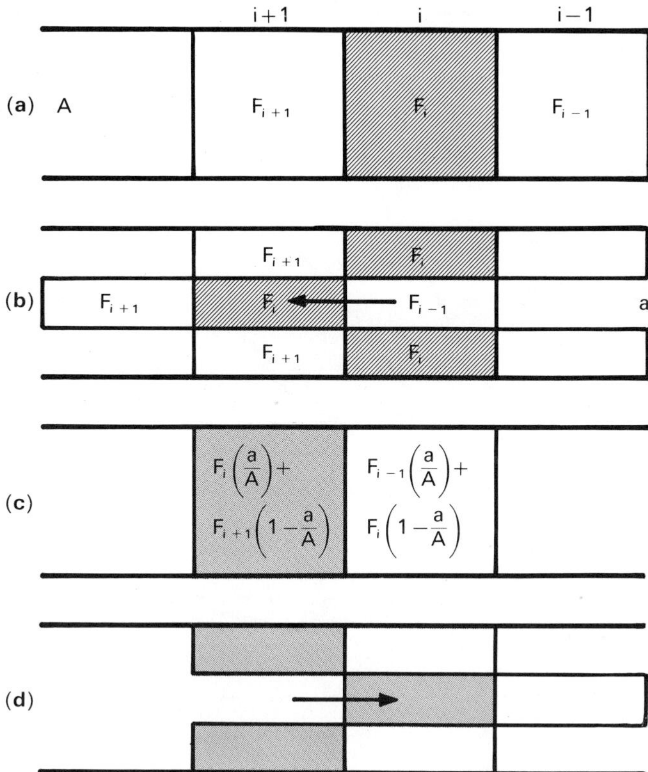

Fig. 4.32. A simple model of axial dispersion along a tube of area A. Compartments which contain different fractions F_i of a dispersing gas are defined (a). Displacement of a central core of area a is assumed (b), followed by perfect lateral mixing by diffusion (c). Reversal of the oscillatory flow (d) completes the cycle.

With a view to modelling CO_2 transfer from the alveoli across a dead space volume $V_D = Axn$ through n compartments separating a reservoir of alveolar gas (fraction F_{ACO_2}) from the atmosphere, we note from eqn (4.34) that the steps in CO_2 fractions between neighbouring compartments are all the same, and write $(F_i - F_{i+1})n = F_{ACO_2}$. Equation (4.35) can then be written in the form

$$\dot{V}_{CO_2} = F_{ACO_2}(A/a - 1)V_T^2 r/V_D. \tag{4.36}$$

If the same dead space were present, the same ventilation would give a conventional CO_2 flux of

$$\dot{V}_{CO_2} = F_{ACO_2}(V_T - V_D)r. \tag{4.37}$$

This very simple model of axial dispersion predicts several of the main features of experimental studies. The work of Jaeger, Kurzweg and Banner

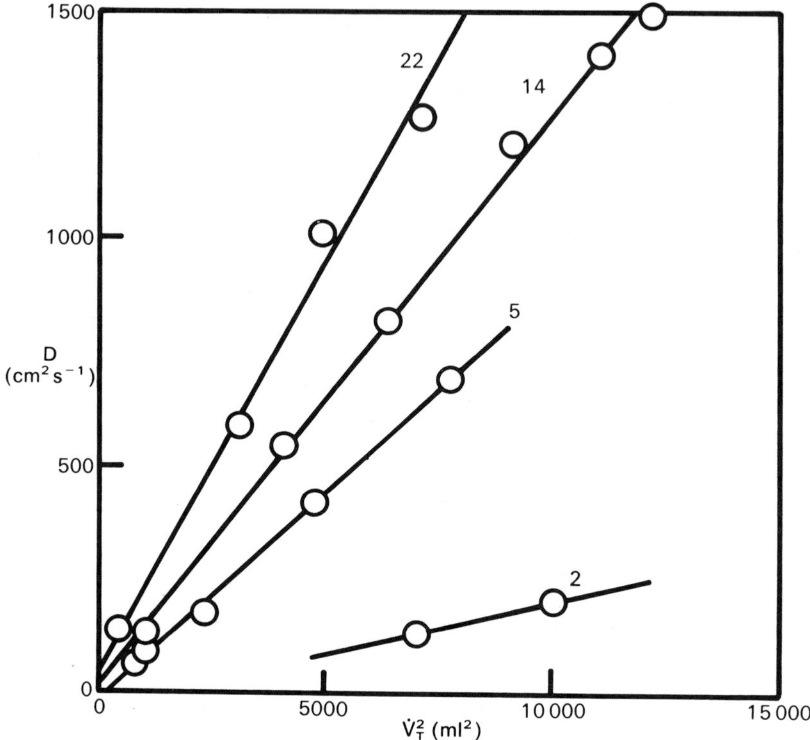

Fig. 4.33. Axial dispersion of oxygen in nitrogen along a circular pipe at four different frequencies of oscillation r(Hz). The diffusion constant D is closely proportional to V_T^2. The gradients are approximately proportional to r. These measurements are consistent with the prediction of eqn (4.36) that a flux is generated which is proportional to $V_T^2 r$. $A = 1.98$ cm². Data from Jaeger, M. J., Kurzweg, U. H., and Banner, M. J. (1984) *Critical Care Medicine* **12**, 708–10.

(Fig. 4.33) provides one example. These authors measured the diffusion coefficient D of oxygen in nitrogen down uniform circular tubes with sinusoidally oscillating flows. They found a linear relationship between D and the product $V_T^2 r$, consistent with our prediction that $\dot{V}_{CO_2}$ is proportional to $V_T^2 r$ (D for our model involving CO_2 would be given by $\dot{V}_{CO_2} L/(A F_{ACO_2}) = (A/a - 1) L V_T^2 r/(A V_D)$, where L is the length of the tube through which axial dispersion is occurring). Diffusion is greatly enhanced by the oscillatory motion, from an expected value in stationary gas of around 0.2 cm² s⁻¹ to over 1000 cm² s⁻¹, a factor of about 5000.

Animal experiments have suggested that the same concept of axial dispersion is applicable to the airways (Fig. 4.34). Ventilation of dogs at frequencies between 100 and 900 cycles min⁻¹ was performed by Carlon et al. to examine the relationship between $\dot{V}_{CO_2}/F_{ACO_2}$ ($=\dot{V}_A$, alveolar ventilation) and

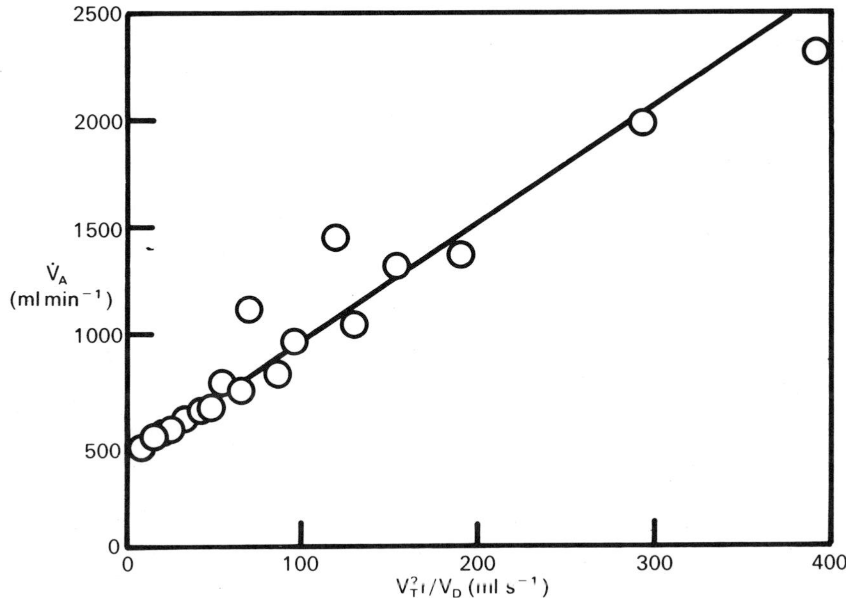

Fig. 4.34. Gas exchange during high frequency ventilation of dogs, plotted as alveolar ventilation against $V_T^2 r/V_D$ (ml sec^{-1}). Frequencies are between 100 and 900 cycles min^{-1}. Equation (4.36) predicts a proportional relationship. Data are from the same source as those in Fig. 4.33.

$V_T^2 r/V_D$. The data are consistent with the linear relationship predicted by eqn (4.36), but with an intercept on the $\dot{V}_A$ axis at 450 ml min^{-1}. It has been suggested that this elevation of gas transfer above expected values may arise from oscillations in the airways generated by the heart independently of the high frequency ventilator.

Axial dispersion clearly occurs and can to some extent be theoretically modelled, but can it contribute significantly to gas exchange during automatic ventilation of the lungs? In their experimental work with oxygen diffusion down tubes (Fig. 4.33), Jaeger, Kurzweg and Banner found their equivalent of our term $(A/a - 1)$ in eqn (4.36) to equal 0.03. For the work of Carlon et al on CO_2 transfer from dogs, the term was 0.05. The ratio ε of gas transfer by axial dispersion to gas transfer by conventional convection can be derived by

$$\varepsilon = (A/a - 1)\frac{V_T^2}{V_D(V_T - V_D)}$$

$$\simeq 0.04 \left/ \left[\frac{V_D}{V_T}\left(1 - \frac{V_D}{V_T} \right) \right] \right. , \qquad (4.38)$$

where the approximate coefficient 0.04 is an average from the experiments mentioned above. Note that ε is predicted by eqn (4.38) to be independent of frequency. For a normal V_D/V_T of around 0.3, ε equals 0.19. This suggests that around 20 per cent of normal CO_2 elimination might be accounted for by axial dispersion. For $V_D/V_T = 0.5$, $\varepsilon = 0.16$. As V_D approaches V_T, ε tends towards infinity; no conventional gas transfer occurs when $V_D = V_T$.

The effectiveness of axial dispersion in high frequency ventilation at maintaining normal gas exchange at tidal volumes less than V_D has been demonstrated in dogs by Kolton (Fig. 4.35). At frequencies above 5 Hz it was found possible to maintain normal F_{ACO_2} with $V_T/V_D < 1$. Figure 4.35 shows that little benefit is gained by increases in frequency above about 15 Hz. At this frequency the ventilation ($\dot{V} = V_T r$) required is around ten times that which would be needed for conventional ventilator settings.

Findings such as those cited here are in broad agreement both with clinical use of high frequency ventilation and with more precise analytic solutions for axial dispersion in relatively simple geometries such as uniform tubes. The anatomical geometry of the airways, with around 23 divisions (Fig. 1.2) is clearly far more complex than a uniform tube. Bifurcations are expected to

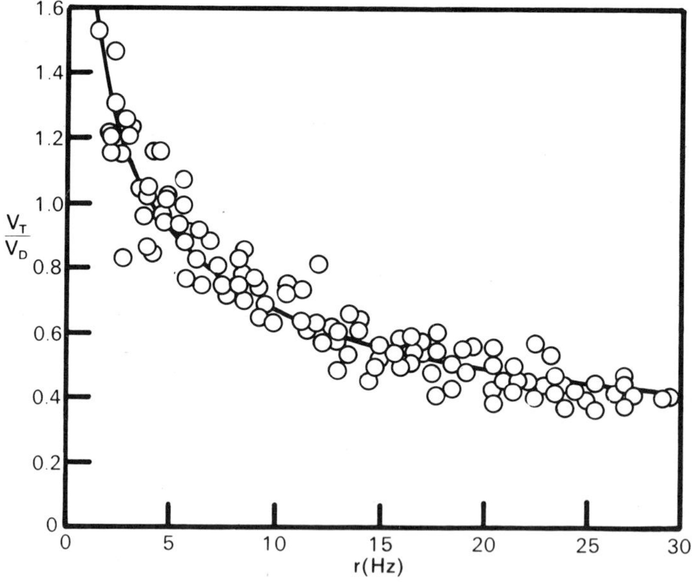

Fig. 4.35. Tidal volume to dead space ratio required at high ventilator frequencies to maintain normal CO_2 levels in dogs. Conventional gas exchange is impossible for $V_T/V_D < 1$, but is achieved in this range for $r > 5$ Hz. Data from Kolton, M. (1984). *Canadian Anaesthetists' Society Journal* **31**, 416–29.

make their own contribution to gas mixing, which more precise models will need to take into account.

We conclude that axial dispersion may well account for errors of around 20 per cent in the analyses of breathing systems using conventional assumptions. Furthermore, gas exchange can be maintained by the use of high frequency ventilation even when the tidal volume is less than the dead space volume. The possible clinical benefits from ventilating patients in such a manner are currently a topic of wide research interest.

Problems

4.1 A patient's ventilation is to be manually controlled at a rate of 10 breaths/min using a Magill breathing system with a fresh gas flow of $15\,l\,min^{-1}$. It is intended to achieve a ventilation of $9\,l\,min^{-1}$ to minimize the elevation of alveolar CO_2 partial pressure which tends to accompany controlled ventilation with this system.

Calculate the minimum volume of reservoir bag which will be adequate for the system assuming that the ratio of inspiratory time to expiratory time is (a) 1:2, (b) 2:1.

4.2 A patient is ventilated during anaesthesia with a Penlon Nuffield 200 ventilator connected to a Bain system as a Type I ventilation system. The ventilatory waveform is plotted in Fig. 4.36. The dead space volume is 300 ml and the patients CO_2 production is $184\,ml\,min^{-1}$. All volumes are measured at ambient conditions.

Use a graphical construction in combination with the given ventilatory waveform to estimate the fraction of CO_2 in expired alveolar gas when the steady fresh gas flow into the system is (a) $6\,l\,min^{-1}$, (b) $12\,l\,min^{-1}$.

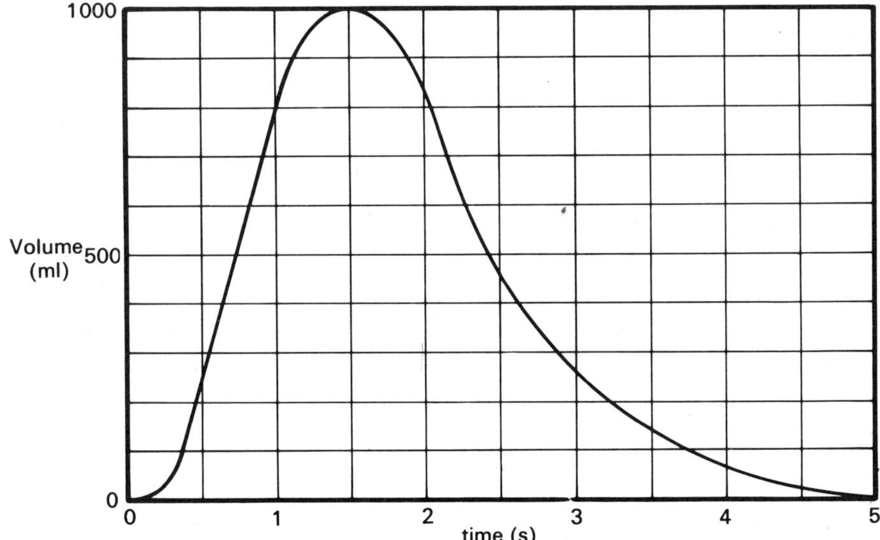

Fig. 4.36

4.3   The theory of Permutt, Mitzner and Weinmann, for high frequency ventilation at tidal volumes V_T close to the dead space volume V_D, predicts the following relationship between CO_2 production $\dot{V}_{CO_2}$, alveolar CO_2 fraction F_{ACO_2}, and respiratory rate r (Permut, S., Mitzner, W., and Weinmann, G. (1985). *Journal of Applied Physiology* **58**, 1956–70.):

$$\dot{V}_{CO_2} = F_{ACO_2} 0.6 n V_D r (V_T/V_D)^{(1 + 0.7/\sqrt{n})}.$$

A patient is ventilated with a system which conforms to this equation. The CO_2 production is 210 ml min^{-1} measured at ambient conditions. Given that $n = 0.3$, $V_D = 170$ ml, and F_{ACO_2} is required to be 0.05, calculate the frequency of ventilation required for the following tidal volumes; (a) $0.7V_D$, (b) V_D, (c) $1.3\ V_D$. For the latter case, what frequency of ventilation would be predicted by conventional theory assuming no axial dispersion?

Further reading

Brauer, L. (1905). Die praktische Durchführung des Ueberdruckverfahrens. *Deutsche Medizinische Wochenschrift* **31**, 1489–92.

Dorrington, K. L. and Lehane, J. R. (1989). Rebreathing during spontaneous and controlled ventilation with T-piece breathing systems: a general solution. *Anaesthesia* (in press).

Chatwin, P. C. (1975). On the longitudinal dispersion of passive contaminant in oscillatory flows in tubes. *Journal of Fluid Mechanics* **75**, 513–27.

Mushin, W. W., Rendell-Baker, L., Thompson, P. W., and Mapleson, W. W. (1980). *Automatic Ventilation of the Lungs* (3rd edn). Blackwell, Oxford. (Includes a directory of ventilator models.)

Sauerbruch, F. (1904). Zur Pathologie des offenen Pneumothorax und die Grundlagen meines Verfahrens zu seiner Ausschattung. *Mitteilungen aus den Grenzgebieten der Medizin und Chirurgie* **13**, 399–482.

Slutsky, A. S. (1984). Mechanisms affecting gas transport during high-frequency oscillation. *Critical Care Medicine* **12**, 713–17.

Tuffier, T. and Hallion, L. (1896). Opérations intrathoraciques avec respiration artificielle par insufflation. *Compte Rendu de Séances de la Société de Biologie* **48**, 951–3.

Waters, D. J. and Mapleson, W. W. (1961). Rebreathing during controlled respiration with various semiclosed anaesthetic systems. *British Journal of Anaesthesia* **33**, 374–81.

Watson, E. J. (1983). Diffusion in oscillatory pipe flow. *Journal of Fluid Mechanics* **133**, 233–44.

Young, J. D. and Dorrington, K. L. (1989) Peak airway pressure during jet ventilation: theory and measurement. *British Journal of Anaesthesia* (in press).

5 Oxygen transfer in extracorporeal lungs

5.1 Introduction

Surgery within the chest was made possible by the introduction of mechanical ventilation of the lungs from the 1890s. The objective of operating inside the heart under direct vision was not realized until the invention of the heart-lung machine. On 6 May 1953 John Gibbon of Philadelphia performed the first successful open heart operation with the use of total cardiopulmonary bypass through a machine. The patient was an 18-year old girl with a large atrial septal defect. She was connected to the apparatus for 45 min and totally dependent on the extracorporeal flow of blood through a pump and an artificial lung for 26 min.

The principle of cardiopulmonary bypass is simple (Fig. 5.1). If sufficiently large cannulae are positioned in the venous and the arterial side of the circulation blood can be diverted from its normal passage through the heart and lungs through a pump and gas exchanger lying outside the body (hence the term *extracorporeal*). If a sufficient flow is maintained and if the transfer of CO_2 and oxygen in the extracorporeal lung are great enough to 'arterialize' the venous blood, life can be maintained without any contribution from the patient's own heart and lungs (Fig. 5.1(b)). It might be thought unnecessary to bypass both the heart and lungs when surgery on the heart alone is planned but because the heart pumps blood round two circulations, the pulmonary and the systemic, bypass of the heart alone would involve a minimum of four cannulations. It has become customary in most bypass procedures to incorporate an artificial lung, as well as a pump to take over the function of the natural heart.

The use of procedures of this kind has increased dramatically since the 1950s. Figure 5.2 gives an estimate of the number of cases involved. Initially cardiopulmonary bypass was performed mainly for the repair of congenital heart defects, like that of Gibbon's first surviving patient. In the 1960s heart valve replacement surgery became established and an upsurge in bypass cases followed. From the 1970s coronary artery bypass surgery has accounted for a large increase in numbers of patients to whom the technology has been applied. In many centres its use is now routine.

Surgery on the heart is not the only setting in which the use of extracorporeal lungs has found a place. As part of the intensive care of patients with failing lungs an artificial lung can be connected temporarily to give a partial or total respiratory support. This form of management is currently only of use in patients whose own lungs are capable of recovery; the use of

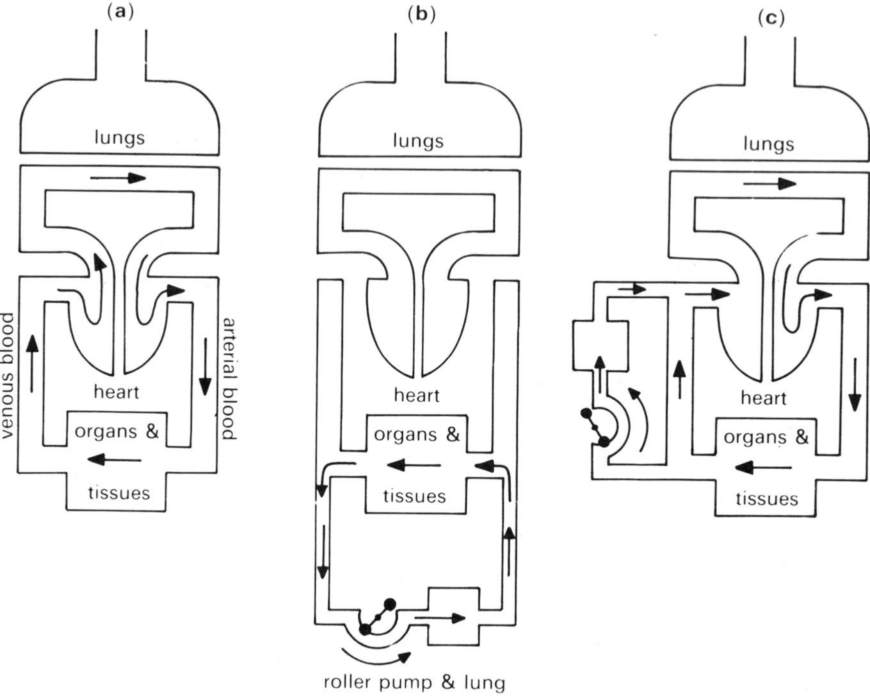

Fig. 5.1. Types of extracorporeal gas exchange. (a) The normal circulation; (b) full cardiopulmonary bypass; (c) vein-to-vein extracorporeal flow involving no bypass of the heart or lungs. Compare Fig. 1.7.

long term artificial lungs remains hypothetical and unlikely in view of the growing success of transplant surgery. Figure 5.1(c) illustrates one mode of connection of an extracorporeal lung which does not involve bypass of the natural lungs or heart. In this arrangement blood is drained from and returned to the venous side of the circulation. Systems have even been devised for achieving high rates of gas transfer using a single cannula, through which the blood flow intermittently changes direction. The lower curve of Fig. 5.2 shows the approximate annual number of cases in which extracorporeal respiratory support has been used. The numbers have been small and variable from year to year. An upsurge since 1980 is accounted for mainly by the promising use of the technique in newborn babies in the USA.

How does an artificial lung work? Gibbon's device contained vertical screens of stainless steel wire mesh down which the blood was caused to flow in a thin film. Oxygen was blown across the surface of these films of blood. Oxygen was taken up by the blood and CO_2 given off by the blood into the gas flow. The pump used to circulate blood comprised of two rollers mounted

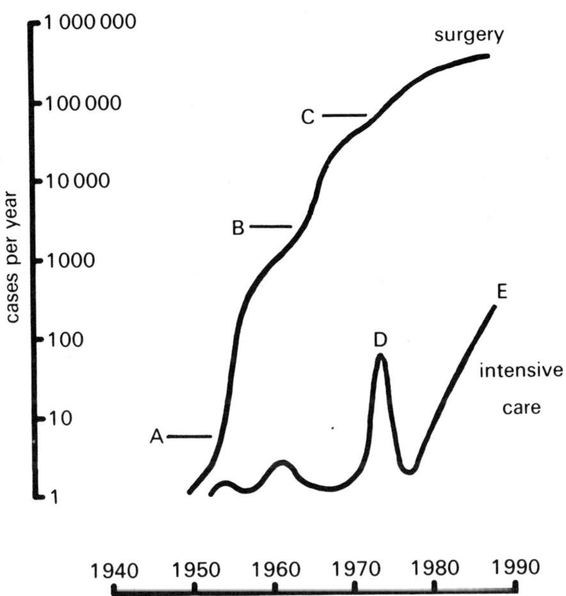

Fig. 5.2. Estimated world numbers of cases per annum in which extracorporeal gas exchange has been used clinically. Letters correspond with introduction of new therapies: A, correction of congenital heart defects; B, heart valve replacements; C, coronary bypass surgery; D, trial in USA of extracorporeal gas exchange in adults with severe lung disease; E, expanding therapy in USA of newborn patients with respiratory failure. Modified from Galletti, P. M. (1984). *American Society for Artificial Internal Organs Journal* **7**, 135–8.

on a revolving arm, and passing over rubber tubing which was clamped in a semicircular position. The rollers moved the blood through the tubing and the blood was unable to flow backwards because there was always at least one roller compressing the tube. This style of 'roller pump' (Fig. 5.1) remains the most commonly used pump to this day, though more durable polymers with better compatibility with blood are now used in place of rubber.

Gibbon's lung involved direct contact between blood and gas, unlike the natural lung in which a membrane is interposed between the two. The direct-contact devices widely used today have bubbles rather than films to achieve gas transfer. By injecting a fine spray of bubbles into flowing blood a large surface area of contact can be achieved within a relatively small device (most modern 'bubblers' are about the size of a domestic coffee percolator). Small bubbles have been found to produce excellent transfer of oxygen but they are not very efficient in terms of CO_2 removal. They may be exceedingly difficult to remove from the blood before it is returned to the patient (a process known as 'defoaming'). Large bubbles are less efficient as far as oxygen transfer is concerned but they are essential for CO_2 elimination. Large bubbles are more easily removed, often by buoyancy alone. Compromises between these opposing specifications have been worked out largely empirically.

Avoidance of direct contact between blood and gas appears to have the theoretical advantage of modelling the natural lungs more closely. The blood–gas interface has long been known to produce damage to plasma proteins, but the interposition of a synthetic membrane raises its own problems. In 1956 Clowes, Hopkins and Neville achieved success in using ethylcellulose and polyethylene membranes of 0.001 in (25 μm) thick to construct a lung for use in dogs. Clinical application of one of their membrane devices was reported in 1958. For adults a sandwich of 50 flat layers of polyethylene was assembled, making a total area of 25 m^2 across which oxygen diffused into and CO_2 diffused out of the blood. Thinner more suitable polymer membranes were to appear later and are now in widespread use. Polypropylene is at present the dominant material for such devices though silicone rubber is also well established.

Membrane lungs which are assembled to form multiple flat layers of blood, then polymer, then gas and so on, suffer from some difficulties in construction. Support of the thin membranes with appropriate spacing to permit blood flow on one side and gas on the other can be difficult to achieve, and leaks must be prevented from the edge of the sandwich by using tight gaskets or sealants. The advent of the thin polymer hollow fibre has popularized a family of 'capillary' lungs in which either blood or gas flows down the centre of each of a bundle of thousands of extremely fine hollow polypropylene fibres. The other phase (gas or blood respectively) flows across and through the bundle of fibres causing oxygen and CO_2 to be transferred by diffusion across the tubular fibre walls. Typical fibre outside diameters are 250 μm with a wall thickness of 25 μm. In the following sections we shall analyse gas transfer for both flat-plate and hollow-fibre geometries of membrane lung.

Adequate exchange of oxygen and CO_2 is clearly one requirement of devices used for extracorporeal respiration. What are the other features required of such a system? The clotting of blood is a major difficulty in the use of extracorporeal circuits. Whenever blood comes into contact with foreign surfaces its clotting mechanism is activated. This can lead not only to the complete seizing up of the blood flow channels but also to *embolism*, the carriage into the patient from the extracorporeal circuit of blood clots which may have devastating consequences such as a stroke. Drugs are usually administered to inhibit clotting, but these in turn may give rise to abnormal bleeding from the patient's own circulation. The drug which is most commonly used for this purpose is heparin.

Swedish researchers have recently discovered a method of covalently bonding heparin to a wide range of materials including most of the polymers used in extracorporeal lungs. This has made it possible for the first time to conduct prolonged extracorporeal gas exchange with little or no heparinization of the blood itself and it is likely to lead to an expansion of the use of these procedures.

Contact between blood and foreign surfaces activates not only the clotting of blood but also numerous other adverse events. *Haemolysis,* the rupture of red cells, is virtually always present. It tends to be a function of turbulence within the blood flow and it is often more related to the type of pump used in the circuit than to the lung itself. Figure 5.3 shows the amount of haemoglobin measured in the plasma of ten anaesthetized dogs, before and during 8 h of extracorporeal gas exchange with a blood flow of 500 ml min^{-1}. Since haemoglobin is normally present mainly in the red cells an increased concentration in plasma gives a measure of the number of red cells undergoing haemolysis. Note that even before commencing extracorporeal blood flow a baseline value of 18 mg dl^{-1} was detected. Since the total blood haemoglobin level in these experiments was around 12 g dl^{-1} and the red cell volume

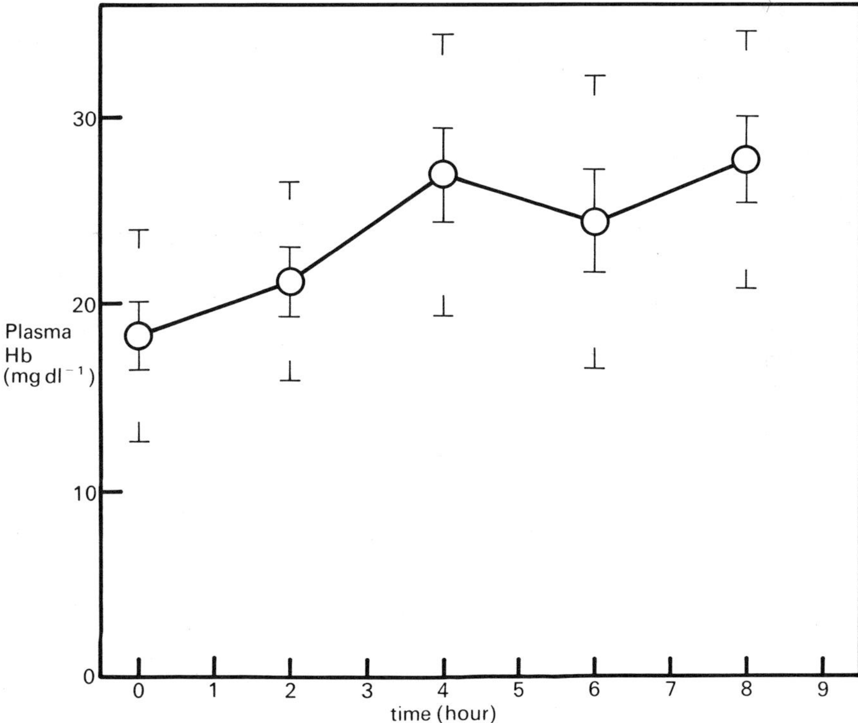

Fig. 5.3. Haemolysis during extracorporeal gas exchange can be quantified by measuring the plasma concentration of haemoglobin (normally held within the red cells). Data for laboratory perfusions with dogs from Gardaz, J.-P. (1988). *Journal of Biomedical Engineering* **10**, 74–81. (Mean ± sem and sd).

(haematocrit) was 35 per cent of the total blood volume, we can deduce that only 0.1 per cent of the haemoglobin is normally in the plasma. The increase in plasma haemoglobin over 8 h at an average rate of around 1 mg dl^{-1} h^{-1} represents a fairly slow rate of increase of this level. Results such as these are commonly observed.

Red cells are not the only ones affected. Platelet function and numbers are almost invariably reduced by extracorporeal circulation, with many platelets becoming deposited on the foreign surfaces of the circuit itself. Figure 5.4 shows typical results, in this case from the same experiments as Fig. 5.3. Part of the early fall in platelet count (to about 84 per cent of its initial value) can be attributed to the dilution of the subjects' blood by the fluid used to prime the circuit, but most is due to other influences.

White cells may also be profoundly affected. In the experiments just described a fall in the number of circulating white cells to 43 per cent at 30 min was seen, followed by a rise to a higher mean level than that preceding the experiment (Fig. 5.5). Explanations for these changes remain far from complete.

Other difficulties with achieving safe extracorporeal gas exchange include sterilization of all components exposed to blood, and avoidance of leaks.

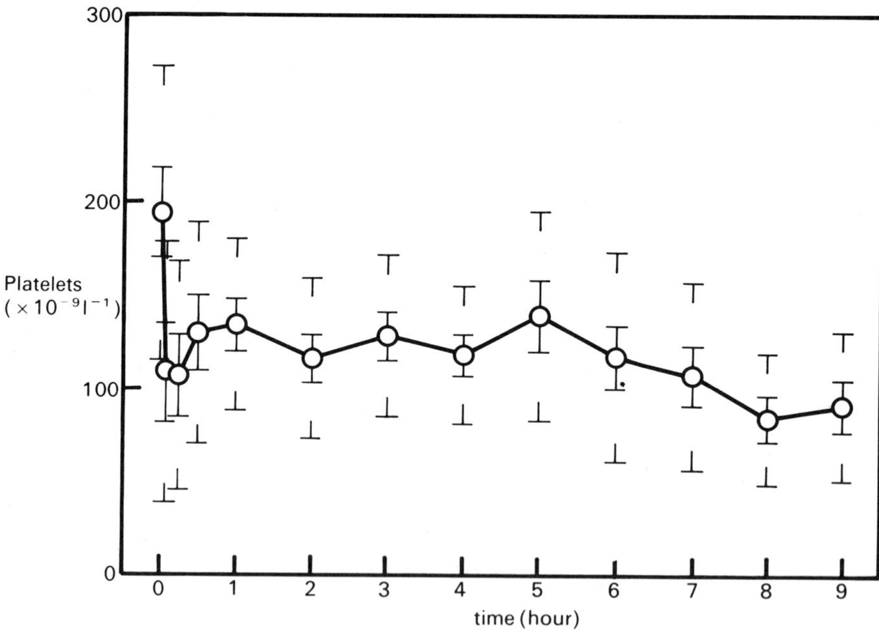

Fig. 5.4. Platelet concentration is depleted by extracorporeal circulation. Data source as Fig. 5.3. (Mean $\pm$ sem and sd).

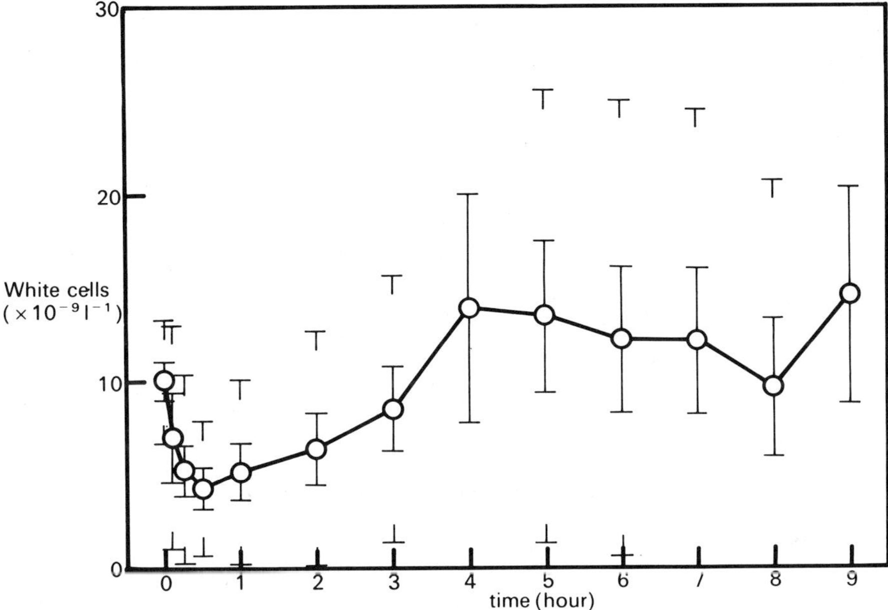

Fig. 5.5. White cell concentration during experimental extracorporeal gas exchange. Data source as Fig. 5.3. (Mean $\pm$ sem and sd).

Blood must not leak out and gas must not leak in. Since many of the polymer membranes used are in fact porous, typically containing micropores of around 0.02 μm diameter, the risk of blowing *gas emboli* into the patient is not restricted only to bubble devices. Great care is needed in the priming of all extracorporeal circuits to eliminate large, potentially lethal, bubbles.

5.2   The parallel plate membrane lung: basic equations

We model membrane lungs constructed from multiple flat polymer membranes, by regarding them as having one upper and one lower membrane between which blood flows in uniform, one-dimensional flow (Fig. 5.6). The membrane inner surfaces lie a distance $2h$ apart. Each membrane has length L, breadth b, and area $A/2 = Lb$. A is the total area of membrane exposed to blood. The membrane thickness is t. Gas flows on the outer surfaces of the membranes across which oxygen and CO_2 are transferred between the blood and gas compartments by diffusion. Coordinates x and y are defined along and normal to the blood channel. $x = 0$ at blood inlet, $x = L$ at the outlet and $y = 0$ at the centreline of the channel.

Consider first an open control volume with dimensions dx by dy, (Fig. 5.6(c)) situated at the site (x, y) shown in Fig. 5.6(b). Imagine this to be a

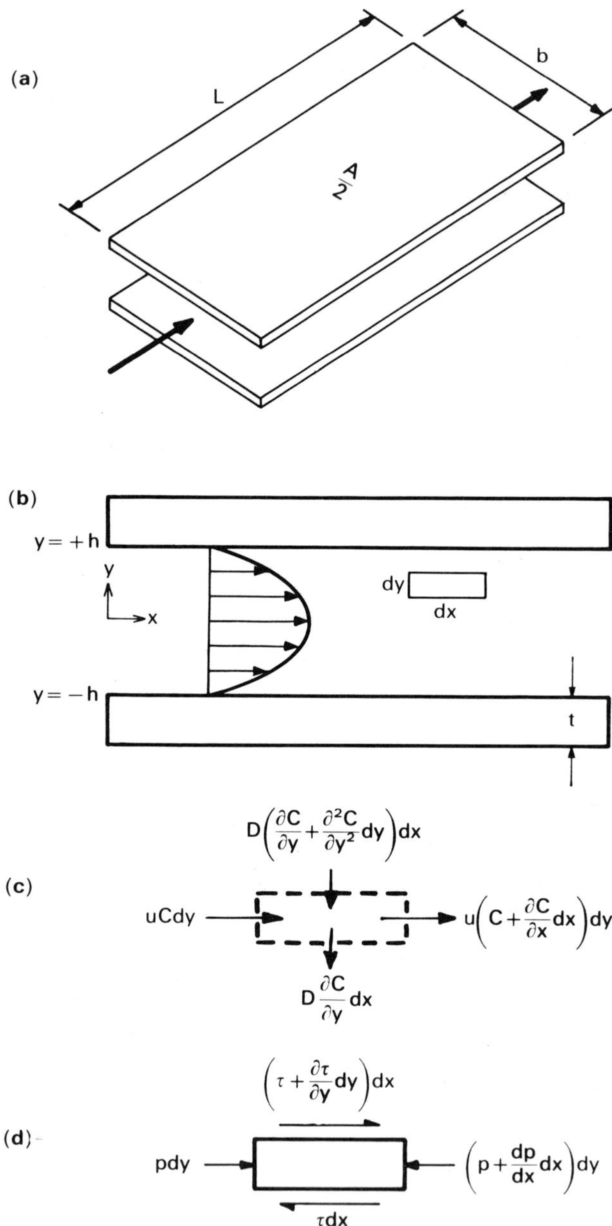

Fig. 5.6. The parallel plate membrane lung modelled (a) with one upper and one lower polymer membrane, between which (b) blood flows in uniform one dimensional flow. An open control volume (c) is used to establish the convection–diffusion equation; a closed control volume (d) facilitates application of the equation of motion.

cage through which blood is flowing in the x direction with velocity u. Blood carrying a gas at concentration C enters at the left-hand end, and thus convects a quantity $uCdy$ into the control volume in unit time. If the concentration at the right-hand side is denoted by $C + (\partial C/\partial x)\,dx$, then the outgoing convection is $u[C + (\partial C/\partial x)dx]dy$.

We shall assume that concentration gradients in the y direction exceed those in x direction so markedly that the inbalance in convection in the x direction in the steady state is accounted for solely by diffusion of the gas in the y direction. Diffusion in the x direction is ignored. For a concentration gradient in the y direction of $\partial C/\partial y$ and a diffusion constant for the gas in blood D, the balance between convection in the x direction and diffusion in the y direction becomes

$$\left[u\left(C + \frac{\partial C}{\partial x}dx \right) - uC \right] = \left[D\left(\frac{\partial C}{\partial y} + \frac{\partial^2 C}{\partial y^2}dy \right) - D\frac{\partial C}{\partial y} \right]dx,$$

or

$$u\frac{\partial C}{\partial x} = D\frac{\partial^2 C}{\partial y^2}. \tag{5.1}$$

The solution of the problem of oxygen and CO_2 transfer in membrane lungs is basically the solution of this convection–diffusion equation. The task may appear simple but attempts to derive appropriate solutions have an involved history dating back to the first attempt by Graetz in 1885 (Graetz, L. (1885). *Annalen der Physik und Chemie*, **25**, 337–57; working in fact with the equivalent axisymmetric problem in radial coordinates).

Solution of eqn (5.1) requires knowledge of the velocity profile across the channel. u is a function of y. We shall ignore entrance effects (change of u with x alone near $x = 0$) and assume uniform fully developed steady flow. The first obstacle we meet is that blood is not a Newtonian fluid (Fig. 5.7). Many fluids approximate closely to the ideal of having a constant viscosity μ and therefore a relationship of proportionality between velocity gradient du/dy and the shear stress τ required to maintain the steady shearing motion:

$$\tau = \mu\frac{du}{dy}. \tag{5.2}$$

Water, for example, displays a viscosity close to $1\ \mathrm{mNs\,m^{-2}}$ (1 centipoise) over a wide range of conditions. Plasma consists of more than 90 per cent water by weight but also contains about 7 per cent by weight of protein. This increases the viscosity in comparison with pure water, but it is the presence in whole blood of around 40 per cent by volume of cells which causes blood viscosity to vary as a function of the shear rate itself.

Figure 5.7 shows this relationship. At low shear rates red cells have a tendency to stack like piles of dinner plates into structures termed 'rouleaux'.

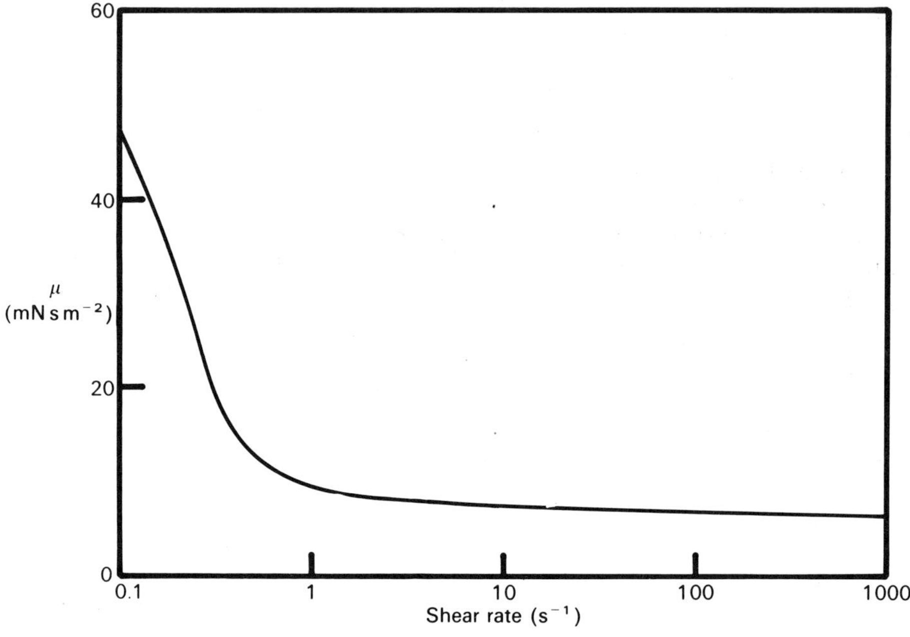

Fig. 5.7. The variation of viscosity of human blood as a function of the rate of shear ($\mathrm{d}u/\mathrm{d}y$). Graph from Trowbridge, E. A. (1984). *Life Support Systems* **2**, 25–38.

The resistance these provide to shearing motion is largely responsible for the rise in viscosity below shear rates of about $1\,\mathrm{s}^{-1}$. The flows we are concerned with here involve shear rates in the range 0–$1000\,\mathrm{s}^{-1}$ and the assumption we shall adopt of Newtonian behaviour must be recognized as one source of error in the modelling of gas transfer.

A further assumption implicit in eqn (5.2), whether or not μ is regarded as constant, is that the blood flow is laminar rather than turbulent. In laminar flow lines of constant y in the blood channel can be regarded as streamlines. Were turbulence to set in this would no longer hold, and the transfer of horizontal momentum by turbulence up and down across lines of constant y would become the main determinant of shear stresses in the flow. Although an equation of the form of eqn (5.2) can still be written for turbulent flow, the interpretation of μ has to be quite different from that adopted for laminar flow.

In membrane lungs flow is usually laminar. We balance the pressure forces and viscous shear forces on a fixed mass of fluid, as depicted in Fig. 5.6(d). For steady uniform flow there is no acceleration and Newton's second law of motion becomes

$$\left(\tau+\frac{\mathrm{d}\tau}{\mathrm{d}y}\mathrm{d}y\right)\mathrm{d}x-\tau\mathrm{d}x=\left(p+\frac{\mathrm{d}p}{\mathrm{d}x}\mathrm{d}x\right)\mathrm{d}y-p\,\mathrm{d}y$$

or

$$\frac{d\tau}{dy} = \frac{dp}{dx}. \tag{5.3}$$

Substitution for τ from eqn (5.2) gives

$$\frac{d^2u}{dy^2} = \frac{1}{\mu}\frac{dp}{dx}. \tag{5.4}$$

For constant μ and dp/dx integration is simple:

$$u = \frac{1}{2\mu}\frac{dp}{dx}y^2 + Ay + B, \tag{5.5}$$

where the integration constants are determined by the boundary condition of zero velocity at the channel walls; $u=0$ for $y=\pm h$:

$$0 = \frac{1}{2\mu}\frac{dp}{dx}h^2 + Ah + B$$

$$0 = \frac{1}{2\mu}\frac{dp}{dx}h^2 - Ah + B$$

or

$$A = 0$$

$$B = -\frac{h^2}{2\mu}\frac{dp}{dx}.$$

Equation (5.5) becomes

$$u = \frac{1}{2\mu}\frac{dp}{dx}(y^2 - h^2). \tag{5.6}$$

It is useful to incorporate a mean velocity $\bar{u}$ in place of the so far unknown dp/dx, and since

$$2h\bar{u} = \int_{-h}^{h} \frac{1}{2\mu}\frac{dp}{dx}(y^2 - h^2)\,dy,$$

$$\bar{u} = -\frac{1}{2\mu}\frac{dp}{dx}\frac{2h^2}{3}, \tag{5.7}$$

and we can then write

$$u = \frac{3}{2}\bar{u}\left[1 - \left(\frac{y}{h}\right)^2\right]. \tag{5.8}$$

This is the widely known parabolic velocity profile of laminar Newtonian flow. Equation (5.7) is one form of an equation originally proposed by Hagen in 1839 then Poiseuille in 1840 to describe the flow of blood down glass tubes.

Our convection–diffusion equation can now be given in a more specific form by substituting eqn (5.8) into eqn (5.1):

$$\frac{3}{2}\bar{u}\left[1-\left(\frac{y}{h}\right)^2\right]\frac{\partial C}{\partial x}=D\frac{\partial^2 C}{\partial y^2}. \tag{5.9}$$

The difficulties of solving eqn (5.9) for oxygen and CO_2 transfer differ in several respects. We tackle oxygen first.

The first problem is that our boundary condition at the wall must inevitably involve the partial pressure P of oxygen in the gas phase, and in the membrane itself, when the relationship for oxygen between C and P is highly non-linear (Fig. 1.8(a)). The second problem resides in our interpretation of the diffusion constant D. Of the total carriage of oxygen in blood depicted in Fig. 1.8(a) a small but very variable percentage is accounted for by dissolved oxygen, whilst most of the total is accounted for by oxygen bound to haemoglobin in the red cells. This larger proportion which is inside the red cells will convect along with the flow of cells, but is not freely available for diffusion. Only the small proportion of oxygen which is physically dissolved in the blood can be regarded as a diffusing species. Since the ratio of dissolved to bound oxygen varies greatly with P, D becomes a complicated function of C. Before tackling these two obstacles we shall define the boundary conditions for the solution.

5.3   The parallel plate membrane lung: boundary conditions

At inlet to the device ($x=0$) the concentration of gas held in the blood will be uniform across the flow section ($-h\leqslant y\leqslant h$). We denote this inlet concentration C_i, and the inlet partial pressure P_i.

$$C(0,\,y)=C_i. \tag{5.10}$$

At the wall ($y=\pm h$) the flux of gas by diffusion across the membrane must equal the flux into (or out of) the blood. Let P_g be the partial pressure of the gas we are considering on the gas side of the membrane. If α_m denotes the *solubility* of the gas in the membrane polymer, then the concentration of the gas in the membrane at the gas side will be $\alpha_m P_g$. Similarly, if P_w is the partial pressure at the inner wall where blood and membrane meet, the membrane concentration there will equal $\alpha_m P_w$. For a diffusion constant D_m of the gas within the membrane, the membrane flux into the blood will be given by $D_m\alpha_m(P_g-P_w)/t$. The boundary condition at the wall is therefore

$$D\frac{\partial C}{\partial y}\bigg|_{y=\pm h}=\pm D_m\alpha_m\frac{(P_g-P_w)}{t}. \tag{5.11}$$

In Fig. (5.8) a comparison is shown between a profile in half of the channel of partial pressure P and concentration C. Note that only P is continuous at

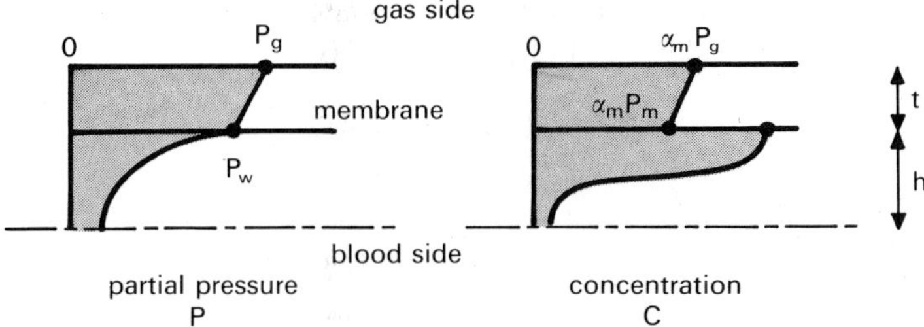

Fig. 5.8. Wall boundary condition for a gas diffusing into blood. Profiles of partial pressure and concentration differ. Only the partial pressure is continuous at the blood–membrane interface (Channel geometry as in Fig. 5.6(b).)

the blood-membrane (and gas-membrane) interface. C is proportional to P within the membrane, but for a gas like oxygen the shapes of the two profiles within the blood are expected to be very dissimilar (see Fig. 1.8(a)).

The question arises whether eqn (5.11) remains applicable to a membrane containing micropores. Pores clearly allow a direct contact between blood and gas over part of the total membrane area and might account for more transfer of gas than the membrane polymer itself. In this situation it will be difficult to attribute meaning to the individual terms D_m, α_m, and t. The term $D_m \alpha_m / t$ is then best regarded as a single coefficient defining the permeability of the membrane to gas transfer.

5.4   The parallel plate membrane lung: advancing front theory

One approach to accommodating a highly non-linear C–P relationship, and to coping with variability of D in eqn (5.9), is that layed down by Lightfoot in 1968 (Lightfoot, E. N. (1968). *American Institute of Chemical Engineers Journal*, **14**, 669–70). Oxygenation of the blood is modelled by dividing the blood flow into two distinct regions (Fig. 5.9). These are separated by an *advancing front* at which there is an abrupt change of concentration from the inlet value C_i to a maximum value C_{max}. This is equivalent to modelling the C–P relationship for oxygen as a curve with a step, as shown in Fig. 5.10.

On the inlet side of the advancing front the blood is homogeneous with respect to both C and P. They take values C_i and P_i. Behind the advancing front the assumption is made that the concentration is C_{max} everywhere but P is not homogeneous; it takes values between P_w at the wall and P_i at the advancing front itself (Fig. 5.9).

What is the rationale for this approach? It must be remembered that the only form of oxygen which is free to diffuse from the wall into the blood is that which is dissolved. For diffusion of dissolved oxygen to occur there must be a gradient in the y direction of dissolved oxygen. Since the concentration

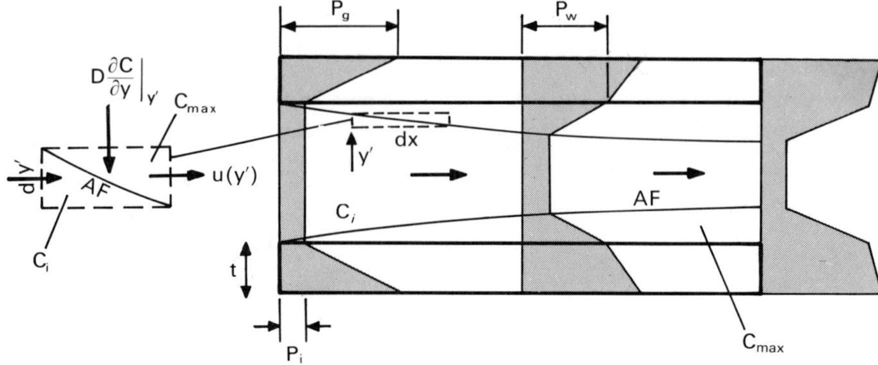

Fig. 5.9. Advancing Front theory for oxygenation of blood. Partial pressure profiles are superimposed on a side view of the blood channel to illustrate the assumption of a linear gradient of partial pressure in the blood lying behind the advancing front (AF).

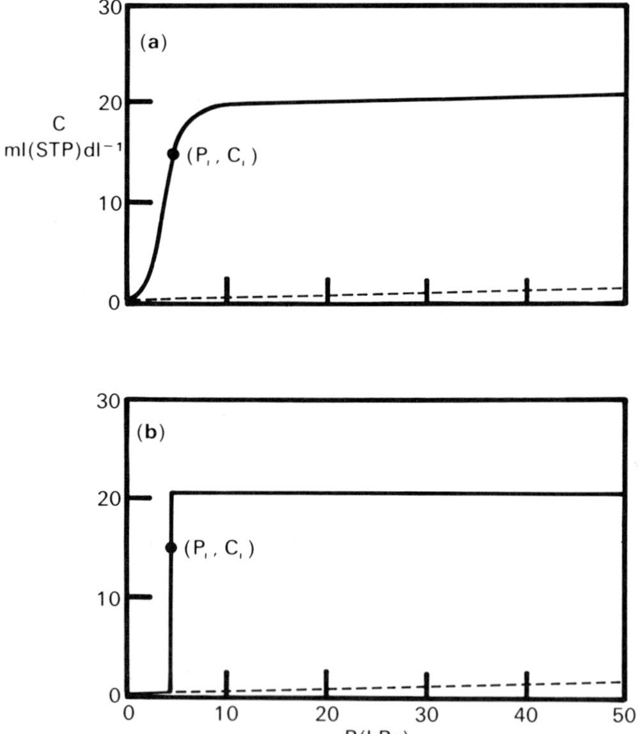

Fig. 5.10. The advancing front theory for oxygenation of blood models the content–partial pressure curve (a) with a step function located at the blood inlet condition P_i, C_i (b). The dashed line represents dissolved oxygen.

of dissolved oxygen is proportional to P (eqn (1.36); the lower straight line in Fig. 5.10(a) and (b)), there must be a gradient in P. If we now make the approximate but simple assumption that the total concentration of oxygen behind the advancing front is equal to the constant C_{max} everywhere, then any oxygen flux normal to the wall within this 'saturated blood' must be a constant which is independent of the distance from the wall. No oxygen can stop off on the way across the saturated region because the total concentration is constant. For such a constant flux of diffusing dissolved oxygen normal to the wall there must be a constant gradient of concentration normal to the wall, and consequently a constant gradient of partial pressure normal to the wall. If y' is the position of the advancing front (Fig. 5.9), the thickness of the 'saturation boundary layer' between the advancing front and the wall is $h-y'$. The gradient in partial pressure is consequently $(P_w-P_i)/(h-y')$ and the gradient in concentration of dissolved oxygen is $\alpha\,(P_w-P_i)/(h-y')$, where α is the solubility coefficient of oxygen in blood. If we let D now signify only the diffusion constant for dissolved oxygen alone then our model predicts an oxygen flux normal to the wall of $D\alpha(P_w-P_i)/(h-y').$*

The appropriate form of the convection–diffusion equation can now be derived. Consider the small open control volume depicted in Fig. 5.9 as straddling the advancing front. Its dimensions are $\mathrm{d}x \times \mathrm{d}y'$. Blood flowing through the stationary control volume changes its oxygen concentration from C_i to C_{max} as it passes through. The balance of convection horizontally and diffusion vertically can therefore be written

$$u(C_{max}-C_i)(-\mathrm{d}y') = D\alpha\frac{(P_w-P_i)}{(h-y')}\,\mathrm{d}x$$

or

$$u\frac{(C_{max}-C_i)}{\mathrm{d}x} = \frac{D\alpha(P_w-P_i)}{(y'-h)\,\mathrm{d}y'}. \tag{5.12}$$

Equation (5.12) is the form of eqn (5.1) which results from our simplification of the problem of oxygen transfer by postulating an advancing front. As it stands the equation cannot be integrated because P_w remains unknown. We determine P_w from the boundary condition at the wall, substituting for the left-hand side of eqn (5.11) the oxygen flux across the saturation boundary layer behind the advancing front:

$$D\alpha\frac{(P_w-P_i)}{(h-y')} = D_m\alpha_m\frac{(P_g-P_w)}{t}. \tag{5.13}$$

---

* D typically takes values in region of $1-2\times10^{-9}\,\mathrm{m^2\,s^{-1}}$.

This equation can be solved directly for P_w:

$$P_w = \left\{ \frac{P_i + P_g\left[\dfrac{D_m\alpha_m(h-y')}{D\alpha t}\right]}{1+\left(\dfrac{D_m\alpha_m(h-y')}{D\alpha t}\right)} \right\}. \tag{5.14}$$

Before using this result to generate a solution to eqn (5.12) we simplify our notation by introducing a dimensionless group of terms known as the wall Sherwood Number Sh_w

$$Sh_w \equiv \frac{D_m\alpha_m h}{D\alpha t}. \tag{5.15}$$

The physical significance of this is readily seen by imagining a stationary layer of blood of thickness h lying adjacent to a membrane of thickness t, through both of which a flux of oxygen Γ is occuring by diffusion (Fig. 5.11). If ΔP_m is the partial pressure drop across the membrane and ΔP_b the partial pressure drop across the layer of blood then

$$\Gamma = D_m\frac{\alpha_m \Delta P_m}{t}, \tag{5.16}$$

and

$$\Gamma = D\frac{\alpha \Delta P_b}{h}. \tag{5.17}$$

The ratio ΔP_m to ΔP_b is therefore

$$\frac{\Delta P_b}{\Delta P_m} = \frac{\Gamma h/(D\alpha)}{\Gamma t/(D_m\alpha_m)} = \frac{D_m\alpha_m h}{D\alpha t} = Sh_w. \tag{5.18}$$

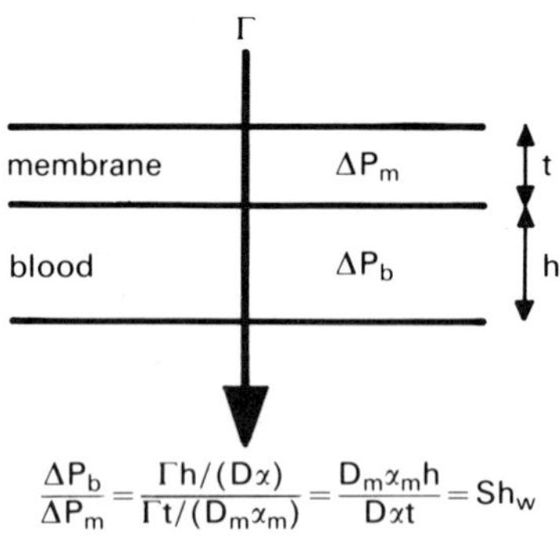

Fig. 5.11. Interpretation of the dimensionless wall Sherwood Number Sh_w (see text).

The wall Sherwood Number can consequently be thought of as a measure of the relative resistance to diffusion of the blood in the channel and the membrane forming the wall. A membrane lung with a low Sh_w suffers from a relatively high membrane resistance to gas transfer. Conversely a lung with high Sh_w is limited mainly by resistance to diffusion in the blood.

Equation (5.14) can be simplified by the use of Sh_w:

$$P_w = \left[\frac{P_i + P_g Sh_w [1 - (y'/h)]}{1 + Sh_w [1 - (y'/h)]} \right]. \tag{5.19}$$

Substituting in eqn (5.12) for P_w from eqn (5.19), and u from eqn (5.8) (rival velocity profiles can be introduced at this stage; see problem 5.1), we get

$$\frac{3}{2}\bar{u}\left[1 - \left(\frac{y'}{h}\right)^2 \right](C_{max} - C_i)\frac{dy'}{dx} = D\alpha\frac{(P_w - P_i)}{(y' - h)}$$

$$= \frac{D\alpha}{(y' - h)}\left\{ \frac{P_i + P_g Sh_w [1 - (y'/h)]}{1 + Sh_w [1 - (y'/h)]} - P_i \right\},$$

or

$$\frac{3}{2}\bar{u}(C_{max} - C_i)\left[1 - \left(\frac{y'}{h}\right)^2 \right]\frac{dy'}{dx} = -\frac{D\alpha Sh_w (P_g - P_i)}{h(1 + Sh_w [1 - (y'/h)])}. \tag{5.20}$$

This is an equation of the form $dy'/dx = f(y')$ which can be integrated to find y' as a function of x. We first separate the variables to achieve y' on the left-hand side and x on the right:

$$\frac{3}{2}\left[1 - \left(\frac{y'}{h}\right)^2 \right]\left\{ 1 + Sh_w\left[1 - \left(\frac{y'}{h}\right) \right] \right\}dy' = -\frac{D\alpha Sh_w (P_g - P_i)}{\bar{u}h(C_{max} - C_i)}dx$$

or

$$\frac{3}{2}\left[(1 + Sh_w) - Sh_w\left(\frac{y'}{h}\right) - (1 + Sh_w)\left(\frac{y'}{h}\right)^2 + Sh_w\left(\frac{y'}{h}\right)^3 \right]d\left(\frac{y'}{h}\right)$$

$$= -\frac{D\alpha Sh_w (P_g - P_i)}{\bar{u}h^2(C_{max} - C_i)}dx. \tag{5.21}$$

At $x = 0$ the advancing front lies at the wall ($y'/h = 1$). Define $y'/h \equiv \eta$ at $x = L$ and integrate eqn (5.21).

$$\int_1^\eta \frac{3}{2}\left[(1 + Sh_w) - Sh_w\left(\frac{y'}{h}\right) - (1 + Sh_w)\left(\frac{y'}{h}\right)^2 + Sh_w\left(\frac{y'}{h}\right)^3 \right]d\left(\frac{y'}{h}\right)$$

$$= -\frac{D\alpha Sh_w (P_g - P_i) L}{\bar{u}h^2(C_{max} - C_i)},$$

or

$$\frac{3}{2}\left[(1+Sh_w)\left(\frac{y'}{h}\right)-\frac{Sh_w}{2}\left(\frac{y'}{h}\right)^2-\frac{(1+Sh_w)}{3}\left(\frac{y'}{h}\right)^3+\frac{Sh_w}{4}\left(\frac{y'}{h}\right)^4\right]_1^\eta$$

$$=-\frac{D\alpha Sh_w(P_g-P_i)L}{\bar{u}h^2(C_{max}-C_i)}.$$

The final result is

$$\left[\frac{5}{8}+\frac{1}{Sh_w}\left(1-\frac{3\eta}{2}+\frac{\eta^3}{2}\right)-\frac{3}{2}\left(\eta-\frac{\eta^2}{2}-\frac{\eta^3}{3}+\frac{\eta^4}{4}\right)\right]=\frac{D\alpha(P_g-P_i)L}{\bar{u}h^2(C_{max}-C_i)}. \tag{5.22}$$

Note that the solution can only be valid for $y' \geqslant 0$, i.e., $\eta \geqslant 0$. Once the advancing fronts meet in the centre of the blood channel there can be no further oxygenation of the blood. The critical channel length L_c is given by

$$\frac{D\alpha(P_g-P_i)L_c}{\bar{u}h^2(C_{max}-C_i)}=\frac{5}{8}+\frac{1}{Sh_w}. \tag{5.23}$$

The precise analytic solution in eqn (5.22) is not in a practically useful form. We have solved for the position of the advancing front as a function of the channel length L, but what we really want to know about is the degree of oxygenation of the blood as a function of L. Figure 5.12 depicts blood leaving the channel.

We define a *fractional saturation change, f,* as a measure of the degree to which blood has been oxygenated during its passage through the lung:

$$f\equiv\frac{C_0-C_i}{C_{max}-C_i}. \tag{5.24}$$

C_0 is the mean outlet concentration of oxygen, sometimes termed the 'cup-

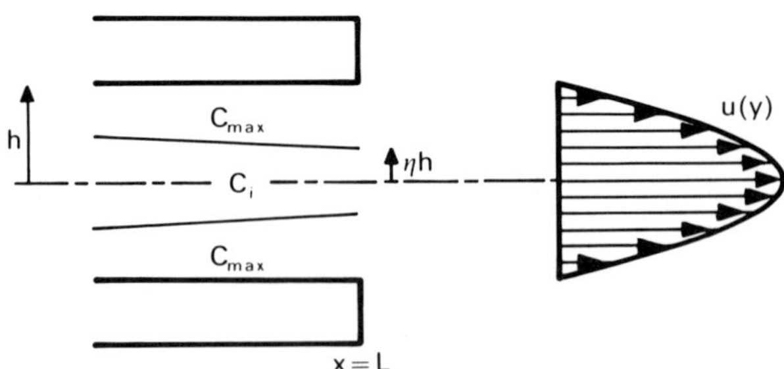

Fig. 5.12. Calculation of the 'cup-mixed' concentration of oxygen in blood at outlet from the membrane lung, where the advancing front lies at a distance ηh from the centreline.

mixed' concentration:

$$C_0 = \frac{\int_0^{\eta h} C_i u \, dy + \int_{\eta h}^{h} C_{max} u \, dy}{\bar{u} h}$$

$$= \frac{3}{2} \int_0^{\eta} C_i (1 - \eta^2) \, d\eta + \frac{3}{2} \int_{\eta}^{1} C_{max} (1 - \eta^2) \, d\eta$$

$$= \frac{3}{2} C_i \left(\eta - \frac{\eta^3}{3} \right) + \frac{3}{2} C_{max} \left(\frac{2}{3} - \eta + \frac{\eta^3}{3} \right). \tag{5.25}$$

By substituting for C_0 from this result into eqn (5.24) we relate f to η directly.

$$f = 1 - \frac{3\eta}{2} + \frac{\eta^3}{2}. \tag{5.26}$$

Equation (5.22) cannot readily be expressed directly in terms of f (though the first bracket on the left-hand side is identical with f). Choosing different values of η, L can be derived from eqn (5.22) and f from eqn (5.26). L and f can then be related graphically. We shall keep to the convention of relating dimensionless variables only and plot f as a function of the dimensionless 'length' L^*, where

$$L^* \equiv \frac{D\alpha(P_g - P_i)L}{\bar{u} h^2 (C_{max} - C_i)}. \tag{5.27}$$

Since we are usually more interested in incorporating blood flow Q_b in analyses than mean velocity $\bar{u}$ and since the total membrane area is of practical importance in design, we express L^* in terms of Q_b and A. From Fig. 5.6 note that $A/2 = Lb$ and $Q_b = 2hb\bar{u}$. Equation (2.27) can be rewritten as

$$L^* = \frac{D\alpha(P_g - P_i)A}{Q_b h (C_{max} - C_i)}. \tag{5.28}$$

The advancing front solution is depicted as a plot of f against L^* in Fig. 5.13. Different values of Sh_w generate different lines. As $Sh_w \to 0$, the second term on the left-hand side of eqn (5.22) dominates the solution which tends towards

$$f = L^* Sh_w. \tag{5.29}$$

This represents the case of very high relative membrane resistance. On the doubly logarithmic plot of Fig. 5.13 this limiting case is represented by a straight line of gradient 1:

$$\log_{10} f = \log L^* + \log Sh_w. \tag{5.30}$$

Solutions for $Sh_w \leqslant 0.1$ correspond very closely to eqn (5.30).

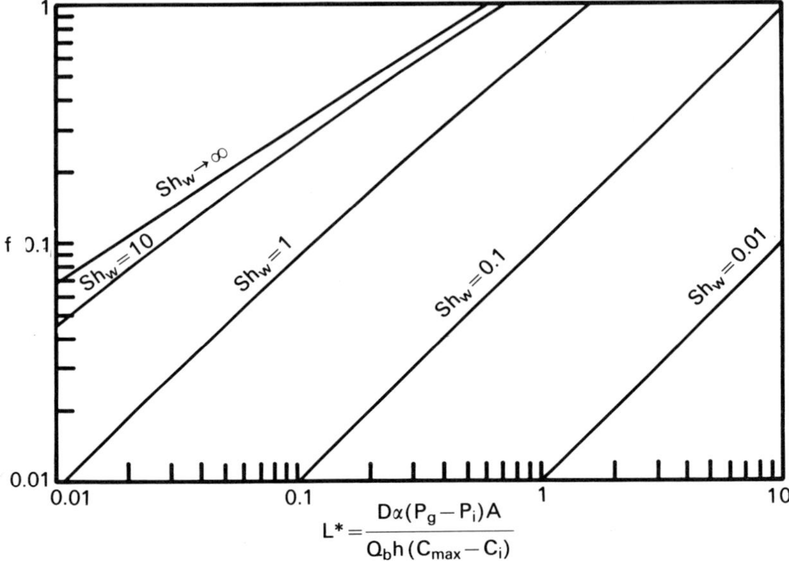

$$L^* = \frac{D\alpha(P_g - P_i)A}{Q_b h(C_{max} - C_i)}$$

Fig. 5.13. Advancing front theory for parallel plate membrane lung. Fractional oxygen saturation change as a function of dimensionless length for different wall Sherwood Numbers (eqns (5.22), (5.27) and (5.28)).

On the basis of work by Vorhees, a comparison of the advancing front theory with experiment has been published by Dorson (In Kenedi 1977), who chose to plot f as a function of our $L^* - f/Sh_w$ (Fig. 5.14) so that theoretical predictions for all values of Sh_w lie on the same line. That this is the case can be seen from eqn (5.22), where $(1 - 3\eta/2 + \eta^3/3)/Sh_w = f/Sh_w$ is one of the terms on the left-hand side, L^* being the right-hand side. Figure 5.14 shows that the measured gas transfer exceeds the theoretical prediction by around 15 per cent over much of the range studied. Dorson was able to show that by modifying assumptions about the dissolved oxygen component the advancing front theory could be brought to within approximately 5 per cent of measured values.

5.5 The hollow fibre membrane lung: advancing front theory

The advancing front theory can be applied to the axisymmetric geometry of a circular tube to yield a solution similar to that for the parallel plate geometry. Figure 5.15 shows the coordinate system we shall use. A single tube has internal radius R, thickness t, and length L (Fig. 5.15(a)). At a distance x from entry to the tube we envisage an advancing front lying a distance r' from the midline (Fig. 5.15(b)). Over a further distance dx along the tube this front

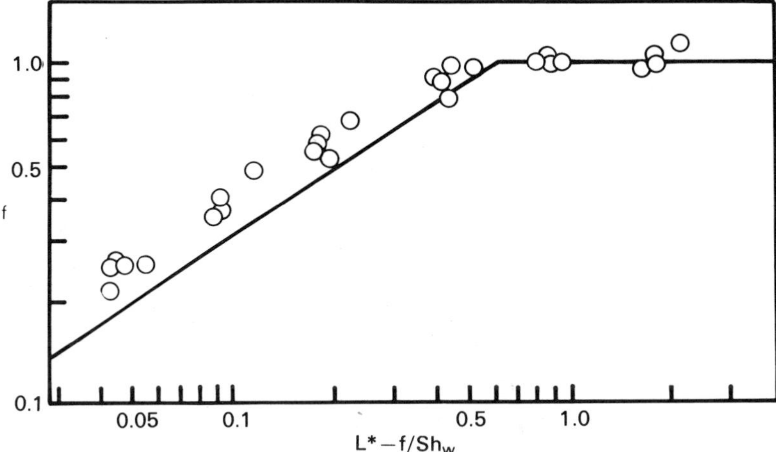

Fig. 5.14. Comparison of eqn (5.22) with measurements of oxygen transfer to blood flowing between parallel plates. Data from Kenedi, R. M. (ed.) (1977). *Artificial Organs*, Chapter 4. Macmillan, New York. Unfortunately no details of membrane material or wall Sherwood Number were given. There is in fact a sparsity of data in the literature for comparison with theory over a wide range of conditions.

advances a distance dr' (negative) towards the midline. Upstream of the front the concentration of oxygen in the blood has the inlet value C_i. The partial pressure is P_i. Downstream of the front the concentration is taken to be a constant C_{max}. As for our previous solution we permit the partial pressure of oxygen behind the advancing front to vary from some value P_w at the wall to P_i at the front.

Recall that the only form of oxygen which diffuses in the blood behind the advancing front is the dissolved oxygen, which has concentration αP where the partial pressure of oxygen is P. Because the total concentration of oxygen (dissolved plus bound) is constant behind the front, the flux of dissolved oxygen which diffuses away from the wall towards the midline must be constant for all values of r greater than r'. Let this flux be Γ per unit length of tube. The appropriate form of Fick's law of steady diffusion becomes

$$\Gamma = 2\pi r \, D\alpha \frac{dP}{dr} \quad (r' \leqslant r \leqslant R). \tag{5.31}$$

Integration gives us the partial pressure profile

$$\int_{r'}^{R} \frac{dr}{r} = \frac{2\pi D\alpha}{\Gamma} \int_{P_i}^{P_w} dP, \tag{5.32}$$

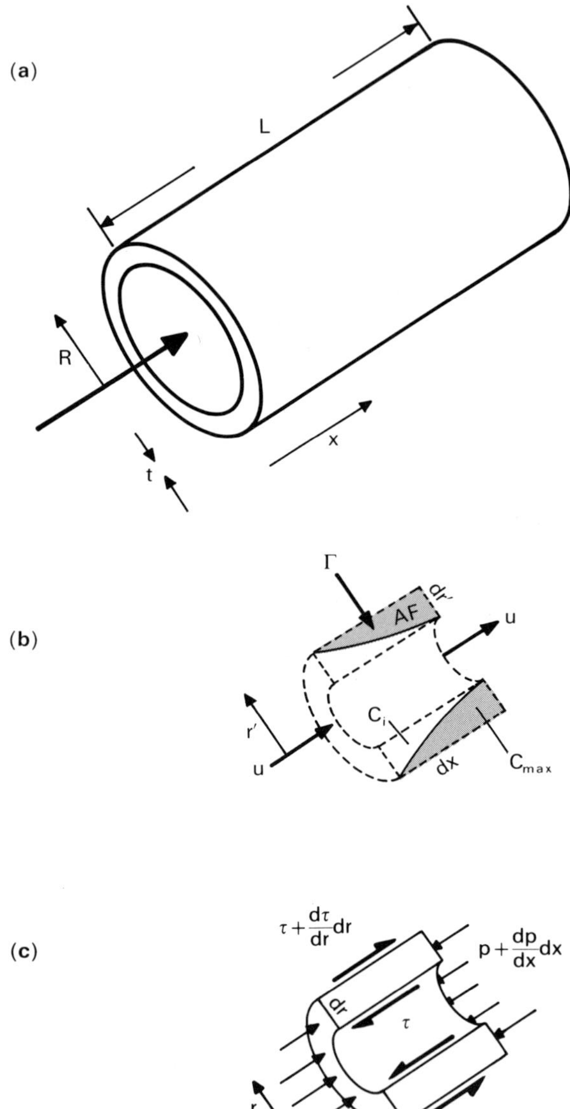

Fig. 5.15. The hollow fibre membrane lung (a). An open control volume (b) is used to establish the convection–diffusion equation at an advancing front (AF); a closed control volume (c) facilitates application of the equation of motion.

or

$$\ln\left(\frac{R}{r'}\right) = \frac{2\pi D\alpha}{\Gamma}(P_{\text{w}} - P_{\text{i}}).\tag{5.33}$$

Writing now the balance for the open control volume of Fig. 5.15(b), of convection in and out and diffusion in, we obtain

$$u(C_{\text{max}} - C_{\text{i}})(2\pi r'\,\mathrm{d}r') = -\Gamma\,\mathrm{d}x$$

$$= \frac{2\pi D\alpha(P_{\text{w}} - P_{\text{i}})}{\ln(r'/R)}\,\mathrm{d}x.\tag{5.34}$$

This is the equivalent equation for the hollow fibre problem to eqn (5.12) for the flat plate geometry. As with the former case we can solve for the position of the advancing front (r') as a function of x if we substitute expressions for u and P_{w} in the convection–diffusion equation.

To derive u we again assume Newtonian behaviour:

$$\tau = \mu\frac{\mathrm{d}u}{\mathrm{d}r},\tag{5.35}$$

where μ, the viscosity, is constant. The balance of shear and pressure forces on an annular element in the steady blood flow is depicted in Fig. 5.15(c):

$$\left(\tau + \frac{\mathrm{d}\tau}{\mathrm{d}r}\mathrm{d}r\right)2\pi(r+\mathrm{d}r)\mathrm{d}x - \tau\,2\pi r\,\mathrm{d}x = \left(p + \frac{\mathrm{d}p}{\mathrm{d}x}\mathrm{d}x\right)2\pi r\mathrm{d}r - p2\pi r\mathrm{d}r,$$

or

$$\frac{\mathrm{d}\tau}{\mathrm{d}r} + \frac{\tau}{r} = \frac{\mathrm{d}p}{\mathrm{d}x}.\tag{5.36}$$

Compare this with eqn (5.3) for flow between parallel plates. The left-hand side of eqn (5.36) can be written $(1/r)\mathrm{d}(\tau r)/\mathrm{d}r$, and substitution from eqn (5.35) gives

$$\frac{\mu}{r}\frac{\mathrm{d}}{\mathrm{d}r}\left(r\frac{\mathrm{d}u}{\mathrm{d}r}\right) = \frac{\mathrm{d}p}{\mathrm{d}x}.\tag{5.37}$$

The velocity profile follows after integration:

$$u = \frac{1}{4\mu}\frac{\mathrm{d}p}{\mathrm{d}x}r^2 + \text{A}\ln r + \text{B},\tag{5.38}$$

where the integration constants are determined by the boundary conditions of zero velocity at the channel wall ($u=0$ for $y=R$) and finite velocity in the midline ($\ln r \to -\infty$ as $r \to 0$ so A must be zero).

$$u = \frac{1}{4\mu} \frac{\mathrm{d}p}{\mathrm{d}x}(r^2 - R^2). \tag{5.39}$$

It is useful to incorporate a mean velocity $\bar{u}$ in place of $\mathrm{d}p/\mathrm{d}x$, and since

$$\pi R^2 \bar{u} = \int_0^R \frac{1}{4\mu} \frac{\mathrm{d}p}{\mathrm{d}x}(r^2 - R^2)2\pi r \mathrm{d}r,$$

$$\bar{u} = -\frac{1}{8\mu} \frac{\mathrm{d}p}{\mathrm{d}x} R^2, \tag{5.40}$$

and we can write

$$u = 2\bar{u}\left[1 - \left(\frac{r}{R}\right)^2\right]. \tag{5.41}$$

Again we confirm the widely known parabolic velocity profile for laminar flow.

To derive P_w in eqn (5.34) we examine the diffusion of oxygen across the membrane. The appropriate form of Fick's law of diffusion is similar to eqn (5.31):

$$\Gamma = 2\pi r D_m \alpha_m \frac{\mathrm{d}P}{\mathrm{d}r} \quad (R \leqslant r \leqslant R+t). \tag{5.42}$$

Integration relates P_g $(r = R + t)$ to P_w $(r = R)$

$$\ln\left(\frac{R+t}{R}\right) = \frac{2\pi D_m \alpha_m}{\Gamma}(P_g - P_w). \tag{5.43}$$

Combine eqns (5.33) and (5.43) to eliminate Γ:

$$\frac{D\alpha(P_w - P_i)}{\ln(R/r')} = \frac{D_m \alpha_m (P_g - P_w)}{\ln[(R+t)/R]}. \tag{5.44}$$

The solution for P_w is

$$P_w = \left\langle \frac{P_i + P_g \left\{ \dfrac{D_m \alpha_m \ln(R/r')}{D\alpha \ln[(R+t)/R]} \right\}}{1 + \left\{ \dfrac{D_m \alpha_m \ln(R/r')}{D\alpha \ln[(R+t)/R]} \right\}} \right\rangle, \tag{5.45}$$

$$= \left[\frac{P_i + P_g \, Sh'_w \ln(R/r')}{1 + Sh'_w \ln(R/r')} \right], \tag{5.46}$$

where $Sh'_w = D_m \alpha_m / \{D\alpha \ln[(R+t)/R]\}$ is a dimensionless wall Sherwood

Number analogous to that introduced for the parallel plate problem (eqn (5.15)).

We are now in a position to solve eqn (5.34) by substituting for u from eqn (5.41), and for P_w from eqn (5.46):

$$2\left[1-\left(\frac{r'}{R}\right)^2\right]r'\,[Sh'_w\ln(r'/R)-1]\,\mathrm{d}r' = \frac{D\alpha(P_g-P_i)}{\bar{u}(C_{max}-C_i)}\,Sh'_w\,\mathrm{d}x,$$

or

$$2\left[-\frac{r'}{R}+Sh'_w\frac{r'}{R}\ln\left(\frac{r'}{R}\right)+\left(\frac{r'}{R}\right)^3-Sh'_w\left(\frac{r'}{R}\right)^3\ln\left(\frac{r'}{R}\right)\right]\mathrm{d}\left(\frac{r'}{R}\right)$$

$$= \frac{D\alpha(P_g-P_i)\,Sh'_w}{\bar{u}R(C_{max}-C_i)}\,\mathrm{d}x. \tag{5.47}$$

We note that two terms take the form $x^n\ln x$ for which the intergral is available:

$$\int x^n\ln x = \frac{x^{n+1}}{n+1}\left(\ln x - \frac{1}{n+1}\right). \tag{5.48}$$

At $x=0$ the advancing front lies at the wall of the tube $(r'/R=1)$. Define $r'/R=\eta$ at $x=L$ and integrate eqn (5.47).

$$\left\{-\left(\frac{r'}{R}\right)^2+Sh'_w\left(\frac{r'}{R}\right)^2\left[\ln\left(\frac{r'}{R}\right)-\frac{1}{2}\right]+\frac{1}{2}\left(\frac{r'}{R}\right)^4\right.$$

$$\left.-\frac{Sh'_w}{2}\left(\frac{r'}{R}\right)^4\left[\ln\left(\frac{r'}{R}\right)-\frac{1}{4}\right]\right\}_1^{\eta} = \frac{D\alpha(P_g-P_i)L}{\bar{u}R^2(C_{max}-C_i)}$$

or

$$\frac{3}{8}+\ln\eta\left(\eta^2-\frac{\eta^4}{2}\right)-\frac{1}{2}\left(\eta^2-\frac{\eta^4}{4}\right)+\frac{1}{Sh'_w}\left(\frac{1}{2}-\eta^2+\frac{\eta^4}{2}\right)$$

$$= \frac{D\alpha(P_g-P_i)L}{\bar{u}R^2(C_{max}-C_i)}. \tag{5.49}$$

We follow our earlier convention of expressing the right-hand side of this equation in terms of the blood flow $Q_b=\pi R^2\bar{u}$ and fibre (inside) surface area $A=2\pi RL$:

$$\frac{3}{4}+2\ln\eta\left(\eta^2-\frac{\eta^4}{2}\right)-\left(\eta^2-\frac{\eta^4}{4}\right)+\frac{1}{Sh'_w}(1-2\eta^2+\eta^4)$$

$$= \frac{D\alpha(P_g-P_i)A}{Q_bR(C_{max}-C_i)} \equiv L'. \tag{5.50}$$

This is the solution for the radial position $\eta(=r'/R)$ of the advancing front at exit from the hollow fibre lung. To relate η to the fractional saturation change f (eqn (5.24)) we note that the cup-mixed oxygen concentration in the blood leaving the hollow fibre is

$$C_0 = \frac{\displaystyle\int_0^{\eta R} C_i u\, 2\pi r\, dr + \int_{\eta R}^{R} C_{max} u\, 2\pi r\, dr}{\bar{u}\pi R^2}$$

$$= 4\int_0^{\eta} C_i(1-\eta^2)\eta\, d\eta + 4\int_{\eta}^{1} C_{max}(1-\eta^2)\eta\, d\eta$$

$$= 2C_i\left(\eta^2 - \frac{\eta^4}{2}\right) + 2C_{max}\left(\frac{1}{2} - \eta^2 + \frac{\eta^4}{2}\right). \tag{5.51}$$

By substituting for C_0 from this result into eqn (5.24) we relate f to η directly.

$$f = 1 - 2\eta^2 + \eta^4. \tag{5.52}$$

Equation (5.50) cannot readily be expressed directly in terms of f (though the last bracket on the left-hand side is identical with f). The relationship between f and L' can be computed from chosen values of η. The result is shown in Fig. 5.16. Note that the solution can only be valid for $r' \geqslant 0$, i.e.,

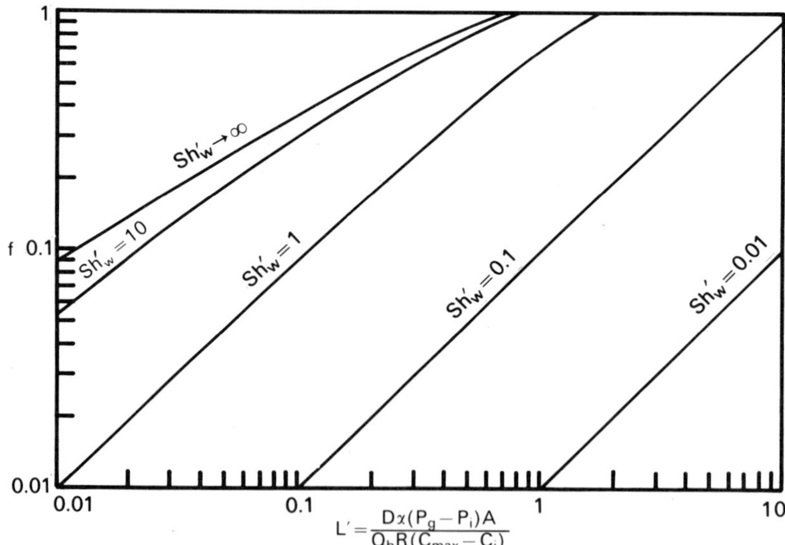

$$L' = \frac{D\alpha(P_g - P_i)A}{Q_b R(C_{max} - C_i)}$$

Fig. 5.16. Advancing front theory for hollow fibre membrane lung. Fractional saturation change as a function of dimensionless length for different wall Sherwood Numbers (eqns (5.50) and (5.52)).

$\eta \geqslant 0$. Once the advancing front merges to a point at the centre of the hollow fibre there can be no further oxygenation of the blood. The critical channel length L_c is given from eqn (5.49) as

$$\frac{D\alpha(P_g - P_i)L_c}{\bar{u}R^2(C_{max} - C_i)} = \frac{3}{8} - \frac{1}{2Sh'_w}. \tag{5.53}$$

This condition represents the point at which the sloping lines meet the horizontal line $f = 1$ in Fig. 5.16.

As $Sh'_w \to 0$, the dominant term on the left-hand side of eqn (5.50) equals f/Sh'_w and the solution tends towards

$$f = L'Sh'_w,$$

or

$$\log_{10} f = \log_{10} L' + \log_{10} Sh'_w. \tag{5.54}$$

This is analogous to eqn (5.30) for the parallel plate case.

In a comparison of the advancing front theory with experiment, Dorson chose to plot f as a function of our $L' - f/Sh'_w$ (Fig. 5.17) so that theoretical predictions for all values of Sh'_w lie on the same line. This can be confirmed from eqn (5.50), where $(1 - 2\eta^2 + \eta^4)/Sh'_w = f/Sh'_w$ is one of the terms on the left-hand side. Figure 5.17 shows that the measured gas transfer tends to exceed the theoretical prediction by around 15 per cent. As with the parallel plate case, Dorson was able to show that by modifying assumptions about

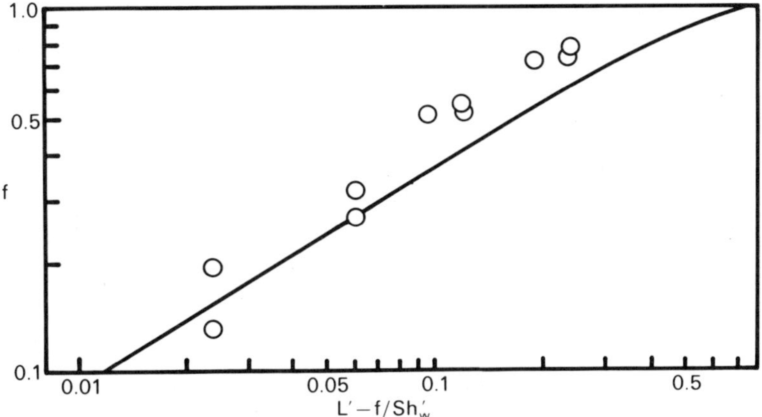

Fig. 5.17. Comparison of eqn (5.50) with measurements of oxygen transfer to blood flowing in a circular hollow tube. Data from Kenedi, R. M. (ed.) (1977). *Artificial Organs*, Chapter 4. Macmillan, New York. The tube material was polytetrafluoroethylene. Similar results for the axisymmetric geometry have been found by other authors.

the dissolved oxygen component the advancing front theory could be brought to within approximately 5 per cent of measured values.

5.6   Other models of oxygen transfer in membrane lungs

The advancing front theory has proved a powerful tool for predicting experimental results to within about 15 per cent. This analytical solution is made possible by simplifying the shape of the C–P curve for oxygen in blood (Fig. 5.10). We represented the curve with a step which permitted us to divide the blood into two quite distinct regions. Another approach of this kind is to represent the curve with a line of constant slope, as in Fig. 5.18. This is chosen to join a point which represents inlet conditions (P_i, C_i) to a point which coincides with the maximum attainable partial pressure P_g. This approach does not generate an analytical solution. Computed solutions have been used by Mikic, Benn and Drinker (Mikic, B. B., Benn, J. A., and Drinker, P. A. (1972). *Annals of Biomedical Engineering* **1**, 212–220) to demonstrate that the constant slope method and the advancing front method can provide close upper and lower bounds on the precise solution to the problem.

   A more sophisticated approach is to use an equation which describes the whole sigmoid form of the $C-P$ relationship for oxygen in blood. An equation which achieves this to a high degree of accuracy is known as the Hill equation:

$$S = \frac{(P_{O_2})^n}{(P_{O_2})^n + (P_{0.5})^n}. \tag{5.55}$$

Here S is the fraction of haemoglobin which is saturated with oxygen and takes values between 0 and 1. $P_{0.5}$ is the partial pressure of oxygen at which

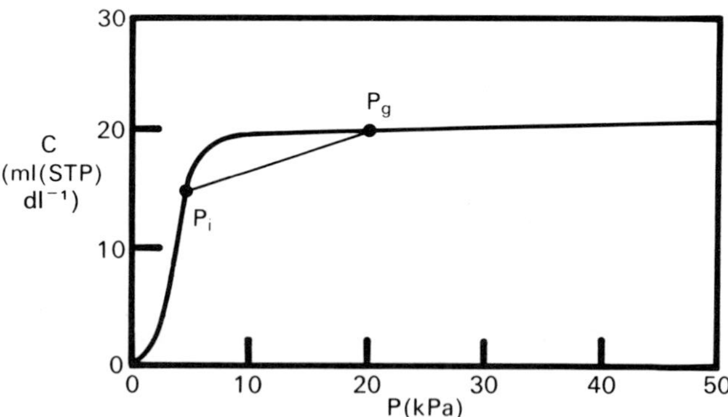

Fig. 5.18. Oxygenation of blood can be modelled by representing the content–partial pressure curve with a line of constant slope which joins inlet conditions (P_i, C_i) to a point which coincides the maximum attainable partial pressure, P_g.

half the haemoglobin is saturated. The parameter n is derived empirically but has interesting theoretical implications.

Consider a hypothetical reaction in which haemoglobin reacts with only one molecule of oxygen to form oxyhaemoglobin:

$$Hb + O_2 \rightleftharpoons HbO_2. \tag{5.56}$$

The equilibrium concentrations of the three species will be related by

$$\frac{[HbO_2]}{[Hb][O_2]} = K, \tag{5.57}$$

where K is the *equilibrium constant* for the reaction. Since the fraction of haemoglobin which is saturated, S, equals $[HbO_2]/[(Hb)+(HbO_2)]$ eqn (5.57) can be written

$$S = \frac{K[Hb][O_2]}{[Hb]+K[Hb][O_2]}$$

$$= \frac{[O_2]}{[O_2]+K^{-1}}. \tag{5.58}$$

The concentration of unbound (dissolved) oxygen in blood equals αP_{O_2} where α is the solubility coefficient. Equation (5.58) can therefore be written

$$S = \frac{(P_{O_2})}{(P_{O_2})+(P_{0.5})}, \tag{5.59}$$

where $P_{0.5} = 1/(\alpha K)$ and S takes the form of eqn (5.55) with $n = 1$.

This behaviour closely models that of *myoglobin* which is a muscle protein capable of binding only one molecule of oxygen. The form of S for this case $n = 1$ is shown in Fig. 5.19.

Consider another hypothetical reaction in which haemoglobin will react with a package of four molecules of oxygen, but never with one, two or three in isolation:

$$Hb + O_2 + O_2 + O_2 + O_2 \rightleftharpoons Hb(O_2)_4. \tag{5.60}$$

The equilibrium constant for this reaction will be given by

$$\frac{[Hb(O_2)_4]}{[Hb][O_2]^4} = K, \tag{5.61}$$

and the resulting expression for S is

$$S = \frac{(P_{O_2})^4}{(P_{O_2})^4+(P_{0.5})^4}. \tag{5.62}$$

This function is also plotted in Fig. 5.19, where the cases $n = 1$ and $n = 4$ are

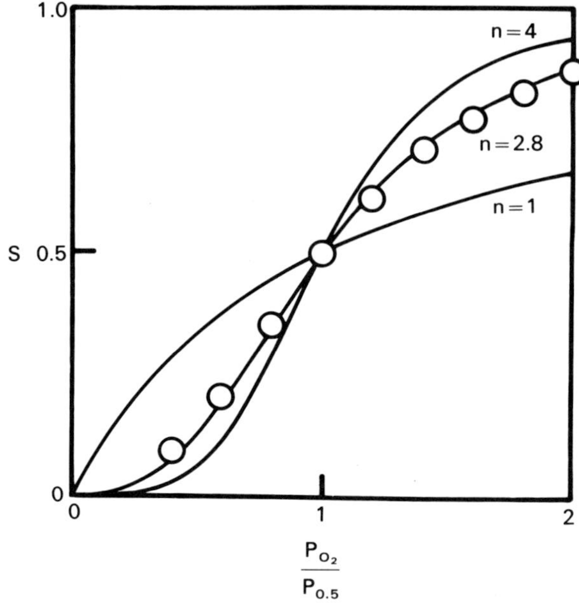

Fig. 5.19. Fractional saturation curves predicted by the Hill eqn (5.55) for different values of n. The case $n = 1$ models the behaviour of myoglobin, which binds a single molecule of oxygen. The case $n = 4$ models the hypothetical case of perfect cooperative binding of four oxygen molecules to haemoglobin. The intermediate case $n = 2.8$ models the measured behaviour as haemoglobin (circles). Data from Nunn, J. F. (1987). *Applied Respiratory Physiology* (3rd edn). p. 264. Butterworths, London. $P_{0.5} = 3.5 \, \text{kPa}$.

compared with measured values of S, and with the case $n = 2.8$ which describes the measured values well.

The significance of the power 2.8 is that it models a degree of cooperation in the bonding of oxygen to haemoglobin, which lies between the extremes of absent and perfect cooperation ($n = 1$ and $n = 4$ respectively). Thus, the binding of one molecule of oxygen encourages the next, and so on. This is another aspect of the haemoglobin molecule by which is adapted for efficient transport of oxygen in the blood.

The use of eqn (5.55) with $n = 2.8$ for modelling of the $C - P$ relationship requires the addition of the dissolved component of oxygen, as well as a measure of the total oxygen binding capacity of haemoglobin:

$$C = \text{Hb} . c \left[\frac{(P_{O_2})^{2.8}}{(P_{O_2})^{2.8} + (P_{0.5})^{2.8}} \right] + \alpha P_{O_2}, \tag{5.63}$$

where Hb is the haemoglobin concentration in blood (typically around $14 \, \text{g} \, \text{dl}^{-1}$), and c is the binding capacity of haemoglobin (typically around $1.35 \, \text{ml} \, (\text{STP}) \, \text{g}^{-1}$). Smeby and Grimsrud (Smeby, L. and Grimsrud, L. (1974).

Medical and Biological Engineering **12,** 698–705) have looked at the use of this approach to calculating oxygen transfer in membrane lungs. Note that in a situation where both oxygen and CO_2 transfer are occurring concurrently, it would be possible to model the Bohr effect by making $P_{0.5}$ in eqn (5.63) itself a function of P_{CO_2}.

Other refinements of the theoretical approach have included attempts to model the non-Newtonian viscosity of blood (Fig. 5.7) and to model non-equilibrium differences between red cells and plasma in oxygen partial pressures.

5.7   Enhancement of oxygen transfer by secondary flow

It is now possible to construct membrane lungs with extremely thin polymer membranes. Both flat-plate and hollow-fibre devices are now manufactured with membranes which are only 25 μm (25×10^{-6} m) thick. Studies on devices such as these have tended to show that the membrane itself offers very little resistance to oxygen transfer. In other words, the appropriate theoretical solutions are for high values of the wall Sherwood Number.

It follows that most of the resistance to transfer of oxygen lies within the blood itself, and in particular in the boundary layer of slowly moving blood which comes to lie next to the membrane and acts as a barrier to further diffusion of oxygen into the flow. This barrier can be broken down by stimulating mixing of the blood as it passes along the channel or tube. The term *secondary flow* is used to describe flow which has a component deviating from the uniform steady flow which we have analysed in this chapter.

Secondary flows can be generated in many ways. True turbulence may be thought of as one kind of secondary flow but is usually deliberately avoided in membrane lungs because it is associated with high rates of haemolysis. The presence of some kind of polymer mesh is sometimes required within the blood channel of a parallel plate device in order to maintain an appropriate spacing between the membranes. Such a 'spacer' can add the benefit of disturbing the otherwise uniform laminar flow and increase oxygen transfer. Secondary flow can be generated in a hollow fibre by winding the fibre into a coil. Centrifugal forces are generated by this configuration and vortices are set up with axes which lie along the tube.

The most effective way of disrupting the oxygen-rich boundary layer originated with Bellhouse in Oxford. (Bellhouse, B. J. *et al.* (1973). *Transactions of the American Society for Artificial Organs* **19,** 72–9.) His approach was to add two modifications to uniform flow between parallel plates. Firstly, a sinusoidally varying backwards and forwards motion was added to the normal mean flow of blood through the channel. Secondly, the formerly flat membranes were moulded to form either grooves or dimples in which vortices could form away from the main stream. This combination leads to repeated

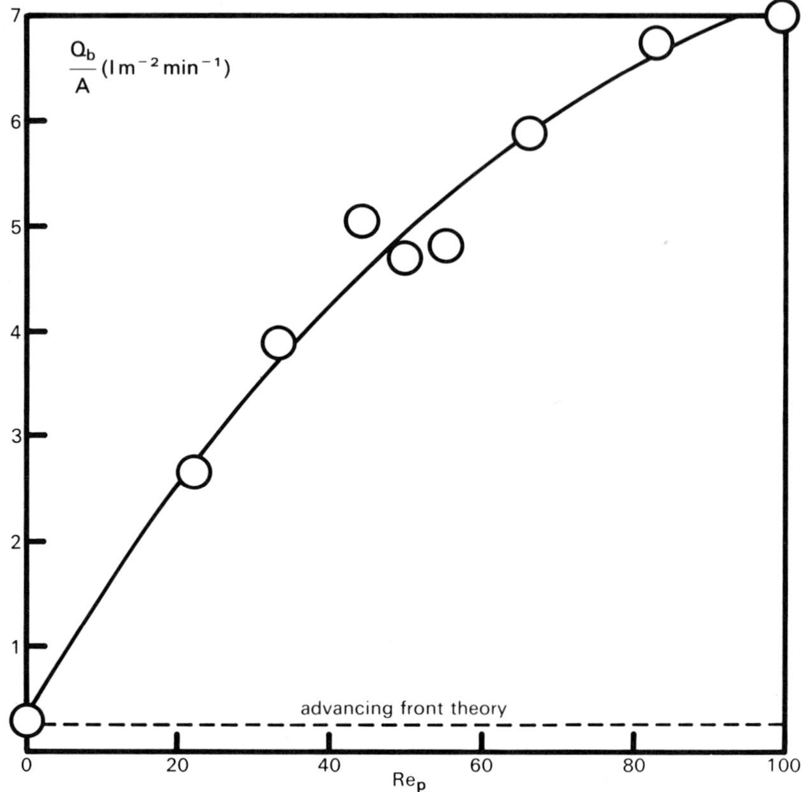

Fig. 5.20. Effect of secondary flow on the oxygen transfer of a membrane lung. The blood flow per m^2 of membrane (plan area) (Q_b/A) was measured for $f = 0.86$, as a function of the intensity of secondary flows generated by pulsation across dimpled membranes, and characterized by a pulsatile Reynolds Number Re_p (see text). Modified from Dorrington, K. L. *et al.* (1985). *Journal of Biomedical Engineering* **7**, 89–99. $(\mu/\rho = 4 \text{ mm}^2 \text{ s}^{-1})$.

formation of vortices in the grooves or dimples, and their ejection from the region close to the membrane with each reversal of the flow. Figure 5.20 shows measurements of the effectiveness of this mechanism.

A membrane lung with dimples (0.4 mm deep, 1.6 mm diameter) was studied to examine the blood flow per m^2 of membrane area (Q_b/A) at which the fractional saturation change f reached 0.86. This measurement of (Q_b/A) was made for various degrees of oscillation of the flow, defined by a pulsatile Reynolds number $Re_p = \rho U h/\mu$, where U was the peak oscillatory flow velocity. Values of Re_p in the range 0–100 corresponded with oscillatory frequencies in the range 0–6 Hz. Figure 5.20 shows that without pulsatile flow the device can only handle a blood flow of $0.2 \, 1 \text{m}^{-2} \text{min}^{-1}$. This is increased within the range studied by around 25 times to $5 \, 1 \text{m}^{-2} \text{min}^{-1}$.

The horizontal dashed line in Fig. 5.20 depicts the estimated (Q_b/A) for uniform steady flow from the advancing front theory with $Sh_w \to \infty$. For $f = 0.86$, Fig. 5.13 gives $L^* = 0.47$. Estimated values for this experiment are $D = 2 \times 10^{-9}\,\mathrm{m^2\,s^{-1}}$; $\alpha = 0.023\,\mathrm{ml\,dl^{-1}.kPa^{-1}}$; $(P_g - P_i) = 89\,\mathrm{kPa}$; $h = 0.3 \times 10^{-3}\,\mathrm{m}$; $C_{max} - C_i = 7\,\mathrm{ml\,dl^{-1}}$. From eqn (5.28) we get

$$\frac{Q_b}{A} \simeq \frac{D\alpha(P_g - P_i)}{L^* h(C_{max} - C_i)}$$

$$= \frac{2 \times 10^{-9} \times 0.023 \times 89}{0.47 \times 0.3 \times 10^{-3} \times 7}$$

$$= 4.15 \times 10^{-6}\,\mathrm{m\,s^{-1}}$$

$$= 0.25\,\mathrm{l\,m^{-2}\,min^{-1}}. \tag{5.64}$$

This agrees well with the measured value for $Re_p = 0$.

Early membrane lungs with uniform laminar flow usually displayed an oxygen transfer rate of around $15\text{--}30\,\mathrm{ml\,m^{-2}\,min^{-1}}$. Note that the figure is given per square metre of membrane. The result of eqn (5.64) coincides with the lower end of this range:

$$\frac{Q_b}{A} \times f \times (C_{max} - C_i) = 0.25\,\mathrm{l\,m^{-2}\,min^{-1}} \times 0.86 \times 7\,\mathrm{ml\,dl^{-1}}$$

$$= 15.05\,\mathrm{ml\,m^{-2}\,min^{-1}}. \tag{5.65}$$

Devices with steady secondary flows generated by internal obstacles have tended to show transfer rates in the range $60\text{--}110\,\mathrm{ml\,m^{-2}\,min^{-1}}$. Active generation of non-steady secondary flows increased this to $200\text{--}400\,\mathrm{ml\,m^{-2}\,min^{-1}}$. In our example (Fig. 5.20), the upper value of $(Q_b/A) = 7\,\mathrm{l\,m^{-2}\,min^{-1}}$ corresponds with an oxygen transfer rate of

$$\frac{Q_b}{A} \times f \times (C_{max} - C_i) = 7\,\mathrm{l\,m^{-2}\,min^{-1}} \times 0.86 \times 7\,\mathrm{ml\,dl^{-1}}$$

$$= 42\,\mathrm{l\,ml\,m^{-2}\,min^{-1}}.$$

If expressed in relation to the true area of membrane $(= 1.35 \times A)$ rather than the plane area (A) the figure becomes $312\,\mathrm{ml\,m^{-2}\,min^{-1}}$.

Problems

5.1   A parallel plate membrane lung is depicted in Fig. 5.21. The following simplifications are adopted in a model which predicts the oxygen transfer properties
(i) the velocity of blood is uniform across the section (*not* parabolic);
(ii) the membranes have negligible resistance to the diffusion of oxygen (Sherwood number $\to \infty$).

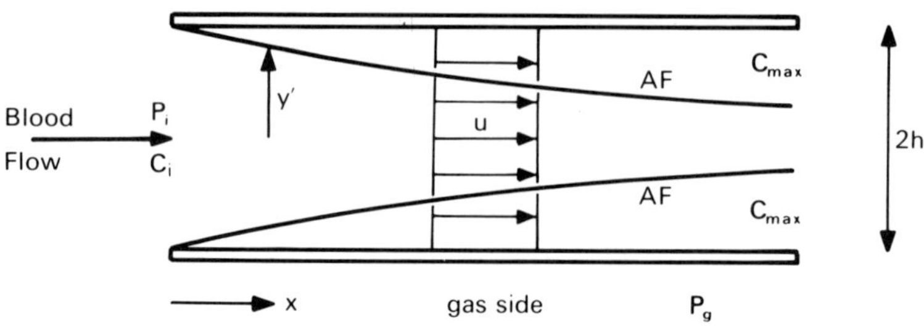

Fig. 5.21

Use the concept of an Advancing Front (AF) behind which the blood is fully saturated with oxygen ($C = C_{max}$) to show that the distance y' of the AF from the midline is a function of the distance x along the plates according to

$$\frac{D\alpha(P_g - P_i)}{uh^2(C_{max} - C_i)}x = \left[\frac{1}{2}\left(\frac{y'}{h}\right)^2 - \left(\frac{y'}{h}\right) + \frac{1}{2}\right].$$

You should assume for this proof that behind the AF there is a constant flux of dissolved oxygen at right angles to the wall; D is the diffusion constant in blood for the dissolved oxygen, α is the solubility coefficient of oxygen in blood, and P_g is the constant gas side partial pressure of oxygen. P_i and C_i are, respectively, the partial pressure and concentration of oxygen in blood entering the device.

If C_0 is the mean (cup-mixed) concentration of oxygen at outlet to the device ($x = L$), we define the fractional increase in saturation f as follows:

$$f \equiv \frac{C_0 - C_i}{C_{max} - C_i}.$$

Show that for this model

$$f = \left[\frac{2D\alpha(P_g - P_i)L}{uh^2(C_{max} - C_i)}\right]^{1/2}.$$

5.2   A designer wishes to compare the relative merits, with regard to oxygen transfer, of a parallel plate membrane lung and a hollow fibre membrane lung. A device is required which handles a blood flow Q_b and provides a high degree of saturation of the blood with oxygen.

Use the results of the Advancing Front Theory for laminar Newtonian flow (eqns (5.23) and (5.53)) to show that when there is negligible membrane resistance to the diffusion of oxygen, the parallel plate area A_1 is related to the hollow fibre area A_2 by

$$\frac{A_1}{A_2} = \frac{5}{6}\left(\frac{R}{h}\right),$$

where R is the fibre inner radius and h is the channel half gap.

If V_1 is the minimum priming volume for the parallel plate design, and V_2 the

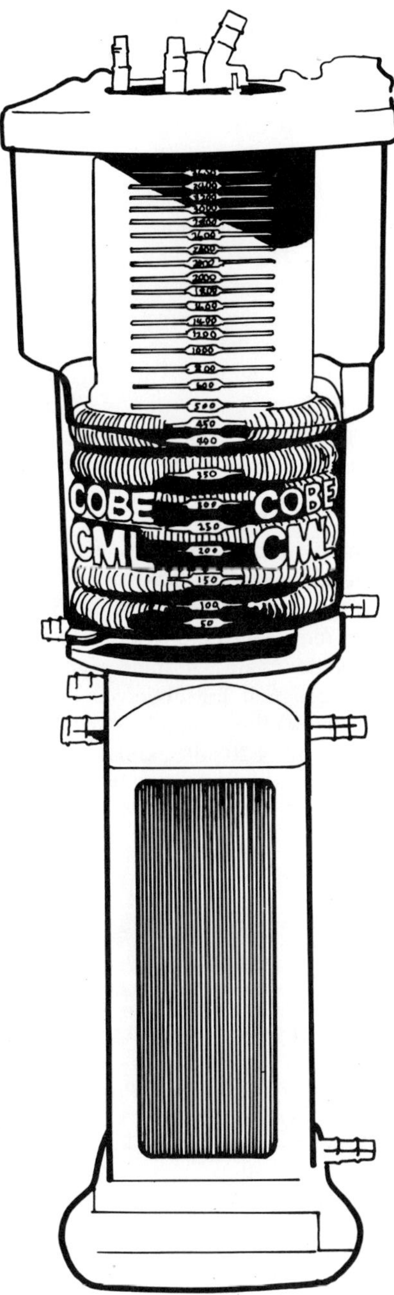

Fig. 5.22

corresponding volume for the hollow fibre design, show that

$$\frac{V_1}{V_2} = \frac{5}{3}.$$

A further design requirement is introduced to the effect that the pressure drops across the laminar blood flow channels in the two cases must be equal. Find the relationship between (A_1/A_2) and the ratio (L_1/L_2) of plate length to fibre length.

5.3   Figure 5.22 shows the Cobe CML membrane lung, which is currently in clinical use for cardiopulmonary bypass. The upper half of the device is composed of a blood reservoir with volume 4 l and containing a metal tube coil heater exchanger. The lower compartment contains two stacks of polypropylene membranes. Each stack has the following configuration: 120 parallel layers of rectangular membrane measuring 11 in by 1.75 in are potted to a total depth of 3 in. Spacers separate the membranes to form alternate blood and gas channels in such a manner that each gas channel has approximately twice the depth of a blood channel.

Estimate in m^2 the total area A of membrane. Assuming that the membrane thickness is negligible as regards this calculation, estimate the blood channel half width h.

The presence of spacing mesh in the blood channel induces steady secondary flows which are likely to result in the advancing front theory underestimating the oxygen transport. Use this theory to provide a lower limit on the likely flow of blood which the device can handle, if it is required to increase the oxygen saturation from 65 per cent to 95 per cent of its maximum value. Assume negligible membrane resistance to oxygen transfer, a diffusion constant for dissolved oxygen of $2 \times 10^{-9}\,m^2\,s^{-1}$, a solubility coefficient of 0.023 ml% kPa^{-1}, an inlet partial pressure of oxygen of 6 kPa, a maximum oxygen concentration of 20 ml%, and a gas-side oxygen partial pressure of 100 kPa. Comment on the probable contribution of secondary flows in the light of this calculation.

Further reading

Clowes, G. H. A., Hopkins, A. L., and Neville, W. E. (1956). An artificial lung dependent upon diffusion of oxygen and carbon dioxide through plastic membranes. *Journal of Thoracic Surgery* **32**, 630–7.

Clowes, G. H. A.. and Neville, W. E. (1958). The membrane oxygenator. In *Extracorporeal Circulation* (ed. J. G. Allen) pp. 81–100. Charles Thomas, Springfield, Illinois.

Cooney, D. O. (1976). *Biomedical Engineering Principles: an Introduction to Fluid, Heat, and Mass Transport Processes*, Chapter 11. Marcel Dekker, New York.

Dorson, W. J. (1970). Oxygenation of blood for clinical applications. In *Blood Oxygenation* (ed. D. Hershey). Plenum Press, New York.

Gibbon, J. H. (1954). Application of a mechanical heart and lung apparatus to cardiac surgery. *Minnesota Medicine* **37**, 171–185.

Lightfoot, E. N. (1974). *Transport Phenomena in Living Systems*. John Wiley & Sons, New York. (Includes a section on direct-contact oxygenation of blood pp. 319–26).

Spaeth, E. E. (1973). Blood oxygenation in extracorporeal devices: theoretical considerations. CRC *Critical Reviews in Bioengineering* **1**, 383–417.

6 Carbon dioxide transfer in extracorporeal lungs

6.1 Introduction

Early theoretical interest in membrane lungs concentrated on the transfer of oxygen. This was because CO_2 transfer was less of a practical problem than oxygen transfer. In the early work of Clowes, Hopkins and Neville (1956. *Journal of Thoracic Surgery*, **32**, 630–7), when sufficient membrane was used to bring the oxygen saturation of blood up to around 85 per cent, the partial pressure of CO_2 was found to be close to the normal value of 5 kPa. Further oxygenation led to lower values of P_{CO_2}. It soon became customary to add CO_2 to the previously pure oxygen which was used to supply membrane lungs to prevent large falls in P_{CO_2} below normal values.

More recently there has been interest in developing membrane lungs which are capable of removing larger than physiological quantities of CO_2 from blood. This has provided a fresh impetus to the use of theoretical models of CO_2 transfer.

In one respect CO_2 transfer is more complicated than oxygen transfer; it exists in blood in *three* separate forms in contrast to the two forms of oxygen (Fig. 1.8). Recall that as CO_2 becomes dissolved in blood much of it diffuses into the red cells, where the enzyme carbonic anhydrase rapidly effects conversion to carbonic acid and consequently bicarbonate (eqn (1.39)). There is also the binding of CO_2 to haemoglobin to form carbamino—CO_2 (eqn (1.40)). In two respects CO_2 transfer is easier to model than oxygen transfer. Firstly, the C–P relationship is more nearly linear over the range of interest. Secondly, the relative proportions of the three forms of CO_2 are less variable and the system can be moderately well modelled by regarding them as one species with an appropriately selected mean diffusion constant D and solubility α.

In chapter 5 we derived the general form of the convection–diffusion equation for uniform flow, with no diffusion in the direction of the flow:

$$u \frac{\partial C}{\partial x} = D \frac{\partial^2 C}{\partial y^2}. \tag{5.1}$$

In this chapter we look for solutions to this equation for the extraction of CO_2 from blood in parallel plate membrane lungs and later examine solutions for the hollow fibre geometry.

6.2   Parallel plate geometry: membrane-limited extraction of CO_2.

Consider the case of a very high membrane resistance to the diffusion of CO_2 such that the gradient in partial pressure across the membrane far exceeds the maximum gradient in partial pressure in the blood itself. Figure 6.1 shows profiles of partial pressure which are consistent with this assumption. Three are depicted: at inlet to the channel, midway along the channel, and at outlet to the channel. The extreme case is shown in which there is no visible gradient of partial pressure across the blood channel. The gas-side partial pressure of CO_2 is P_g. In the blood both P and C are regarded as primarily functions of x, $P(x)$ and $C(x)$. The gradient in CO_2 concentration across the membrane becomes $\alpha_m (P(x) - P_g)/t$, and we can integrate eqn (5.1) directly:

$$\int_{-h}^{h} u \frac{dC(x)}{dx} \, dy = -2 D_m \alpha_m \frac{(P(x) - P_g)}{t}, \tag{6.1}$$

or

$$\frac{dC(x)}{dx} = -\frac{D_m \alpha_m (P(x) - P_g)}{\bar{u} h t}. \tag{6.2}$$

The right-hand side of eqn (6.1) represents the integral with respect to y of the right-hand side of eqn (5.1)

$$\int_{-h}^{h} D \frac{\partial^2 C}{\partial y^2} \, dy = \left[D \frac{\partial C}{\partial y} \right]_{-h}^{h}. \tag{6.3}$$

$$= \text{flux of } CO_2 \text{ into blood at upper wall } +$$

$$\text{flux of } CO_2 \text{ into blood at lower wall.}$$

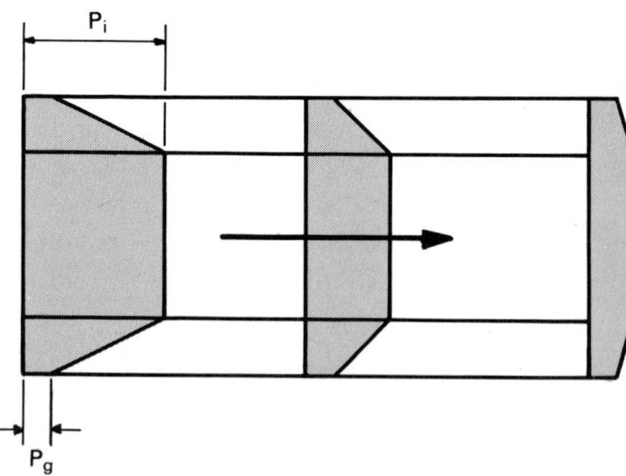

Fig. 6.1. Parallel plate geometry: membrane-limited extraction of CO_2. Partial pressure profiles for CO_2 are depicted in which there is a large gradient across the membrane but no visible gradient across the blood channel.

Each of these two terms is equated with D_m times the concentration gradient across the wall. The solution (6.2) is therefore derived by assuming that C and P vary insignificantly with respect to y as far as the left-hand side of eqn (5.1) is concerned, but vary significantly with respect to y as far as the right-hand side of eqn (5.1) is concerned.

Equation (6.2) can be integrated, either analytically or numerically, using a variety of expressions to describe the C–P relationship for CO_2 (Fig. 1.9). We adopt the simple model of linearizing the curve in the region of interest, and write

$$C = \alpha P + \beta. \tag{6.4}$$

Figure 6.2 depicts this linearization. The choice of gradient and intercept for this equation can usefully be made according to the blood inlet condition (P_i)

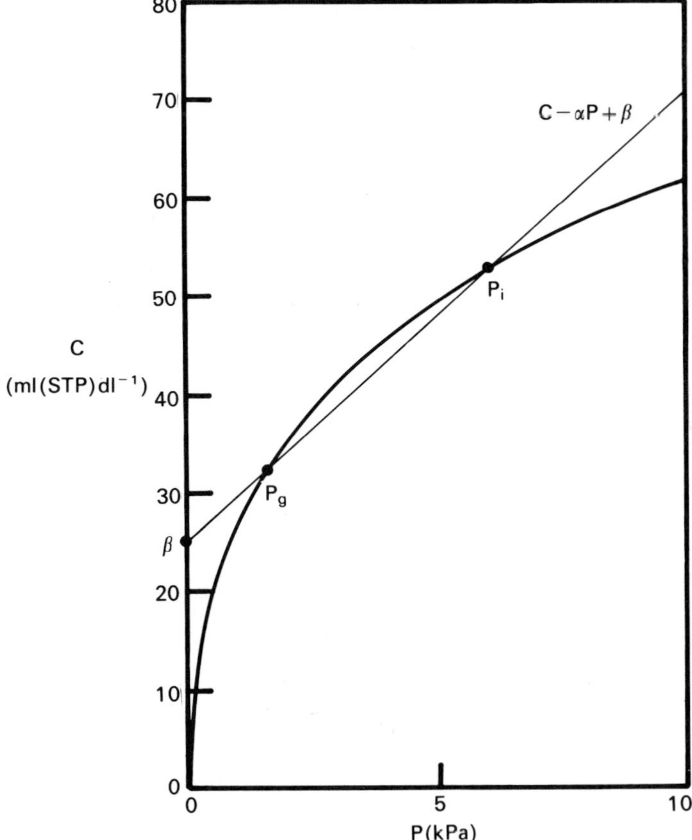

Fig. 6.2. Linearization of the C–P relationship for CO_2 (eqn 6.4).

and the degree to which blood is expected to be depleted of CO_2. For example, if blood is expected to approach gas partial pressure P_g closely then the line can be chosen to intercept at both P_i and P_g, as shown in Fig. 6.2.

Substitute eqn (6.4) into (6.2):

$$\frac{dP(x)}{dx} = -\frac{D_m \alpha_m (P(x) - P_g)}{\alpha \bar{u} h t}. \tag{6.5}$$

Integration with respect to x gives

$$\int_{P_i}^{P_o} \frac{dP(x)}{(P(x) - P_g)} = \int_0^L -\frac{D_m \alpha_m}{\alpha \bar{u} h t} \, dx, \tag{6.6}$$

or

$$\frac{P_o - P_g}{P_i - P_g} = \exp\left(-\frac{D_m \alpha_m L}{\alpha \bar{u} h t}\right). \tag{6.7}$$

P_o is the outlet partial pressure of CO_2 in blood.

Convention defines a dimensionless partial pressure change during CO_2 transfer, θ, analogous to f for oxygen transfer

$$\theta \equiv \frac{P_i - P_0}{P_i - P_g}. \tag{6.8}$$

θ takes values between 0 and 1. In terms of θ, eqn (6.7) takes the form

$$\theta = 1 - \exp\left(-\frac{D_m \alpha_m L}{\alpha \bar{u} h t}\right). \tag{6.9}$$

As for oxygen transfer, we prefer to express our solution in terms of the blood flow Q_b and the total membrane area A. Recall (Fig. 5.6) that $A/2 = Lb$ and $Q_b = 2hb\bar{u}$. Equation (6.9) can be written as

$$\theta = 1 - \exp\left(-\frac{D_m \alpha_m A}{\alpha Q_b t}\right). \tag{6.10}$$

The dimensionless wall Sherwood Number

$$Sh_w = \frac{D_m \alpha_m h}{D \alpha t} \tag{5.15}$$

has the same physical significance as described in chapter 5. In terms of Sh_w, eqn (6.10) becomes

$$\theta = 1 - \exp\left(-Sh_w \frac{DA}{hQ_b}\right). \tag{6.11}$$

The wall Sherwood number is a measure of the relative resistance to diffusion of a stationary layer of blood of thickness h, compared with a

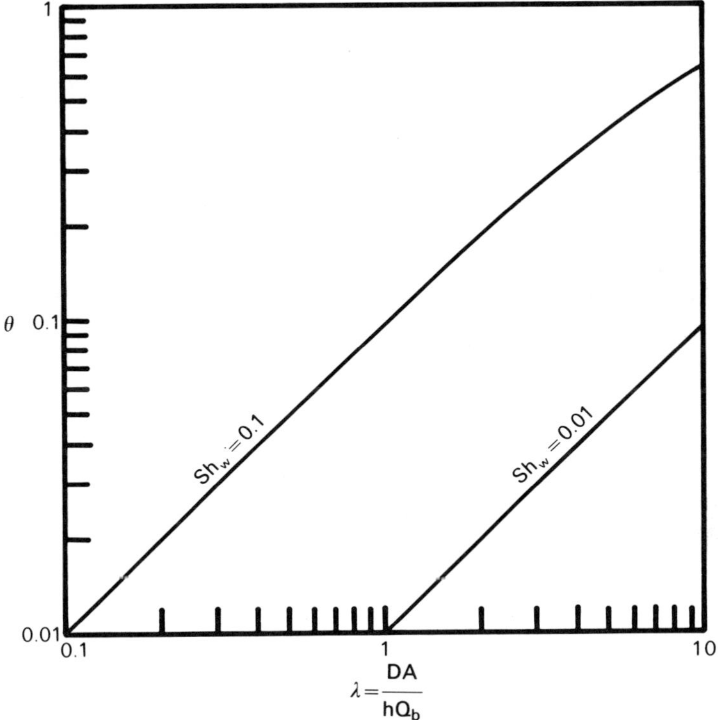

Fig. 6.3. Parallel plate membrane lung. CO_2 transfer predicted for low wall Sherwood Numbers ($Sh_w \ll 1$) by an approximate analytical solution (eqn 6.11).

membrane of thickness t (Fig. 5.11). In deriving eqn (6.11) we have assumed a high relative membrane resistance (Fig. 6.1). We consequently expect this solution to model the system only for low values of Sh_w. Figure 6.3 is a doubly logarithmic plot of θ as a function of $DA/(hQ_b)$, which we can usefully regard as a dimensionless length λ for the membrane lung:

$$\lambda \equiv \frac{DA}{hQ_b}. \tag{6.12}$$

$$\theta = 1 - \exp(-Sh_w \lambda).$$

Solutions are plotted for two values for which $Sh_w \ll 1$.

Note that eqn (6.11) has been derived without specifying a velocity profile across the blood channel. We shall see later in this chapter that a numerical solution to eqn (5.1), for the case of a parabolic velocity profile, agrees well with the analytical solution for $Sh_w \ll 1$.

6.3   Parallel plate membrane lung: approximate solution for intermediate membrane resistance to CO_2 transfer

The solution to the convection–diffusion eqn (5.1) can be explored using the method of *separation of variables*. We assume that at least part of the solution takes the form of a product of a function of x and a function of y:

$$C = X(x)\,Y(y). \tag{6.13}$$

We examine to what extent such a solution can satisfy the form of the convection–diffusion equation for a Newtonian fluid

$$\frac{3}{2}\bar{u}\left[1 - \left(\frac{y}{h}\right)^2\right]\frac{\partial C}{\partial x} = D\,\frac{\partial^2 C}{\partial y^2}. \tag{5.9}$$

Since

$$\frac{\partial C}{\partial x} = Y(y)\,\frac{\mathrm{d}X(x)}{\mathrm{d}x}$$

and

$$\frac{\partial^2 C}{\partial y^2} = X(x)\,\frac{\mathrm{d}^2 Y(y)}{\mathrm{d}y^2},$$

eqn (5.9) can be written in the form

$$\frac{3h^2\bar{u}}{2D}\frac{1}{X}\frac{\mathrm{d}X}{\mathrm{d}x} = \frac{1}{[1 - (y/h)^2]\,Y}\frac{\mathrm{d}^2 Y}{\mathrm{d}(y/h)^2}. \tag{6.14}$$

X is now shorthand for $X(x)$ and Y for $Y(y)$.

The left-hand side of eqn (6.14) is a function only of x and the right-hand side is a function only of y. x and y are independent variables. Consequently, if a solution of the form of eqn (6.13) exists, each side must equal some constant. We choose this to be a negative number $(-\gamma^2)$ so that X turns out to be a credible decreasing, rather than increasing, function of x:

$$\frac{3h^2\bar{u}}{2D}\frac{\mathrm{d}X}{X} = -\gamma^2\,\mathrm{d}x$$

or

$$X = X_0 \exp\left(-\frac{2D}{3h^2\bar{u}}\gamma^2 x\right). \tag{6.15}$$

Y is the solution to the differential equation

$$\frac{\mathrm{d}^2 Y}{\mathrm{d}(y/h)^2} + \gamma^2\,[1 - (y/h)^2]\,Y = 0. \tag{6.16}$$

We need a solution which is symmetrical about $y = 0$. One trivial solution is obtained by setting $\gamma^2 = 0$ and integrating to give $C = $ constant. An example of a non-trivial solution to eqn (6.16) is for $\gamma^2 = 1$

$$Y = Y_0 \exp\left[-\frac{1}{2}\left(\frac{y}{h}\right)^2\right]. \tag{6.17}$$

C is given by X times Y:

$$C = C_0 \exp\left(-\frac{2D}{3h^2\bar{u}}x\right)\exp\left[-\frac{1}{2}\left(\frac{y}{h}\right)^2\right], \tag{6.18}$$

where $C_0 = X_0 Y_0$. Equation (6.18) suffers the disadvantage that C tends to zero as $x \to \infty$. Solutions for different values of γ can be added in series (see eqn (6.54) to follow) and so this inadequacy can be overcome by adding a constant, C_g, to the right-hand side. Set $C_g = \alpha P_g + \beta$. C_g is then the CO_2 concentration which would be reached for blood in equilibrium with a gas partial pressure P_g of CO_2. Equation (6.18) becomes

$$(C - C_g) = C_0 \exp\left(-\frac{2D}{3h^2\bar{u}}x\right)\exp\left[-\frac{1}{2}\left(\frac{y}{h}\right)^2\right]. \tag{6.19}$$

What physical situation does this solution represent?
Consider first the membrane boundary condition

$$D\left.\frac{\partial C}{\partial y}\right|_{y=\pm h} = \pm D_m \alpha_m \frac{(P_g - P_w)}{t}. \tag{5.11}$$

Differentiation of eqn (6.19) gives the flux of CO_2 leaving blood at the wall as

$$D\left.\frac{\partial C}{\partial y}\right|_{y=\pm h} = \mp \frac{DC_0}{h}\exp\left(-\frac{1}{2}\right)\exp\left(\frac{-2D}{3h^2\bar{u}}x\right). \tag{6.20}$$

The concentration at the wall C_w is given by eqn (6.19):

$$(C_w - C_g) = C_0 \exp\left(-\frac{1}{2}\right)\exp\left(\frac{-2D}{3h^2\bar{u}}x\right). \tag{6.21}$$

It follows from eqns (6.20) and (6.21) that for all x the wall flux and wall concentration are related by

$$D\frac{\partial C}{\partial y} = \mp D\frac{(C_w - C_g)}{h} \tag{6.22}$$

For this property of our trial solution (eqn (6.19)) to concord with the boundary condition (eqn (5.11)) we require only that

$$D\frac{(C_w - C_g)}{h} = D_m \alpha_m \frac{(P_w - P_g)}{t}. \tag{6.23}$$

Recalling the assumed linear relationship between C and P (eqn (6.4)), we find that eqn (6.23) is satisfied only if

$$\frac{D_\mathrm{m}\alpha_\mathrm{m}h}{D\alpha t} = 1. \tag{6.24}$$

We recognize this collection of terms to be the wall Sherwood Number, and note that the solution can only be valid for the case $Sh_\mathrm{w} = 1$. This represents the situation in which the resistance to diffusion of the membrane equals that of a stationary layer of blood of thickness h. In other word, CO_2 transfer is limited about equally by the membrane and the blood.

The solution in eqn (6.19) satisfies the wall boundary condition exactly if $Sh_\mathrm{w} = 1$. It does not, however, satisfy the condition of uniform concentration at inlet

$$C(0, y) = C_\mathrm{i}, \tag{5.10}$$

since eqn (6.19), for $x = 0$, gives

$$C - C_\mathrm{g} = C_0 \exp\left[-\frac{1}{2}\left(\frac{y}{h}\right)^2 \right], \tag{6.25}$$

which is a function of y.

Figure 6.4 depicts partial pressure profiles for this solution, at inlet, midway along the channel, and at exit to the channel. The non-uniformity at inlet is from a maximum concentration of $C_\mathrm{g} + C_0$ in the midline to $C_\mathrm{g} + 0.607\,C_0$ at the wall. The mean concentration at any section $\bar{C}$ is given by

$$\bar{C} - C_\mathrm{g} = I\,C_0 \exp\left(\frac{-2Dx}{3h^2\bar{u}}\right), \tag{6.26}$$

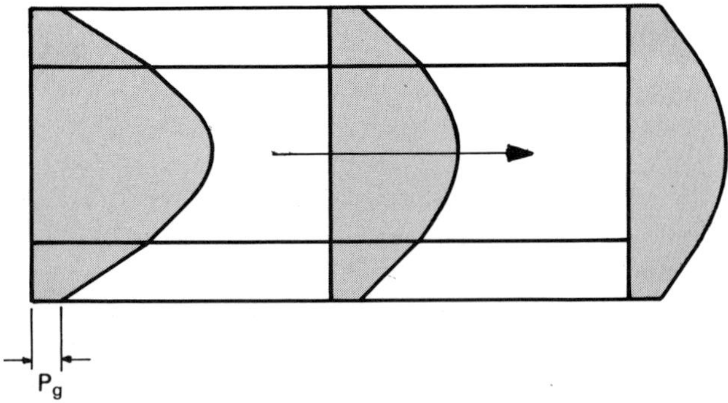

Fig. 6.4. Parallel plate membrane lung: approximate solution for the case $Sh_\mathrm{w} = 1$. Partial pressure profiles for CO_2 are depicted for a single term solution to the convection–diffusion equation, with separated variables (eqn 6.19). The solution satisfies the wall boundary condition exactly if $Sh_\mathrm{w} = 1$ but it fails to conform to the inlet condition of a uniform concentration.

where

$$I \equiv \frac{1}{2h} \int_{-h}^{+h} \exp\left[-\frac{1}{2}\left(\frac{y}{h}\right)^2 \right] dy. \tag{6.27}$$

Using the dimensionless partial pressure change θ (eqn 6.8) we can now express the overall performance for this solution:

$$\theta = \frac{I C_0 - I C_0 \exp\left(-\frac{2DL}{3h^2\bar{u}} \right)}{I C_0}$$

or

$$\theta = 1 - \exp\left(-\frac{2}{3} \times \frac{DA}{hQ_b} \right), \tag{6.28}$$

where L and $\bar{u}$ have been replaced by A and Q_b as in eqn (6.10).

Equation (6.28) is plotted in Fig. (6.5). We shall see later in this chapter that this approximate solution agrees well with a precise numerical solution to

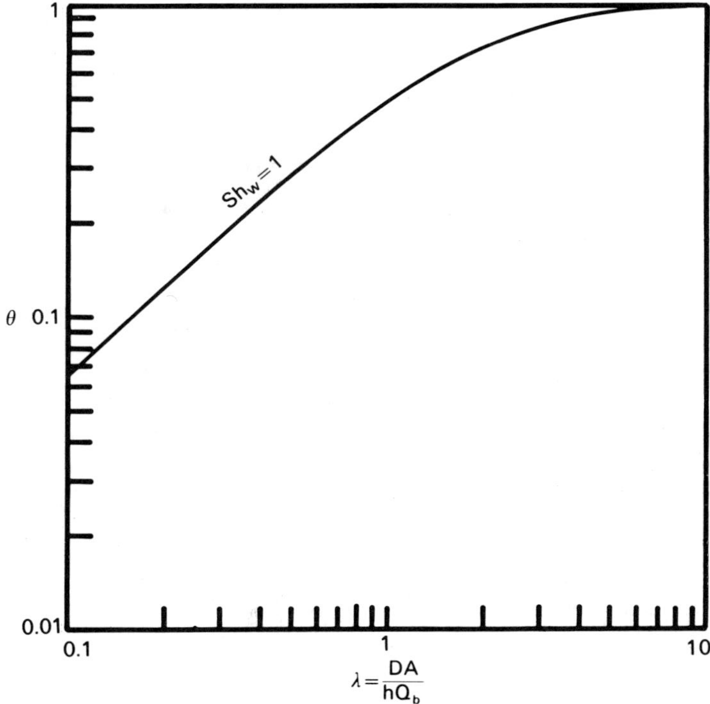

Fig. 6.5. Parallel plate membrane lung. CO_2 transfer predicted for $Sh_w = 1$ by an approximate analytical solution (eqn 6.28).

eqn (5.9) for the case $Sh_w = 1$. We shall also see that a general solution which conforms to the inlet boundary condition of uniform CO_2 concentration across the blood channel can be expressed as the sum of an infinite series of terms, each of which takes the form $X(x) Y(y)$.

6.4   Parallel plate membrane lung: approximate solution for the case of low membrane resistance to CO_2 transfer

In this section we examine the case of CO_2 removal from blood across membranes which offer minimal resistance to the diffusion of CO_2. Figure 6.6 depicts the partial pressure profiles we envisage for this situation. The relatively high resistance to diffusion of the blood is expected to give rise to two fairly distinct zones within the blood. In the centre of the channel the blood inlet conditions (P_i, C_i) are likely to remain undisturbed for a considerable distance into the channel. At the side of the channel we envisage a *mass transfer boundary layer* within which the concentration of CO_2 falls from around C_i to a low value at the wall. The edge of this boundary layer will advance into the flow from the wall at increasing distance down the channel, and it is depicted by two fine lines in Fig. 6.6.

We shall artificially define a mass transfer boundary layer of thickness $\delta(x)$ at the inner edge of which the CO_2 concentration equals C_i exactly. We shall also limit our model to the extreme case of zero membrane resistance so that the concentration at the outer edge of the boundary layer equals C_g ($= \alpha P_g + \beta$; $Sh_w \to \infty$).

Our approach to a solution for this special case is one commonly adopted in boundary layer problems in which an exact solution is difficult to obtain.

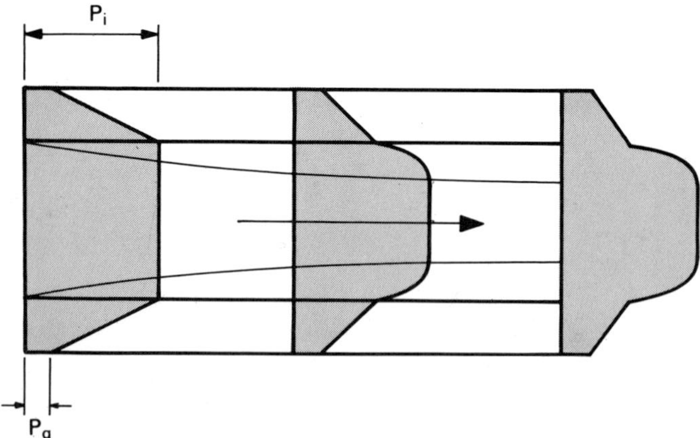

Fig. 6.6. Parallel plate membrane lung: approximate solution for the case $Sh_w \to \infty$. Partial pressure profiles are envisaged in which a mass transfer boundary layer lies next to the wall and an undisturbed core of blood with inlet CO_2 concentration flows in the centre of the channel.

The method hinges on writing a polynomial (in this case cubic) approximation to the variation of CO_2 concentration within the mass transfer boundary layer. The polynomial function is written for simplicity in such a way that this concentration profile (and therefore also the partial pressure profile) has a constant shape for all values of x. Only the thickness δ of the boundary layer changes.

Consider the following general cubic function as an approximation to the concentration profile at the lower wall of the channel

$$C = C_1 + C_2\left(\frac{y+h}{\delta}\right) + C_3\left(\frac{y+h}{\delta}\right)^2 + C_4\left(\frac{y+h}{\delta}\right)^3. \tag{6.30}$$

Note that, since y is measured from the channel centre line, the wall coordinate $y = -h$ coincides with $(y+h)/\delta = 0$, and the inner edge of the boundary layer coincides with $(y+h)/\delta = 1$. The four coefficients in eqn (6.30) can be determined by ensuring that the concentration profile satisfies four important conditions:

(i) At the inner edge of the boundary layer $C = C_i$:

$$C_i = C_1 + C_2 + C_3 + C_4. \tag{6.31}$$

(ii) At the wall $C = C_g$:

$$C_g = C_1. \tag{6.32}$$

(iii) At the wall, where $u = 0$, eqn (5.1) requires

$$\partial^2 C/\partial y^2 = 0:$$

$$2C_3/\delta = 0. \tag{6.33}$$

(iv) At the inner edge of the boundary layer there is no flux in the y direction ($D\,\partial C/\partial y = 0$):

$$C_2 + 2C_3 + 3C_4 = 0. \tag{6.34}$$

The solution to eqns (6.31–6.34) is

(i) $C_1 = C_g$
(ii) $C_2 = (3/2)(C_i - C_g)$
(iii) $C_3 = 0$
(iv) $C_4 = -(1/2)(C_i - C_g).$
$$\tag{6.35}$$

Equation (6.30) becomes

$$C = C_g + \frac{(C_i - C_g)}{2}\left[3\left(\frac{y+h}{\delta}\right) - \left(\frac{y+h}{\delta}\right)^3\right], \tag{6.36}$$

or

$$\frac{C_i - C}{C_i - C_g} = 1 - \frac{3}{2}\left(\frac{y+h}{\delta}\right) + \frac{1}{2}\left(\frac{y+h}{\delta}\right)^3. \tag{6.37}$$

Because this concentration profile is only on approximation it will be incapable of satisfying accurately the convection–diffusion eqn (5.1) at every value of y within the boundary layer. The rational approach we adopt is therefore to satisfy the convection–diffusion balance for the whole thickness of the boundary layer.

Figure 6.7 depicts a segment of the mass transfer boundary layer on the lower wall of the channel, of length dx, at a distance x from the channel inlet. Profiles of CO_2 partial pressure are shaded. The integrated form of the convection–diffusion equation takes the form

$$\frac{d}{dx} \int_{y=-h}^{y=\delta-h} u(y)\,C\,dy - u(\delta-h)\,C_i\,\frac{d\delta}{dx} = D\,\frac{\partial C}{\partial y}\bigg|_{\delta-h} - D\,\frac{\partial C}{\partial y}\bigg|_{-h}. \quad (6.38)$$

In words:

$$\begin{pmatrix} \text{cd flux} - \text{ab flux by} \\ \text{convection} \end{pmatrix} - \begin{pmatrix} \text{bc flux by} \\ \text{convection} \end{pmatrix} = \begin{pmatrix} \text{flux across bc and ad by} \\ \text{diffusion} \end{pmatrix}$$

Note that the first term on the right-hand side is zero according to condition (iv) above.

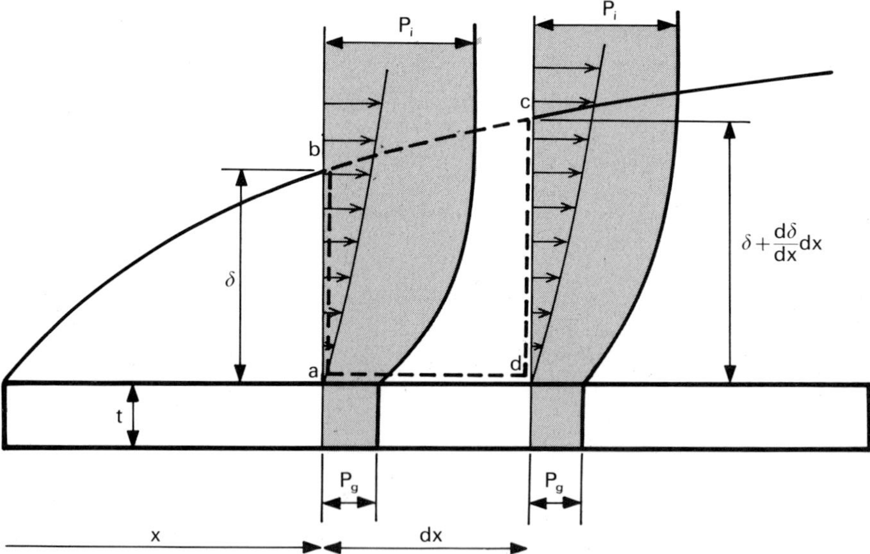

Fig. 6.7. Mass transfer boundary layer of thickness δ on lower wall of parallel plate membrane lung, used to derive an approximate solution to CO_2 transfer for the case $Sh_w \to \infty$. Partial pressure profiles are shaded. Velocity profiles are defined by arrows.

Substitute for C from eqn (6.37) into eqn (6.38):

$$\frac{\mathrm{d}}{\mathrm{d}x}\int_{-h}^{\delta-h} u(y)\left\{C_i - (C_i - C_g)\left[1 - \frac{3}{2}\left(\frac{y+h}{\delta}\right) + \frac{1}{2}\left(\frac{y+h}{\delta}\right)^3\right]\right\}\mathrm{d}y$$

$$- u(\delta - h)C_i\frac{\mathrm{d}\delta}{\mathrm{d}x} = -\frac{3D}{2\delta}(C_i - C_g). \tag{6.39}$$

Since

$$\frac{\mathrm{d}}{\mathrm{d}x}\int_{-h}^{\delta-h} u(y)\,C_i\,\mathrm{d}y = u(\delta - h)\,C_i\frac{\mathrm{d}\delta}{\mathrm{d}x}, \tag{6.40}$$

eqn (6.39) can be written in the simpler form

$$\frac{\mathrm{d}}{\mathrm{d}x}\int_{-h}^{\delta-h} u(y)\left[1 - \frac{3}{2}\left(\frac{y+h}{\delta}\right) + \frac{1}{2}\left(\frac{y+h}{\delta}\right)^3\right]\mathrm{d}y = \frac{3D}{2\delta}. \tag{6.41}$$

Substitute for $u(y)$ from eqn (5.8) and integrate:

$$\frac{\mathrm{d}}{\mathrm{d}x}\left(\frac{h\delta^2}{5} - \frac{\delta^3}{24}\right) = \frac{Dh^2}{\delta\bar{u}} \tag{6.42}$$

or

$$\left(\frac{2h\delta^2}{5} - \frac{3\delta^3}{24}\right)\frac{\mathrm{d}\delta}{\mathrm{d}x} = \frac{Dh^2}{\bar{u}}. \tag{6.43}$$

Equation (6.43) can be integrated to give δ as a function of L:

$$\frac{2}{15}\left(\frac{\delta}{h}\right)^3 - \frac{1}{32}\left(\frac{\delta}{h}\right)^4 = \frac{DL}{\bar{u}h^2} = \frac{DA}{hQ_b}. \tag{6.44}$$

Equation (6.44) gives us the thickness of the mass transfer boundary layer in relation to the length of the wall. We wish to relate θ to L, and can do so by first relating θ to δ. From eqs (6.8) and (6.37), noting that C is linearly related to P (Fig. 6.2), we write

$$\theta = \frac{1}{2h\bar{u}}\int_{-h}^{h} u(y)\left(\frac{C_i - C}{C_i - C_g}\right)\mathrm{d}y$$

$$= \frac{1}{h\bar{u}}\int_{-h}^{\delta-h} \frac{3\bar{u}}{2}\left[1 - \left(\frac{y}{h}\right)^2\right]\left[1 - \frac{3}{2}\left(\frac{y+h}{\delta}\right) + \frac{1}{2}\left(\frac{y+h}{\delta}\right)^3\right]\mathrm{d}y. \tag{6.45}$$

Integration yields

$$\theta = \frac{3}{10}\left(\frac{\delta}{h}\right)^2 - \frac{1}{16}\left(\frac{\delta}{h}\right)^3. \tag{6.46}$$

Note from eqns (6.41) and (6.45) that

$$\frac{d\theta}{dx} = \frac{3D}{2\delta\bar{u}h},$$

(6.47)

a relationship which is consistent with eqns (6.44) and (6.46).

The solution expressed in eqns (6.44) and (6.47) is plotted in Fig. 6.8. We shall show later in the chapter that the agreement with a precise numerical solution for $Sh_w \to \infty$ is excellent. We can only expect the solution to be useful for $(\delta/h) \leqslant 1$, since when δ becomes equal to h the mass transfer boundary layers of our model meet on the channel centre line. The corresponding values of plotted variables are

$$\theta = 0.24$$

(6.48)

$$\frac{DA}{hQ_b} = 0.10.$$

(6.49)

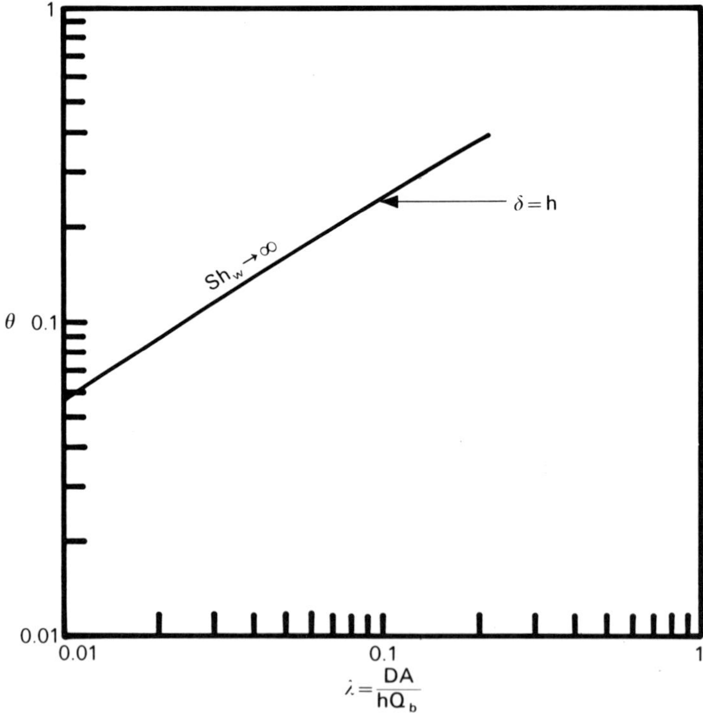

Fig. 6.8. Parallel plate membrane lung. CO_2 transfer predicted for $Sh_w \to \infty$ by an approximate analytical solution (eqns 6.44 and 6.46). Compare with Fig. 6.5. The arrow depicts the upper value of θ for which the solution is appropriate (see text).

The solution is therefore only credible for low degrees of CO_2 transfer in which θ remains in the lower third of its range 0–1.

For $(\delta/h) \leqslant 1$ eqns (6.44) and (6.46) approximate closely to the relationship

$$\theta = \frac{3}{10}\left(\frac{15DA}{2hQ_b}\right)^{2/3}. \tag{6.50}$$

This is consistent with the doubly logarithmic plot in Fig. 6.8 being an almost straight line with gradient 2/3.

6.5   Parallel plate membrane lung: general solution for CO_2 transfer

In this section we show how a general solution to the convection–diffusion eqn (5.9) can be approached. We have seen that a solution of the form $C = X(x)\,Y(y)$ exists if it satisfies the equations

$$X = X_0 \exp\left(-\frac{2D}{3h^2\bar{u}}\gamma^2 x\right) \tag{6.15}$$

$$\frac{d^2 Y}{d(y/h)^2} + \gamma^2 [1 - (y/h)^2]\,Y = 0 \tag{6.16}$$

It follows that a series of such solutions, each with a different X_0 and γ will also satisfy the convection–diffusion equation. For, if

$$C = C_1 + C_2 + \ldots + C_j + \ldots C_n, \tag{6.51}$$

and each term C_j satisfies the equation

$$\frac{3}{2}\bar{u}\left[1 - \left(\frac{y}{h}\right)^2\right]\frac{\partial C_j}{\partial x} = D\frac{\partial^2 C_j}{\partial y^2}, \tag{6.52}$$

then

$$\frac{3}{2}\bar{u}\left[1 - \left(\frac{y}{h}\right)^2\right]\frac{\partial}{\partial x}(C_1 + C_2 + \ldots + C_n) = D\frac{\partial^2}{\partial y^2}(C_1 + C_2 + \ldots + C_n),$$
$$\tag{6.53}$$

or

$$\frac{3}{2}\bar{u}\left[1 - \left(\frac{y}{h}\right)^2\right]\frac{\partial C}{\partial x} = D\frac{\partial^2 C}{\partial y^2}. \tag{5.9}$$

To summarize, a general solution takes the form

$$C = \sum_{j=1}^{j=n} X_{0j}\, Y_j(y)\exp\left(-\frac{2D}{3h^2\bar{u}}\gamma_j^2 x\right), \tag{6.54}$$

where

$$\frac{d^2 Y_j}{d(y/h)^2} + \gamma_j^2 [1 - (y/h)^2]\,Y_j = 0. \tag{6.55}$$

It is useful to take the term $C = C_g$ (a constant) corresponding to $\gamma_j = 0$ over to the left-hand side of eqn (6.54) and write

$$(C - C_g) = \sum_{j=1}^{j=n} X_{0j}\, Y_j(y)\exp\left(-\frac{2D}{3h^2\bar{u}}\,\gamma_j^2 x\right), \tag{6.56}$$

insisting henceforth that $\gamma_j \neq 0$.

The inlet boundary condition (eqn (5.10)) requires the concentration of CO_2 at $x = 0$ to be independent of y. From eqn (6.56) we see that this amounts to

$$(C_i - C_g) = \sum_{j=1}^{j=n} X_{0j}\, Y_j(y). \tag{6.57}$$

Our second boundary condition relates to the membrane surface (eqn (5.11)). Here the CO_2 flux leaving the blood must equal the flux diffusing through the membrane. Equation (6.56) becomes

$$D \sum_{j=1}^{j=n} X_{0j}\,\frac{dY_j(y)}{dy}\exp\left(-\frac{2D}{3h^2\bar{u}}\,\gamma_j^2 x\right) =$$

$$\mp \frac{D_m\alpha_m}{\alpha t} \sum_{j=1}^{j=n} X_{0j}\, Y_j(y)\exp\left(-\frac{2D}{3h^2\bar{u}}\,\gamma_j^2 x\right)\Bigg|_{y=\pm h}, \tag{6.58}$$

which reduces to

$$\frac{dY_j(y)}{d(y/h)} = \mp\, Sh_w\, Y_j(y)\Bigg|_{y=\pm h}. \tag{6.59}$$

It is useful to regard Y as a function of a dimensionless channel half-width $\eta \equiv y/h$, $Y(\eta)$, rather than as a function of y alone. Since $\eta = \pm 1$ where $y = \pm h$ we may write eqn (6.59) in the succinct form

$$\left.\begin{aligned} Y'(1) &= -\,Sh_w\, Y(1) \\ Y'(-1) &= Sh_w\, Y(-1), \end{aligned}\right\} \tag{6.60}$$

where Y' denotes $dY/d(y/h)$, that is $dY/d\eta$.

Our problem has been transformed to the following form: we are trying to find a series of functions $Y_j(\eta)$, each associated with its own number γ_j (called an *eigenvalue* from the German eigen = own), and obeying the differential equation

$$Y_j''(\eta) + \gamma_j(1 - \eta^2)\, Y_j(\eta) = 0, \tag{6.61}$$

where $Y_j''(\eta)$ is shorthand for the first term in eqn (6.55). $Y_j(\eta)$ must also satisfy a boundary condition at $\eta = \pm 1$ (eqn (6.60)), and be such that a sum of a certain multiple of each of the functions is equal to a constant for all values of η:

$$\sum_{j=1}^{j=n} X_{0j}\, Y_j(\eta) = \text{constant}, \tag{6.62}$$

as in eqn (6.57).

It is possible to proceed by writing the function $Y_j(\eta)$ as a polynomial*

$$Y(\eta) = a_0 + a_1\eta^2 + a_2\eta^4 + \ldots + a_n\eta^{2n} + \ldots$$

$$= \sum_n a_n\eta^{2n}, \tag{6.63}$$

choosing only even powers of η to ensure that we satisfy the requirement for symmetry about $\eta = 0$. Since

$$Y''(\eta) = 2a_1 + 12a_2\eta^2 + \ldots + 2n(2n-1)a_n\eta^{2(n-1)} + \ldots$$

$$= \sum_n 2n(2n-1)a_n\eta^{2(n-1)}, \tag{6.64}$$

our differential eqn (6.61) is satisfied only if the following *recurrence* relation holds true

$$2n(2n-1)a_n + \gamma^2(a_{n-1} - a_{n-2}), \tag{6.65}$$

with $a_1 = -\gamma^2 a_0/2$ (i.e., $a_{-1} \equiv 0$).

Next we impose the wall condition on our polynomial $Y(\eta)$. Since

$$Y'(\eta) = 2a_1\gamma + 4a_2\eta^3 + \ldots + 2na_n\eta^{2n-1} + \ldots, \tag{6.66}$$

eqn (6.60) yields

$$Sh_w = -\frac{\sum_n 2na_n}{\sum_n a_n} \quad (=f(\gamma)). \tag{6.67}$$

In parenthesis we have noted that this wall Sherwood Number itself turns out to be a function $f(\gamma)$ of the eigenvalue γ. Conversely, for a known value of Sh_w, the eigenvalues will be the roots (solutions) to eqn (6.67).

Various processes of 'trial and error' and numerical computation have been used to find the roots to eqn (6.67), using values of a_n computed from eqn (6.65). Brown has computed the first ten eigenvalues for the case $Sh_w \to \infty$ (Brown, G. M. (1960). *American Institute of Chemical Engineers Journal*, **6**, 179–83). These are listed in Table 6.1.

Once γ_j has been found, its corresponding *eigenfunction* $Y_j(\eta)$ can be constructed from the recurrence relation (eqn (6.65)). This being complete, it remains to deduce the coefficients X_{0j} which determine what proportion of the whole solution is made up by each eigenfunction.

Consider now the effect of multiplying both sides of eqn (6.57) by $(1-\eta^2)Y_k(\eta)$ and integrating with respect to η from $\eta = -1$ to $\eta = 1$:

$$(C_i - C_g)\int_{-1}^{1}(1-\eta^2)Y_k(\eta)d\eta = \sum_{j=1}^{j=n}X_{0j}\int_{-1}^{1}(1-\eta^2)Y_j(\eta)Y_k(\eta)d\eta. \tag{6.68}$$

* from here on we omit the subscript j from some equations for clarity.

Table 6.1. *The first ten eigen values for the solution to CO_2 removal from blood flowing between parallel membranes (see text). $Sh_w \to \infty$.*

j	γ_j
1	1.682
2	5.670
3	9.668
4	13.668
5	17.667
6	21.667
7	25.667
8	29.667
9	33.667
10	37.667

We shall show below that the integral on the right-hand side of this equation is zero whenever $j \neq k$. This leaves only one coefficient X_{0k} in the equation and thereby provides the necessary solution

$$X_{0k} = (C_i - C_g)\frac{\int_{-1}^{1}(1 - \eta^2)\,Y_k(\eta)\,\mathrm{d}\eta}{\int_{-1}^{1}(1 - \eta^2)\,Y_k^2(\eta)\,\mathrm{d}\eta}, \qquad (6.69)$$

from which X_{0k} can be computed because $Y_k(\eta)$ is already known (eqns (6.63) and (6.65)). The solution is then complete and it remains only to evaluate a sufficiently large number of terms (each with an eigenvalue γ_j, an eigenfunction $Y_j(\eta)$, and a coefficient X_{0j}) to yield the accuracy demanded for the problem in hand.

Before completing this section we examine the integral on the right-hand side of eqn (6.68). From eqn (6.61) we deduce that

$$\int_{-1}^{1}\gamma_j^2(1 - \eta^2)\,Y_j(\eta)\,Y_k(\eta)\,\mathrm{d}\eta = \int_{-1}^{1}Y_j''(\eta)\,Y_k(\eta)\,\mathrm{d}\eta, \qquad (6.70)$$

and similarly

$$\int_{-1}^{1}\gamma_k^2(1 - \eta^2)\,Y_k(\eta)\,Y_j(\eta)\,\mathrm{d}\eta = \int_{-1}^{1}Y_k''(\eta)\,Y_j(\eta)\,\mathrm{d}\eta. \qquad (6.71)$$

Subtract eqn (6.71) from (6.70):

$$(\gamma_j^2 - \gamma_k^2) \int_{-1}^{1} (1 - \eta^2)\, Y_j(\eta)\, Y_k(\eta)\, \mathrm{d}\eta = \int_{-1}^{1} [\, Y_j''(\eta)\, Y_k(\eta) - Y_k''(\eta)\, Y_j(\eta)\,]\, \mathrm{d}\eta.$$

$$(6.72)$$

Using the method of integration by parts*, the right-hand side (RHS) of eqn (6.72) can be expanded

$$\mathrm{RHS} = [\, Y_j'(\eta)\, Y_k(\eta) - Y_k'(\eta)\, Y_j(\eta)\,]_{-1}^{1}$$

$$- \int_{-1}^{1} [\, Y_j'(\eta)\, Y_k'(\eta) - Y_k'(\eta)\, Y_j'(\eta)\,]\, \mathrm{d}\eta,$$

where the last term is equal to zero. Equation (6.72) becomes

$$(\gamma_j^2 - \gamma_k^2) \int_{-1}^{1} (1 - \eta^2)\, Y_j(\eta)\, Y_k(\eta)\, \mathrm{d}\eta = [\, Y_j'(\eta)\, Y_k(\eta) - Y_k'(\eta)\, Y_j(\eta)\,]_{-1}^{1}.$$

$$(6.73)$$

At the wall ($\eta = \pm 1$) the boundary conditions given in eqn (6.60) obtain; eqn (6.73) yields

$$(\gamma_j^2 - \gamma_k^2) \int_{-1}^{1} (1 - \eta^2)\, Y_j(\eta)\, Y_k(\eta)\, \mathrm{d}\eta$$

$$= [- Sh_\mathrm{w}\, Y_j(1)\, Y_k(1) + Sh_\mathrm{w}\, Y_k(1)\, Y_j(1)]$$

$$- [Sh_\mathrm{w}\, Y_j(-1)\, Y_k(-1) - Sh_\mathrm{w}\, Y_k(-1)\, Y_j(-1)]$$

$$= 0, \qquad\qquad\qquad\qquad\qquad\qquad\qquad (6.74)$$

for all j and k, whether equal or not. Since when $j \neq k$ it is also true that $(\gamma_j^2 - \gamma_k^2) \neq 0$ we see that for all cases in which j is different from k

$$\int_{-1}^{1} (1 - \eta^2)\, Y_j(\eta)\, Y_k(\eta)\, \mathrm{d}\eta = 0; \quad j \neq k, \qquad (6.75)$$

as used above in the derivation of eqn (6.69).

The method described in this section can be used to derive 'exact' solutions to the parallel plate convection–diffusion problem by simple but laborious computation. Colton et al. (Colton, C. K. *et al.* (1971). *American Institute of Chemical Engineers Journal* **17**, 773–81.) present graphically the necessary eigenvalues over a wide range of wall Sherwood Numbers.

Other methods have been used for computing solutions to the convection–diffusion problem. Recently, Mayes has used the *method of lines*

$$* \int_{a}^{b} u\, \frac{\mathrm{d}v}{\mathrm{d}x}\, \mathrm{d}x = [uv]_{a}^{b} - \int_{a}^{b} v\, \frac{\mathrm{d}u}{\mathrm{d}x}\, \mathrm{d}x$$

to present results for CO_2 transfer in which account was taken of two complicating factors which we have not so far attempted to model (Mayes, P. J. D., Khoo, G. T., and Gaylor, J. D. S. (1986). *Life Support Systems*, **4**, suppl. 1, 37–47). Firstly, the *C–P* relationship for CO_2 (Fig. 6.2) was modelled by a curvilinear function rather than a straight line. Secondly, two different species of CO_2 were permitted different coefficients of diffusion. One species was taken to be the dissolved CO_2; the second species was taken to include both bicarbonate and carbamino forms.

The method also generates the solution to the convection-diffusion problem for a linear *C–P* relationship with one species of CO_2, as used extensively in this chapter. Mayes has kindly given permission for these results to be plotted in Fig. 6.9 and recorded more extensively in Table 6.2.

Comparisons in Fig. 6.9 between the three approximate analytical solutions derived earlier, and the computed solution show fair agreement. In Fig. 6.10 measurements of CO_2 transfer in a membrane lung are compared with the numerical solutions. The data is obtained from a device with a dimpled membrane (see legend) for which the preceding theory is expected to give an approximate description in the case of steady flow (filled circles).

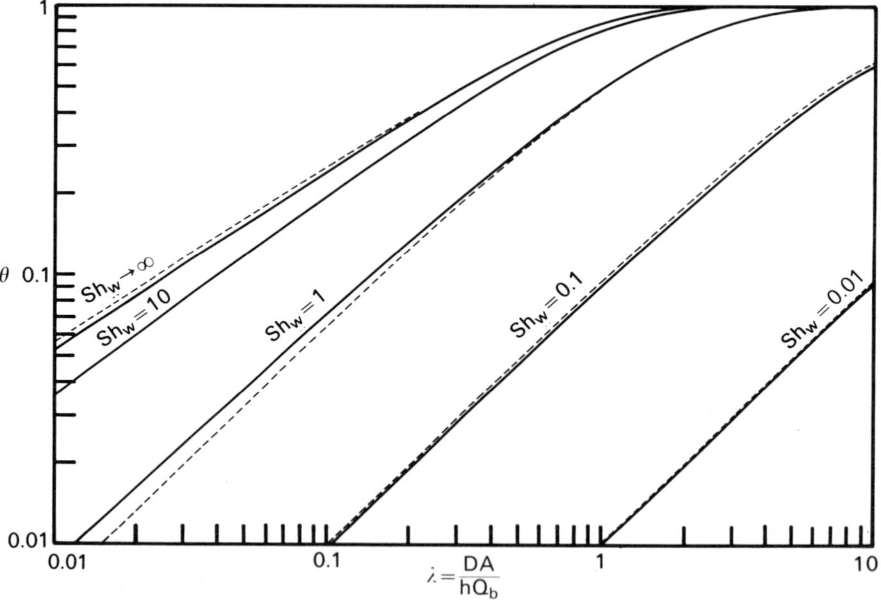

Fig. 6.9. Parallel plate membrane lung. Numerical solution (solid lines) to CO_2 transport, as in Table 6.2. The approximate analytical solutions from Fig. 6.3, 6.5 and 6.8 are plotted for comparison (dashed lines).

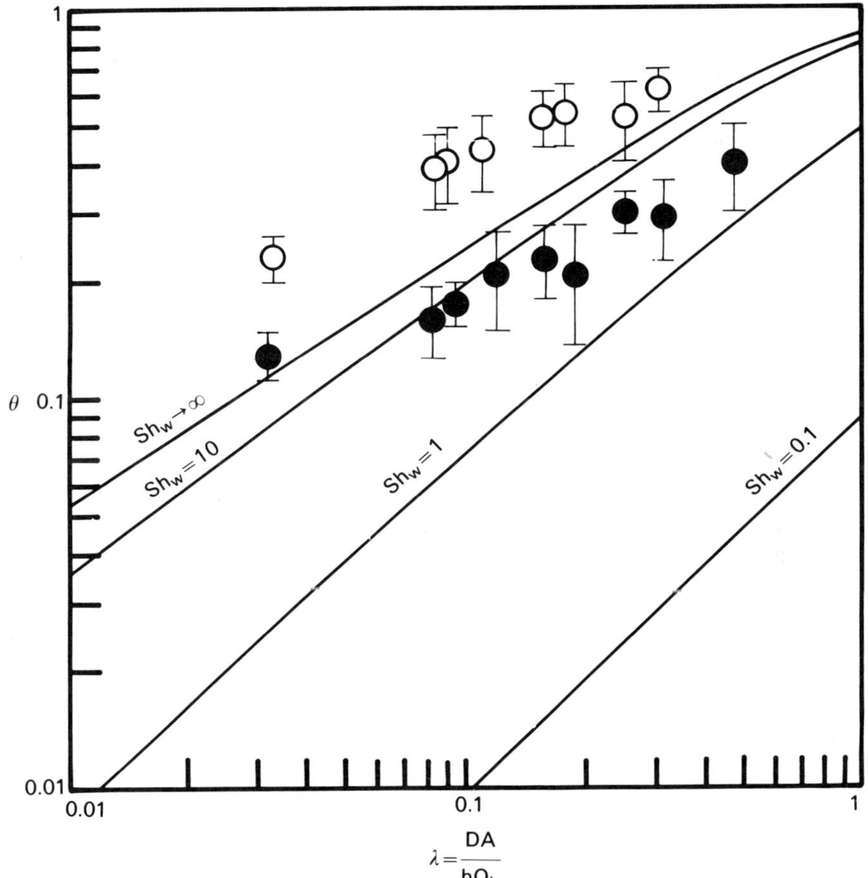

Fig. 6.10. Measurements of CO_2 transfer for a membrane lung under conditions of steady flow ●, and of oscillatory flow ○ with a pulsatile Reynolds number of 99 (see Fig. 5.20 and 6.11). These in vivo data are for a parallel plate lung constructed with dimpled membranes with minimum separation ($2h$) 0.6 mm, mean separation 1.0, and a ratio of true membrane area to plan area (A) of 1.35. The numerical solution (solid lines) from Table 6.2 is expected to reflect the performance of this system for the steady flow case, and indicates a mean value of Sh_w around 5. D has been taken to be 1.5×10^{-3} mm^{2}s^{-1}. Error bars denote $\pm$ sample standard deviations. For membrane conformation see Dorrington, K. L. *et al.* (1985). *Journal of Biomedical Engineering* **7**, 89–99, Fig. 1.

Measurements are consistent with a mean wall Sherwood Number of around 5. This suggests that the blood resistance to CO_2 transfer is more important than the membrane resistance.

This conclusion is consistent with the finding that the CO_2 transfer can be markedly increased by introducing secondary flows, as was found to be the case for oxygen transfer (Fig. 5.20). In Fig. 6.10 the data for CO_2 transfer in

Table 6.2. *Parallel plate membrane lung. Computed solutions to eqn (5.9) subject to boundary conditions (5.10) and (5.11) and a linearized C–P relationship (Fig. 6.2). θ is tabulated a function of (2/3) $[DA/(hQ_b)]$ for ten values of Sh_w. Data kindly provided by Dr. P. J. D. Mayes according to computation using the method of lines.*

$\frac{2}{3}\left(\frac{DA}{hQ_b}\right)$	Sh_w							Sh_w		
	∞	100	20	10	3.33	2	1	0.1	0.05	0.01
0.001	0.0151	0.0138	0.0102	0.00768	0.00381	0.00253	0.00137	0.00015	0.00007	0.00001
0.002	0.0239	0.0223	0.0174	0.0136	0.00717	0.00486	0.00269	0.00030	0.00015	0.00003
0.003	0.0313	0.0294	0.0236	0.0188	0.0103	0.00708	0.00397	0.00044	0.00022	0.00004
0.004	0.0378	0.0358	0.0292	0.0237	0.0133	0.00924	0.00522	0.00059	0.00030	0.00006
0.005	0.0438	0.0416	0.0344	0.0282	0.0162	0.0113	0.00646	0.00074	0.00037	0.00007
0.006	0.0494	0.0471	0.0394	0.0326	0.0190	0.0134	0.00769	0.00089	0.00045	0.00009
0.007	0.0547	0.0523	0.0441	0.0367	0.0218	0.0154	0.00890	0.00103	0.00052	0.00010
0.008	0.0598	0.0572	0.0486	0.0407	0.0244	0.0174	0.0101	0.00118	0.00059	0.00012
0.009	0.0646	0.0619	0.0529	0.0445	0.0271	0.0194	0.0113	0.00132	0.00067	0.00013
0.010	0.0693	0.0664	0.0570	0.0483	0.0296	0.0213	0.0125	0.00147	0.00074	0.00015
0.020	0.109	0.106	0.0935	0.0815	0.0533	0.0395	0.0238	0.00293	0.00148	0.00030
0.030	0.143	0.138	0.124	0.110	0.0747	0.0563	0.0347	0.00437	0.00222	0.00045
0.040	0.172	0.168	0.152	0.136	0.0945	0.0721	0.0452	0.00581	0.00295	0.00060
0.050	0.199	0.194	0.177	0.160	0.113	0.0873	0.0554	0.00725	0.00369	0.00075
0.060	0.224	0.219	0.201	0.182	0.131	0.102	0.0653	0.00868	0.00442	0.00090

0.070	0.248	0.242	0.223	0.203	0.148	0.116	0.0750	0.0101	0.00515	0.00105
0.080	0.270	0.265	0.245	0.223	0.165	0.130	0.0846	0.0115	0.00588	0.00120
0.090	0.291	0.286	0.265	0.243	0.181	0.143	0.0939	0.0129	0.00661	0.00134
0.100	0.312	0.306	0.285	0.262	0.196	0.156	0.103	0.0144	0.00734	0.00149
0.200	0.483	0.476	0.450	0.421	0.333	0.274	0.189	0.0284	0.0146	0.00298
0.300	0.610	0.603	0.576	0.545	0.446	0.375	0.267	0.0422	0.0218	0.00447
0.400	0.706	0.700	0.673	0.643	0.539	0.461	0.336	0.0558	0.0289	0.00596
0.500	0.779	0.772	0.748	0.719	0.617	0.536	0.399	0.0692	0.0360	0.00744
0.600	0.833	0.828	0.806	0.779	0.681	0.600	0.457	0.0824	0.0430	0.00892
0.700	0.874	0.869	0.850	0.826	0.735	0.655	0.508	0.0954	0.0500	0.0104
0.800	0.905	0.901	0.885	0.864	0.780	0.703	0.555	0.108	0.0569	0.0119
0.900	0.929	0.925	0.911	0.893	0.817	0.744	0.597	0.121	0.0638	0.0133
1.000	0.946	0.943	0.931	0.916	0.848	0.780	0.636	0.133	0.0706	0.0148
2.000	0.997	0.996	0.995	0.992	0.976	0.950	0.866	0.249	0.136	0.0294
3.000	1.00	1.00	1.00	0.999	0.996	0.989	0.951	0.349	0.197	0.0438
4.000	1.00	1.00	1.00	1.00	0.999	0.997	0.982	0.436	0.254	0.0580
5.000	1.00	1.00	1.00	1.00	1.00	0.999	0.993	0.511	0.307	0.0719
6.000	1.00	1.00	1.00	1.00	1.00	1.00	0.998	0.576	0.356	0.0857
7.000	1.00	1.00	1.00	1.00	1.00	1.00	0.999	0.633	0.401	0.0992
8.000	1.00	1.00	1.00	1.00	1.00	1.00	1.00	0.682	0.443	0.113
9.000	1.00	1.00	1.00	1.00	1.00	1.00	1.00	0.724	0.483	0.126
10.000	1.00	1.00	1.00	1.00	1.00	1.00	1.00	0.761	0.519	0.139

the presence of secondary flows lies well to the left of that for steady flows and in excess of the maximum transfer which can be achieved with steady flow between perfectly flat membranes ($Sh_w \to \infty$). The data for steady flow will transpose approximately onto that with secondary flows with a horizontal shift in Fig. 6.10 representing a factor between 5 and 6. In other words, the same transfer can be achieved with secondary flows when using only about 20 per cent of the membrane area which is needed for the steady flow case.

Figure 6.11 looks at this behaviour in another way. Here measurements have been made of the blood flow per square metre of membrane from which

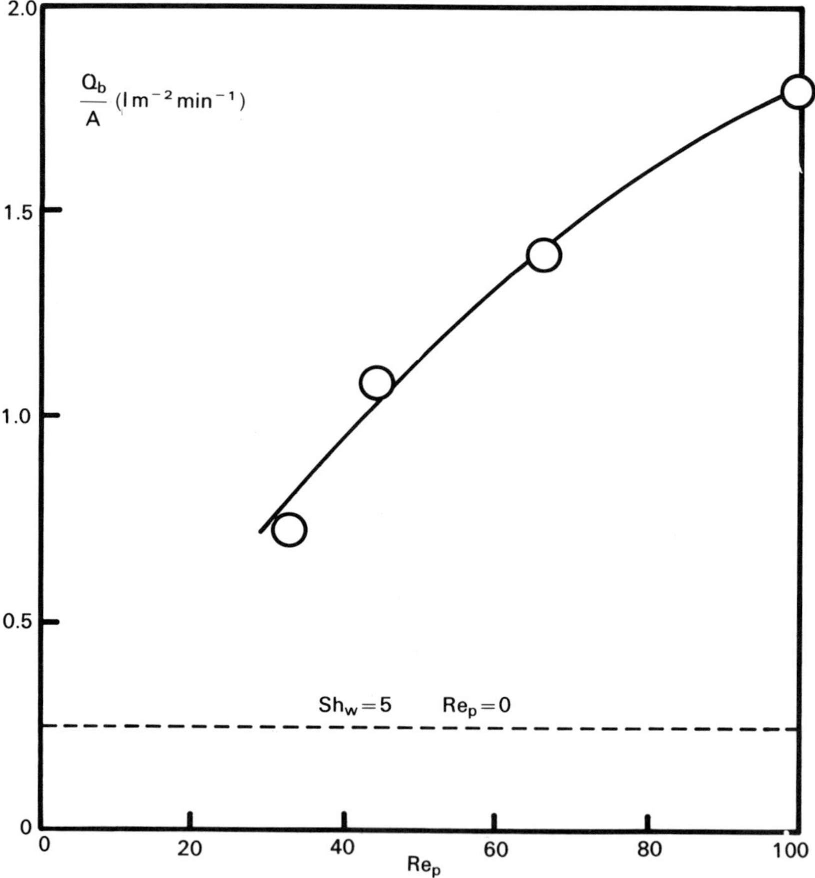

Fig. 6.11. Effect of secondary flow on the CO_2 transfer of a membrane lung of the kind represented in Fig. 6.10. The blood flow per m^2 of membrane plan area was measured for a CO_2 extraction of 190 ml (STP) dl^{-1} of blood, as a function of the pulsatile Reynolds number. Data source as Fig. 5.20.

190 ml (STP) of CO_2 per dl of blood can be removed, at various pulsatile Reynold's numbers. This high degree of CO_2 extraction corresponds with $\theta \simeq 0.8$ on a linearized form of the C–P plot (Fig. 6.2). For $Sh_w = 5$ the numerical solution (Table 6.2) gives $(2/3)(DA/hQ_b) \simeq 0.8$ from which we calculate $(Q_b/A) \simeq 0.25\,\mathrm{l\,min}^{-1}$. This result is shown by the dashed line in Fig. 6.11. It is consistent with our finding from Fig. 6.10 that $Re_p = 99$ decreases the required area by a factor of around 5 compared with the steady flow case ($Re_p = 0$).

6.6   Hollow fibre membrane lung

For a tube the convection–diffusion equation takes the form

$$u(r)\frac{\partial C}{\partial r} = D\frac{1}{r}\frac{\partial}{\partial r}\left(r\frac{\partial C}{\partial r}\right). \tag{6.76}$$

For laminar flow we have already derived the velocity profile (eqn (5.41)) and eqn (6.76) becomes

$$2u\left[1-\left(\frac{r}{R}\right)^2\right]\frac{\partial C}{\partial r} = D\frac{1}{r}\frac{\partial}{\partial r}\left(r\frac{\partial C}{\partial r}\right), \tag{6.77}$$

where R is again the inner radius of the tube (see Fig. 5.15).

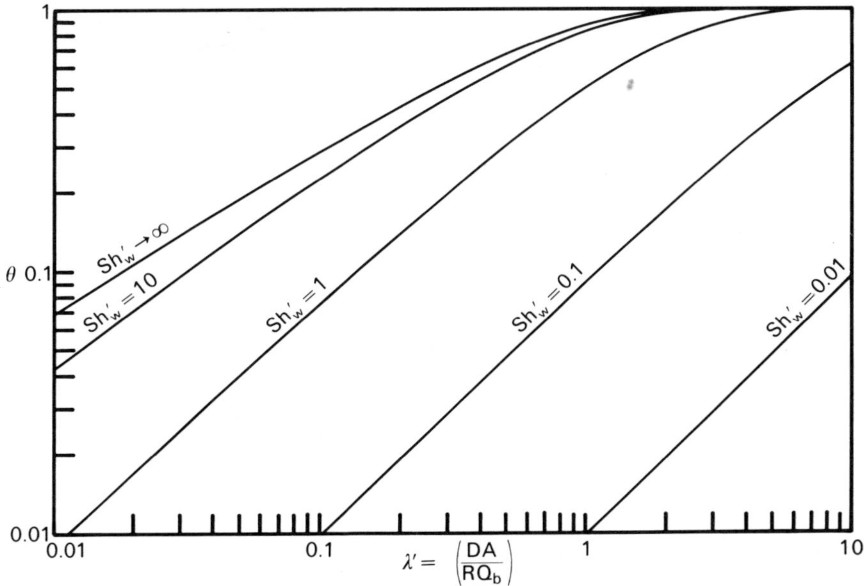

Fig. 6.12. Hollow fibre membrane lung. Numerical solution to CO_2 transport as in Table 6.3.

Table 6.3. *Hollow fibre membrane lung. Computed solution to eqn* (6.77) *subject to the boundary conditions* $C(0, r) = C_i[\theta(0, r) = 0]$ *and* $D(\partial C/\partial r) = \alpha R Sh'_w(P_g - P)|_{r = R} \cdot (\partial\theta/\partial(r/R) = Sh'_w(1 - \theta)|_{r = R})$. θ *is tabulated as a function of* $(1/4)\,[DA/(RQ_b)]$ *for ten values of* Sh'_w. *Data kindly provided by Dr P. J. D. Mayes according to computation using the method of lines.*

$\frac{1}{4}\left(\dfrac{DA}{RQ_b}\right)$	∞	100	20	10	3.33	2	1	0.1	0.05	0.01
0.001	0.0382	0.0352	0.0264	0.0200	0.0100	0.00669	0.00365	0.00040	0.00020	0.00004
0.002	0.0597	0.0559	0.0443	0.0350	0.0188	0.0128	0.00712	0.00079	0.00040	0.00008
0.003	0.0772	0.0730	0.0595	0.0481	0.0269	0.0186	0.0105	0.00118	0.00060	0.00012
0.004	0.0926	0.0880	0.0732	0.0601	0.0346	0.0242	0.0138	0.00158	0.00079	0.00016
0.005	0.107	0.102	0.0856	0.0712	0.0419	0.0296	0.0170	0.00197	0.00099	0.00020
0.006	0.119	0.114	0.0973	0.0816	0.0490	0.0349	0.0202	0.00236	0.00119	0.00024
0.007	0.131	0.126	0.108	0.0916	0.0559	0.0401	0.0234	0.00275	0.00139	0.00028
0.008	0.143	0.137	0.119	0.101	0.0626	0.0451	0.0265	0.00314	0.00158	0.00032
0.009	0.154	0.148	0.129	0.110	0.0691	0.0501	0.0296	0.00352	0.00178	0.00036
0.010	0.164	0.158	0.138	0.119	0.0754	0.0549	0.0326	0.00391	0.00198	0.00040
0.020	0.249	0.242	0.219	0.194	0.133	0.100	0.0617	0.00777	0.00394	0.00080
0.030	0.316	0.309	0.283	0.256	0.182	0.140	0.0889	0.0116	0.00590	0.00120
0.040	0.372	0.365	0.338	0.309	0.226	0.178	0.115	0.0154	0.00785	0.00159
0.050	0.421	0.414	0.386	0.356	0.267	0.212	0.139	0.0192	0.00979	0.00199
0.060	0.465	0.458	0.430	0.398	0.305	0.245	0.163	0.0229	0.0117	0.00239
0.070	0.505	0.497	0.469	0.437	0.340	0.276	0.186	0.0267	0.0137	0.00279
0.080	0.541	0.534	0.505	0.473	0.373	0.305	0.208	0.0304	0.0156	0.00318

0.090	0.574	0.567	0.539	0.506	0.404	0.333	0.229	0.0341	0.0175	0.00358
0.100	0.605	0.597	0.570	0.537	0.433	0.359	0.250	0.0378	0.0194	0.00398
0.200	0.810	0.805	0.782	0.755	0.654	0.571	0.478	0.0739	0.0384	0.00794
0.300	0.909	0.905	0.890	0.870	0.789	0.713	0.563	0.109	0.0570	0.0119
0.400	0.956	0.954	0.944	0.931	0.871	0.807	0.666	0.142	0.0753	0.0158
0.500	0.979	0.978	0.972	0.963	0.921	0.871	0.745	0.174	0.0932	0.0197
0.600	0.990	0.989	0.986	0.981	0.952	0.913	0.805	0.205	0.111	0.0236
0.700	0.995	0.945	0.993	0.990	0.971	0.942	0.851	0.235	0.128	0.0275
0.800	0.998	0.997	0.996	0.995	0.982	0.961	0.886	0.264	0.145	0.0314
0.900	0.999	0.999	0.998	0.997	0.989	0.974	0.913	0.291	0.161	0.0352
1.000	0.999	0.999	0.999	0.998	0.993	0.983	0.934	0.318	0.178	0.0390
2.000	1.00	1.00	1.00	1.00	1.00	1.00	0.996	0.535	0.324	0.0765
3.000	1.00	1.00	1.00	1.00	1.00	1.00	1.00	0.683	0.444	0.113
4.000	1.00	1.00	1.00	1.00	1.00	1.00	1.00	0.783	0.543	0.147
5.000	1.00	1.00	1.00	1.00	1.00	1.00	1.00	0.852	0.624	0.181
6.000	1.00	1.00	1.00	1.00	1.00	1.00	1.00	0.899	0.691	0.213
7.000	1.00	1.00	1.00	1.00	1.00	1.00	1.00	0.931	0.746	0.243
8.000	1.00	1.00	1.00	1.00	1.00	1.00	1.00	0.953	0.791	0.273
9.000	1.00	1.00	1.00	1.00	1.00	1.00	1.00	0.968	0.828	0.301
10.00	1.00	1.00	1.00	1.00	1.00	1.00	1.00	0.978	0.858	0.328

Approximate solutions to eqn (6.77) can be approached in the same manner we have used for the parallel plate geometry (see, for example, Problem 6.2). They can be usefully expressed in the form

$$\theta = f(\lambda'), \tag{6.78}$$

where

$$\lambda' \equiv \frac{DA}{RQ_b}, \tag{6.79}$$

and the appropriate form of the wall Sherwood number is

$$Sh'_w = \frac{D_m \alpha_m}{D\alpha \ln[(R+t)/R]}. \tag{6.80}$$

The computed solution for this case is plotted in Fig. 6.12 and presented more extensively in Table 6.3.

Problems

6.1   The ability of a membrane lung to remove CO_2 from blood is described by the equation

$$\theta = \frac{3}{10}\left(\frac{15DA}{2hQ_b}\right)^{2/3},$$

where θ is the dimensionless partial pressure change ($\theta \equiv (P_i - P_o)/(P_i - P_g)$; subscript i refers to inlet blood, o to outlet blood and g to the gas side). The membrane lung has two parallel plates each of area $A/2$, spaced a distance $2h$ apart, and receives a blood flow Q_b, D, the diffusion constant for CO_2 in blood here equals $2 \times 10^{-3}\ \text{mm}^2\,\text{s}^{-1}$.

The membrane lung is to be used to remove the CO_2 produced by a patient who is consuming 250 ml (STP) per min of oxygen, and it is intended to use a blood flow of either $1\ \text{l min}^{-1}$ or $5\ \text{l min}^{-1}$. Calculate the areas of membrane required to achieve this at these two flows, given that $P_g = 0$, $P_i = 6\ \text{kPa}$, $h = 0.2$ mm, R (respiratory quotient) $= 0.8$, and that the concentration C of CO_2 in blood is related to its partial pressure by

$$C = \alpha P + \beta,$$

where $\alpha = 4.5\ \text{ml (STP) dl}^{-1}\,\text{kPa}^{-1}$ and $\beta = 25\ \text{ml (STP) dl}^{-1}$.

What is the minimum volume of blood needed to prime the device in each of the two cases considered?

6.2   Derive the CO_2 transfer for a hollow fibre membrane lung, in the limiting case of a very high membrane resistance, analogous to eqn (6.11) for the parallel plate case.

6.3   A hollow fibre membrane lung is required to take over all the respiratory gas exchange of a patient who is consuming 250 ml (STP) min^{-1} of oxygen and has a respiratory exchange ratio of 1. It is intended to use a bundle of polypropylene fibres of length 30 cm, with blood flowing inside the fibres, which have an internal diameter 200 μm.

Using the advancing front theory for oxygen transfer (eqn (5.50)) and the computed solution for CO_2 transfer given in Table 6.3 (Fig. 6.12) compare the numbers of fibres required for the two tasks of oxygen transfer and CO_2 transfer. The following values should be used: D for oxygen and CO_2 equals 2×10^{-3} mm^2 s^{-1}; $Q_b = 5$ l min^{-1}; P_i for both oxygen and CO_2 equals 6 kPa; C_i for oxygen equals 14 ml (STP) dl^{-1}; $C_{max} = 20$ ml (STP) dl^{-1}; $P_g = 90$ kPa (pure oxygen); α for oxygen equals 0.023 ml (STP) dl^{-1} kPa^{-1}; $Sh'_w \to \infty$ for both gases; CO_2 dissociation relationship as in Problem 6.1.

What are the respective membrane areas associated with the computed numbers of fibres?

Further reading

Dorson, W. J. and Vorhees, M. (1974). Limiting models for the transfer of CO_2 and O_2 in membrane oxygenators. *Transactions of the American Society for Artificial Internal Organs* **20**, 219–26.

Gaylor, J. D. S. (1988). Membrane oxygenators: current developments in design and application. *Journal of Biomedical Engineering* **10**, 541–7.

Kay, J. M. and Nedderman, R. M. (1985). *Fluid Mechanics and Transfer Processes*. Cambridge University Press, Cambridge. (Mass transfer in laminar and turbulent flows, Chapters 16 and 17.)

Kooijman, J. M. (1973). Laminar heat or mass transfer in rectangular channels and in cylindrical tubes for fully developed flow: comparison of solutions obtained for various boundary conditions. *Chemical Engineering Science* **28**, 1149–60.

Mook, P. H., Wong, P., Wildevuur, C. R. H., Mayes, P. J. D., and Gaylor, J. D. S. (1983). Comparative performance of microporous polypropylene membrane lungs for CO_2 removal at low blood flow rates. *Transactions of the American Society for Artificial Internal Organs* **29**, 215–19.

Tanishita, K., Ujihira, M., Watabe, A., Nakano, K., Richardson, P. D., and Galletti, P. M. (1985). Design features of serpentine tube membrane lung for ECCO$_2$R. *Transactions of the American Society for Artificial Internal Organs* **31**, 622–6. (Induction of secondary flows in a tube to enhance CO_2 transfer.)

Answers to problems

2.1 $\dot{V}_{FG} \geqslant 6000 \text{ ml min}^{-1}$

2.2 $F_{O_2} = 0.37$

2.3 $A = 6.42 \text{ mm}^2$
$a/A = 0.017$
$q = 5.20 \text{ cm H}_2\text{O}$
$r = -0.095 \text{ cm H}_2\text{O min l}^{-1}$
$s = -0.043 \text{ cm H}_2\text{O min}^2 \text{l}^{-2}.$

(Note: in deriving pressures in $\text{cm H}_2\text{O}$ it is assumed that the density of water is 1000 kg m^{-3} and that the acceleration due to gravity is 9.816 m s^{-2})

2.4 $\dot{V}_{FG} = 6385 \text{ ml min}^{-1}$
Error = 3.9 per cent

3.1 $p_{sat} = 22.3 \text{ kPa}$
splitting ratio = 13.1
$c_p = 0.973 \text{ kJ kg}^{-1} \text{K}^{-1}$
3.85 per cent isoflurane

3.2 1.41 per cent enflurane

3.3 $p_0 = 1.435 \times 10^{17}$ $(p_{sat} = 58.57 \text{ kPa})$
At $40\,^{\circ}\text{C}$:
$$p_{sat} \text{ (Antoine)} = 122.6 \text{ kPa}$$
$$p_{sat} \text{ (Dupré)} = 97.9 \text{ kPa}$$

At $-20\,^{\circ}\text{C}$
$$p_{sat} \text{ (Antoine)} = 8.81 \text{ kPa}$$
$$p_{sat} \text{ (Dupré)} = 15.49 \text{ kPa}$$

4.1 (a) 1.4 litre
(b) 1.9 litre

4.2 (a) $F_{ECO_2} = 0.048$
(b) $F_{ECO_2} = 0.029$

4.3 (a) 5.16 Hz
(b) 2.29 Hz
(c) 1.26 Hz and 1.37 Hz

5.2 $\left(\dfrac{L_1}{L_2}\right)\left(\dfrac{A_1}{A_2}\right) = \dfrac{5\sqrt{10}}{9}$

5.3 $A = 2.98 \text{ m}^2$
$h = 0.21 \text{ mm}$
$Q_b = 1.12 \text{ l min}^{-1}$

268

6.1 $A = 0.86\,\text{m}^2$ $(Q_b = 1\,\text{l}\,\text{min}^{-1})$

     $A = 0.39\,\text{m}^2$ $(Q_b = 5\,\text{l}\,\text{min}^{-1})$

     Prime volume $= 172$ ml $(Q_b = 1\,\text{l}\,\text{min}^{-1})$

     Prime volume $= 77$ ml $(Q_b = 5\,\text{l}\,\text{min}^{-1})$

Note that both A and prime volume are inversely proportional to $\sqrt{Q_b}$.

6.2 $\theta = 1 - \exp\left(-Sh'_w\,\dfrac{DA}{RQ_b}\right)$

where

$$Sh'_w = D_m \alpha_m / (D\alpha \ln\left[(R + t)/R\right])$$

as for eqn (5.46).

6.3   Oxygen: 31 600 fibres

             5.95 m²

     CO_2:   1100 fibres.

             0.21 m²

Index

270